NUCLEAR CARDIAC IMAGING

NUCLEAR CARDIAC IMAGING

Companion Atlas

SIXTH EDITION

Ami E. Iskandrian and Fadi G. Hage

OXFORD
UNIVERSITY PRESS

OXFORD
UNIVERSITY PRESS

Oxford University Press is a department of the University of Oxford. It furthers the University's objective of excellence in research, scholarship, and education by publishing worldwide. Oxford is a registered trade mark of Oxford University Press in the UK and certain other countries.

Published in the United States of America by Oxford University Press
198 Madison Avenue, New York, NY 10016, United States of America.

CIP data is on file at the Library of Congress
ISBN 978–0–19–752143–4

DOI: 10.1093/med/9780197521434.001.0001

Printed by Integrated Books International, United States of America

CONTENTS

CONTRIBUTORS

Wael A. AlJaroudi, MD, EMBA, FACC, FASNC
Professor of Medicine
Wellstar Health Medical College of Georgia
Augusta, Georgia, USA

Ahmed Aljizeeri, MBBS
King Abdulaziz Cardiac Center, Riyadh, Kingdom of Saudi Arabia
King Saud bin Abdulaziz University for Health Sciences—Riyadh, Kingdom of Saudi Arabia
King Abdullah International Medical Research Center—Riyadh, Kingdom of Saudi Arabia

Mouaz H. Al-Mallah, MD, Msc
Beverly B. and Daniel C. Arnold Distinguished Chair,
Professor of Cardiology, Houston Methodist Academic Institute and Professor of Medicine, Weill Cornell Medicine.
Director, Cardiovascular PET, Houston Methodist DeBakey Heart and Vascular Center, Houtson, Texas, USA

Efstathia Andrikopoulou, MD, MBA, FACC
Assistant Professor of Medicine, Cardiovascular Disease,
University of Alabama at Birmingham,
Birmingham, AL, USA

Kathryn J. Ascah
Division of Cardiology, University of Ottawa Heart Institute, Ottawa, Ontario, Canada

Roberta Assante, MD, PhD
Department of Advanced Biomedical Sciences, School of Medicine, University of Naples Federico II, Naples, Italy

Jeroen J. Bax, MD, PhD
Department of Cardiology, Leiden University Medical Centre, Leiden, The Netherlands

Rob S. B. Beanlands, MD, FRCP(C), FACC, MASNC, FCCS
Deputy Director General, University of Ottawa Heart Institute
Professor of Medicine—Division of Cardiology and
Distinguished Chair in Cardiovascular Imaging Research
University of Ottawa, Ontario, Canada

Pradeep Bhambhvani, MD
Professor of Radiology
The University of Alabama at Birmingham
Birmingham, Alabama, USA

John P. Bois, MD
Associate Professor of Medicine, Mayo Clinic, Rochester, Minnesota, USA

Jamieson M. Bourque, MD, MHS
Professor of Medicine and Radiology, Medical Director of Nuclear Cardiology and the Stress Laboratory, Medical Director of Echocardiography, University of Virginia, Charlottesville, Virginia, USA

Paco E. Bravo, MD
Divisions of Nuclear Medicine and Cardiothoracic Imaging, Department of Radiology, and Division of Cardiology, Department of Medicine, Hospital of the University of Pennsylvania, Philadelphia, Pennsylvania, USA

Juliana Brenande de Oliveira Brito
Division of Cardiology, University of Ottawa Heart Institute, Ottawa, Ontario, Canada

Ronny R. Buechel, MD
Deputy Director and Professor,
University Hospital Zurich, Department of Nuclear Medicine, Cardiac Imaging, Zurich, Switzerland

Panithaya Chareonthaitawee, MD
Professor of Medicine, Director of Nuclear Cardiology, Mayo Clinic, Rochester, Minnesota, USA

Ji Chen, PhD
Head of Engineering, Acelerate
San Francisco Bay Area

Timothy F. Christian, MD, MPA
DeMatteis Research Center/St Francis Hospital, Roslyn, New York, USA

Alberto Cuocolo
Department of Advanced Biomedical Sciences, School of Medicine, University of Naples Federico II, Naples, Italy

Robert A. deKemp, PhD
Head Imaging Physicist, University of Ottawa Heart Institute, Ottawa, Ontario, Canada

Victoria Delgado, MD, PhD
Department of Cardiology, Leiden University Medical Centre, Leiden, The Netherlands

Ana Carolina do A. H. de Souza, MD, PhD
Cardiovascular Imaging Program, Brigham and Women's Hospital, Harvard Medical School, Boston, Massachusetts, USA

Vasken Dilsizian, MD
Chief, Division of Nuclear Medicine, Department of Diagnostic Radiology and Nuclear Medicine, University of Maryland School of Medicine, Baltimore, Maryland, USA

Maurizio Dondi, MD
Division of Human Health, International Atomic Energy Agency, Vienna, Austria

Sharmila Dorbala, MD, MPH
Director of Nuclear Cardiology, Professor of Radiology, Brigham and Women's Hospital, Harvard Medical School, Boston, Massachusetts, USA

Rami Doukky, MD, MSc, MBA, FASNC
Chairman, Division of Cardiology
Cook County Health,
Chicago, Illinois, USA

W. Lane Duvall, MD, FASNC
Director of Nuclear Cardiology, Hartford Hospital, Hartford, CT, USA

Andrew J. Einstein, MD, PhD, FACC, FAHA, MASNC, MSCCT, FSCMR
Professor of Medicine (in Radiology)
Director, Nuclear Cardiology, Cardiac CT, and Cardiac MRI
Director, Advanced Cardiac Imaging Fellowship
Seymour, Paul and Gloria Milstein Division of Cardiology, Department of Medicine, Columbia University Irving Medical Center/NewYork-Presbyterian Hospital
New York, New York, United States of America

Soraya El Ghannudi, MD, PhD
Departments of Radiology and Nuclear Medicine, Nouvel Hôpital Civil—University Hospitals of Strasbourg, Strasbourg, France

Daniel C. Fisher, MD
Director, Stress Nuclear Laboratory, Bellevue Hospital, New York, USA

Oliver Gaemperli, MD, FESC
Professor, Consultant Cardiologist, HeartClinic Zurich AG, Hirslanden Hospital, Zurich, Switzerland, EU

James R. Galt, PhD
Professor of Radiology and Imaging Sciences, Emory University School of Medicine, Atlanta, Georgia, USA

Ernest V. Garcia, PhD, FASNC
Professor of Radiology and Imaging Sciences (Retired)
Emory University School of Medicine, Atlanta, Georgia, USA

Valeria Gaudieri, MD, PhD
Department of Advanced Biomedical Sciences, School of Medicine, University of Naples Federico II, Naples, Italy

Henry Gewirtz, MD[†]
Professor of Medicine, Harvard Medical School
Boston, Massachusetts, USA

Alessia Gimelli, MD, FESC
Head of Nuclear Cardiology Lab, Imaging Department, Fondazione Toscana Gabriele Monasterio, Pisa, Italy

Javier Gomez, MD
Division of Cardiology, Cook County Health,
Chicago, Illinois. USA

Martha Grogan, MD
Associate Professor of Medicine, Department of Cardiovascular Medicine, Mayo Clinic, Rochester, Minnesota, USA

Fadi G. Hage, MD, FACC, FAHA, FSCCI, MASNC
Professor of Medicine, Cardiovascular Disease, University of Alabama at Birmingham and the Birmingham VA Medical Center, Birmingham, Alabama, USA

Matthew E. Harinstein, MD, MBA
SVP, COO, Associate CMO, UPMC International, Associate Professor of Medicine, University of Pittsburgh School of Medicine, Pittsburgh, Pennsylvania, USA

Anastasia M. Hartzes, PhD
Department of Biostatistics, University of Alabama at Birmingham, Birmingham, Alabama, USA

Robert C. Hendel, MD, MACC, MASNC
Professor of Medicine and Radiology, Tulane University School of Medicine, New Orleans, Louisiana, USA

Milena J. Henzlova, MD, PhD
Mount Sinai Medical Center
New York, NY, USA

Alessio Imperiale, MD, PhD
Department of Nuclear Medicine and Molecular Imaging, Institut de Cancérologie de Strasbourg Europe (ICANS), Strasbourg, France

Ami E. Iskandrian, MD, MACC, MASNC
Professor Emeritus
Heersink School of Medicine, University of Alabama at Birmingham
Birmingham Alabama, USA

Philipp A. Kaufmann, MD
Professor and Chairman, Department of Nuclear Medicine, University Hospital Zurich, Zurich, SZ

Ran Klein
Imaging Physicist, The Ottawa Hospital
Ottawa, Ontario, Canada

Riccardo Liga, MD, PhD, FESC
University of Pisa and University Hospital of Pisa, Pisa, Italy

Saurabh Malhotra, MD, MPH
Director of Advanced Cardiac Imaging, Cook County Health, Chicago, Illinois, USA

Brian A. Mc Ardle, MD
Clinical Assistant Professor, University of British Columbia, Victoria, British Columbia, Canada

Sean R. McMahon
Division of Cardiology, Hartford Hospital, Hartford Heart and Vascular Institute, Hartford, CT, USA

Robert J. H. Miller, MD, FRCPC, FACC
Clinical Associate Professor, University of Calgary, Calgary, Alberta, Canada

Charity J. Morgan, PhD
Professor, The University of Alabama at Birmingham
Birmingham, AL, USA

Paul H. Murphy, PhD
Professor Emeritus of Radiology, Baylor College of Medicine, Houston, Texas, USA

Arnold C. T. Ng, MBBS, PhD
Department of Cardiology, Princess Alexandra Hospital, University of New South Wales, Australia

Pilar Orellana, MD
Nuclear Medicine and Diagnostic Imaging Section, Division of Human Health, International Atomic Energy Agency, Vienna, Austria

Diana Paez, MD, MSc, Ed.
Head of the Nuclear Medicine and Diagnostic Imaging Section, Division of Human Health, International Atomic Energy Agency, Vienna, Austria

Minnsun K. Park, MD
Cardiology Fellow, Tulane University School of Medicine, New Orleans, Louisiana, USA

Sara L. Partington, MD
Assistant Professor of Clinical Medicine, Hospital of the University of Pennsylvania and Children's Hospital of Philadelphia, Philadelphia, Pennsylvania, USA

Amalia Peix, MD, MSc, PhD
Nuclear Cardiologist, Master in Cardiac Magnetic Resonance Francisco Vittoria University Spain, Institute of Cardiology and Cardiovascular Surgery, La Habana, Cuba

Lawrence M. Phillips, MD
Associate Professor of Medicine, Leon H. Carney Division of Cardiology, NYU Grossman School of Medicine, New York USA

Steven Port, MD
AdvocateAuroraHealth, Aurora Cardiovascular Services, Milwaukee, Wisconsin, USA

Steven Promislow, MD, FRCPC
Assistant Professor of Medicine
Department of Internal Medicine, Section of Cardiology
University of Manitoba
Winnipeg, Manitoba, Canada

Jennifer M. Renaud, MSC
Research Scientist, INVIA Medical Imaging Solutions, Ann Arbor, Michigan, USA

David G. Rosenthal, MD, FACC, FHRS
Swedish Medical Center,
Seattle, Washington, USA

Benjamin Rotstein, PhD
Associate Professor and Scientist
University of Ottawa and University of Ottawa Heart Institute, Ottawa, Ontario, Canada

Elona Rrapo Kaso, MD
Division of Cardiovascular Medicine and the Cardiac Imaging Center, Departments of Medicine and Radiology, University of Virginia Health System, Charlottesville, Virginia, USA

Terrence D. Ruddy, MD, FRCPC, FACC, FAHA, FCCS, FSNMMI, MASNC
Consulting Cardiologist, Division of Cardiology, Professor of Medicine and Radiology,University of Ottawa Heart Institute, Ottawa, Ontario, Canada

Raymond Russell, MD, PhD, MASNC, FACC
Professor of Medicine, Institution Alpert Medical School of Brown University, Providence, Rhode Island, USA

Mehran M. Sadeghi, MD
Professor of Medicine (Cardiology), Yale School of Medicine, New Haven, Connecticut, USA
Physician, VA Connecticut Healthcare System, West Haven, Connecticut, USA

Heinrich R. Schelbert, MD, PhD
Department of Molecular and Medical Pharmacology, David Geffen School of Medicine at UCLA, University of California at Los Angeles, Los Angeles, California, USA

Thomas H. Schindler, MD, PhD
Professor of Radiology and Medicine; Mallinckrodt Institute of Radiology, Division of Nuclear Medicine, Washington University in Saint Louis, School of Medicine, Saint Louis, Missouri, USA

Daniel Shpilsky, MD
Division of Cardiology, University of Pittsburgh Medical Center, Pittsburgh, Pennsylvania, USA

Gursukhmandeep S. Sidhu, MD
University of Illinois Chicago,
Chicago, Illinois, USA

Piotr J. Slomka, PhD
Departments of Medicine (Division of Artificial Intelligence in Medicine), Imaging and Biomedical Sciences Cedars-Sinai Medical Center, Los Angeles, CA, USA

Gary R. Small
Division of Cardiology, University of Ottawa Heart Institute, Ottawa, Ontario, Canada

Prem Soman, MD, PhD
Professor of Medicine, and Clinical and Translational Science, University of Pittsburgh Medical Center, Pittsburgh, Pennsylvania, USA

Viviany R. Taqueti, MD, MPH
Cardiovascular Imaging Program, Brigham and Women's Hospital and Cardiology Division, VA Boston Healthcare, Harvard Medical School, Boston, Massachusetts, USA

Sina Tavakoli, MD, PhD
Assistant Professor and Chief of the Division of Cardiothoracic Imaging, Department of Radiology, University of Pittsburgh, Pittsburgh, Pennsylvania, USA

Gregory S. Thomas, MD, MPH, FACC, MASNC
MemorialCare Health System, Fountain Valley, California, USA; Division of Cardiology, University of California, Irvine, California, USA

Mark I. Travin, MD, FACC, MASNC
Division of Nuclear Medicine, Professor of Clinical Radiology and Clinical Medicine, Montefiore Medical Center. Albert Einstein College of Medicine, Bronx, New York, USA

Ines Valenta, MD
Research Associate; Mallinckrodt Institute of Radiology, Washington University in Saint Louis, School of Medicine, Saint Louis, Missouri, USA

William A. Van Decker, MD
Professor of Medicine, Lewis Katz School of Medicine at Temple University, Philadelphia, Pennsylvania, USA

Venkatesh Ravi, MD, FACC, FHRS
Clinical Cardiac Electrophysiologist, Adjunct Clinical Assistant Professor, Saint Francis Health System, Tulsa, Oklahoma, USA, Chicago, Illinois, USA

Joao V. Vitola, MD, PhD
Quanta Diagnóstico & Terapia, Curitiba, Brazil

Frans J. Th. Wackers, MD, PhD
Professor Emeritus of Diagnostic Radiology and Medicine (Cardiology), Yale University School of Medicine, New Haven, Connecticut, USA

L. Samuel Wann, MD
Clinical Professor of Cardiovascular Medicine, University of New Mexico Santa Fe, New Mexico

R. Glenn Wells
Division of Cardiology, University of Ottawa Heart Institute, Ottawa, Ontario, Canada

Christiane Wiefels, MD, PhD
Assistant Professor of Medicine, Department of Medicine, Division of Nuclear Medicine, University of Ottawa, Canada

Keiichiro Yoshinaga, MD, PhD[†]
Team leader at the Department of Molecular Imaging and Theragnostic, National Institute of Radiological Sciences, Chiba, Japan

Emilia Zampella
Department of Advanced Biomedical Sciences, School of Medicine, University of Naples Federico II, Naples, Italy

Barry L. Zaret, MD[†]
Robert W. Berliner Professor Emeritus of Internal Medicine (Cardiology), Yale University School of Medicine, New Haven, Connecticut, USA

1.

NUCLEAR CARDIOLOGY

HISTORY AND MILESTONES

Barry L. Zaret and Frans J. Th. Wackers

QUESTIONS

1. The first nuclear studies involving the cardiovascular system were performed in the laboratory of:
   a. Pierre Curie
   b. Paul Cannon
   c. Herman Blumgart
   d. Joseph Kriss
2. Exercise myocardial perfusion studies were first performed in:
   a. 1970s
   b. 1980s
   c. 1990s
   d. 2000–2010
3. Based on physical and biologic properties, it was shown that conventional SPECT studies were best performed with:
   a. Tc-99m
   b. Tl-201
   c. K-43
   d. Rb-82
4. The impact of noninvasive imaging on outcomes was first rigorously defined by:
   a. Echocardiography
   b. CT scanning
   c. Nuclear cardiology
   d. MRI

ANSWERS

1c, 2a, 3a, 4c

2.

RADIATION PHYSICS AND RADIATION SAFETY

Paul H. Murphy and James R. Galt

QUESTIONS

1. Some radionuclides used in nuclear cardiology decay by electron capture. Following electron capture, which of the following may be emitted?
   a. Characteristic x-rays
   b. Gamma rays
   c. Characteristic x-rays and gamma rays
   d. Positrons

2. Attenuation of ^{99m}Tc 140 keV photons passing through soft tissue is primarily due to which of the following?
   a. Bremsstrahlung
   b. Compton scatter
   c. Photoelectric effect
   d. Pair production

3. How long will it take for activity in a patient to be reduced by half after administration of a radiopharmaceutical that has a physical half-life of 3 days and a biologic half-life of 10 days?
   a. 2.3 days
   b. 3.0 days
   c. 13.0 days
   d. 30 days

ANSWERS

1c. Electron capture requires that an inner-shell electron be captured by the nucleus. The electron and a proton are converted to a neutron and a neutrino. This leaves an inner-shell electron vacancy and usually leaves the nucleus with excess energy. Therefore, characteristic x-rays and gamma rays may be emitted. Positron emission is a competing process with electron capture. In a given decay either positron emission or electron capture will take place, not both.

2b. The primary interaction of high-energy photons in soft tissue is Compton scatter. This is true for 50 keV x-rays, 511 keV annihilation photons, and everything in between. Photoelectric effect occurs primarily in the detectors (collimator, crystal) and bone (in lower-energy x-rays). Pair production requires a photon with enough energy to create an electron/positron pair (1,022 keV). Bremsstrahlung is the process where a high-energy electron or beta particle passes near a nucleus, loses energy, and emits x-rays.

3a. The time required will be the effective half-life and will be determined by the equation:

$$T_{eff} = \frac{(T_p * T_b)}{(T_p + T_b)} = \frac{(3*10)}{(3+10)} = \frac{30}{13} = 2.3\ days$$

where T_{eff} = effective half-life, T_p = physical half-life, and T_b = biologic half-life.

Also note that the T_{eff} will always be less than either T_p or T_b. Only answer a. could possibly be correct.

3.

SPECT AND PET INSTRUMENTATION

CONVENTIONAL AND NEW

James R. Galt, Ernest V. Garcia, and Ji Chen

QUESTIONS

1. If all other collimator parameters are the same, a collimator with shorter holes will be characterized by which of the following?
   a. Finer spatial resolution and lower sensitivity
   b. Finer spatial resolution and higher sensitivity
   c. Poorer spatial resolution and lower sensitivity
   d. Poorer spatial resolution and higher sensitivity
2. Solid-state detectors have been implemented in both SPECT and PET systems. What distinguishes solid-state systems from conventional systems?
   a. Use of solid-state detectors in place of scintillation crystals
   b. Use of solid-state detectors in place of photomultiplier tubes (PMTs)
   c. Elimination of collimation
   d. High-sensitivity camera designs
3. If the thickness of the myocardial wall varies around the circumference of a SPECT short axis slice, counts in the slice will:
   a. Depend solely on the attenuation pattern
   b. Vary with the thickness and the tracer concentration
   c. Prevent the determination of wall thickening in gated SPECT
   d. Always be higher in the lateral wall than the septal wall.

ANSWERS

1d. The diameter and length of each hole in a collimator defines the angle subtended by the hole. The wider the angle, the higher the sensitivity (more activity is seen through the hole). The wider the angle, the poorer the resolution.

2b. A solid-state device is, by definition, a device that does not use vacuum tubes. PMTs are vacuum tubes. Some solid-state detectors utilize scintillation. Collimation and the sensitivity have nothing to do with whether the device is solid-state or not. Some sort of collimation (mechanical or electronic) is required for all imaging of high-energy photons.

3b. If the size or thickness of an object is small compared to the resolution of the imaging system, brightness in the image will vary with the size or thickness due to the partial volume effect. Full-width-at-half-maximum resolution of SPECT is 10 to 15 mm. Thus, the thickness of the myocardium is a factor in the maximum counts. This may complicate the interpretation of gated SPECT images since the myocardium appears brighter in areas where it is thicker and dimmer in areas where thinner, but it will not prevent the determination of wall thickening. The lateral wall often appears brighter than the septal wall in myocardial perfusion SPECT because it has less attenuation in most cases (not related to thickness).

4.

KINETICS OF CONVENTIONAL AND NEW CARDIAC RADIOTRACERS

Ran Klein, Robert A. deKemp, Benjamin Rotstein, and Keiichiro Yoshinaga

QUESTIONS

1. For a cardiac tracer that is taken up and trapped in the myocardium, the optimal time for uptake imaging is:
   a. Immediately with tracer administration
   b. As soon as significant clearance from the blood is achieved
   c. No later than one physical half-life after administration
   d. When metabolism and washout are mostly exhausted
2. Which of the following tracer kinetic properties are advantageous for a cardiac tracer?
   a. Fast metabolism
   b. Affinity to hemoglobin
   c. Avid hepatic uptake
   d. Free diffusion across the cellular membrane
3. Patient motion is detrimental to quantifying physiologic function with dynamic PET because it:
   a. Alters the physiologic state of the patient
   b. Promotes tracer washout
   c. Introduces errors to image-sampled time–activity curves
   d. Introduces inaccuracies in extraction correction

ANSWERS

1b. Once the tracer has been cleared from the blood, myocardium-to-blood contrast is high and there is high activity to achieve good count statistics.

2d. Free diffusion across the cellular membrane is favorable to producing high first-pass uptake to the myocardium. Metabolites, hemoglobin binding, and hepatic uptake can all lead to poor myocardium-to-background contrast.

3c. When the patient moves, regions of interest that are used to sample tracer activity concentrations from the image may not consistently align with the anatomy for all time frames, resulting in erroneous time–activity curves.

5.

RADIONUCLIDE ANGIOGRAPHY

Steven Port

QUESTIONS

1. A 59-year-old man sustained an acute anterior STEMI and was successfully treated with emergent PCI of the mid LAD coronary artery. His risk factors included mild hypertension treated with amlodipine 5 mg daily, smoking, and obesity (BMI 42.0). A routine post-PCI, contrast-enhanced echocardiogram was performed the day after his event but was of poor quality due to his body habitus. The calculated LVEF was 34%. He was discharged on guideline-directed medical therapy including metoprolol, lisinopril, aspirin and clopidogrel, and 1 week later you re-evaluated the patient in the outpatient cardiology clinic for routine post-MI care. There were no symptoms and no signs of congestive heart failure. The heart rate was 62 and blood pressure 146/82. An ERNA was requested for evaluation of wall motion and LVEF.

   Refer to the images. Of the following, which course of treatment would you pursue for the patient?
   a. Continue the regimen and re-evaluate blood pressure in 2 weeks.
   b. Discontinue his lisinopril and initiate sacubitril/valsartan therapy
   c. Refer the patient to electrophysiology for ICD therapy.
   d. Refer the patient to endocrinology to consider SGLT2 inhibitor therapy.

2. A request for an ERNA is received from an ordering provider who indicated that both RV and LV ejection fractions were important. Of the following, which would be the most efficient protocol to provide the requested results?
   a. Change to a FPRNA and process both the RV and LV phases.
   b. Acquire a planar ERNA for both RV and LV ejection fractions.
   c. Acquire a gated first-pass study and a subsequent planar ERNA.
   d. Acquire a SPECT ERNA for both RV and LV ejection fractions.

3. Refer to the images. Of the following, which is the most appropriate qualitative interpretation?
   a. Normal RV and LV size and normal LV and RV systolic function
   b. Dilated RV with normal RV function and normal LV size and function
   c. Dilated RV with decreased function and normal LV size and function
   d. RVEF measurement is underestimated. The study should be reprocessed.

4. Refer to the images. Which of the following best describes LV wall motion and function?
   a. A shows normal LV size, paradoxical septal motion, and a normal LVEF.
   b. B shows a dilated LV, a dyskinetic septum and apex, and a reduced LVEF.
   c. A shows normal LV size, dyskinetic septum and apex, and a reduced LVEF.
   d. B shows a dilated LV, paradoxical septal and apical motion, and a reduced LVEF.

5. Refer to the images. Which of the following best characterize LV synchrony?
   a. Panel A: Bandwidth 45, SDθ 20; Panel B: Bandwidth 150, SDθ 12
   b. Panel A: Bandwidth 90, SDθ 8; Panel B: Bandwidth 45, SDθ 30
   c. Panel A: Bandwidth 45, SDθ 8; Panel B: Bandwidth 90, SDθ 30
   d. Panel A: Bandwidth 120, SDθ 12; Panel B: Bandwidth 150, SDθ 30

ANSWERS

1a. The SPECT ERNA shows an apical/septal infarct with a reduced LVEF of 38%. The patient has not experienced any CHF nor any dysrhythmia. As such, the patient does not qualify for sacubitril/valsartan therapy, which is approved for patients with reduced LVEF and congestive heart failure. ICD therapy would be indicated were the LVEF less than 35%. The SGLT2 inhibitors or gliflozins are a class of compound that is indicated in patients with a reduced LVEF and CHF and who are already treated with an ACE-I or ARB, a beta-blocker, and an RAS inhibitor such as spironolactone. Consequently, no other change than addressing the elevated blood pressure is necessary based on the ERNA and clinical data.[1,2]

2d. FPRNA can be used to measure both RV and LV ejection fractions, but to get enough data for an accurate RVEF, one must prolong the injection bolus to increase the number of available beats. Extending the bolus, however, runs the risk of a high background count during processing of the LV phase, which would overestimate the LVEF. RVEF is consistently underestimated on planar ERNA when compared to gated FPRNA or SPECT ERNA. The combination of a gated FPRNA followed by a planar ERNA is certainly an acceptable protocol for the requested data. Gated FPRNA was appropriate prior to the advent of tomographic ERNA. It is more difficult to perform and results in two datasets for processing. SPECT ERNA is, therefore, the more efficient protocol.

3c. Interpreting physicians must develop the ability to visually estimate size and function of the ventricles on ERNA or, for that matter, on any imaging modality. Automated and semi-automated programs for measurement of chamber sizes and function are not fail-safe, and the physician must know when to reprocess the data. In this case, the RV is unequivocally dilated and shows reduced function. LV size and function are clearly normal. Answer d is incorrect because the visual assessment of RV function suggests a reduced EF. Compare the RV size and function in this case to the RV size and function in Question 1.

4b. Panel A shows a dilated LV, which should be obvious by comparison to the RV. There is typical paradoxical septal motion, characterized by early inward motion of the septum and then motion toward the RV as the lateral wall contracts late. LVEF is unequivocally reduced. Panel B shows a dilated LV, again obvious when compared to the RV. The septum and apex are dyskinetic, showing bulging toward the RV throughout the cardiac cycle. LVEF is clearly reduced.

5c. The image in Panel A shows extremely uniform onset of mechanical contraction in both the LV and RV, indicating very normal intraventricular and interventricular synchrony, which would best be characterized by a narrow bandwidth and a small SDθ. Panel B shows inhomogeneous onset of contraction in the LV, which is best characterized by a large bandwidth and associated large SDθ.

REFERENCES

1. McMurray JJ, Pakcer M, Desai M et al. Angiotensin-neprolysin inhibition versus enalapril in heart failure. *N Engl J Med.* 2014;371:993–1004.
2. Packer M, Anker SD, Butler J, et al. Cardiovascular and Renal Outcomes with Empagliflozin in Heart Failure. *N Engl J Med.* 2020;383:1413–1424.

6.

GATED SPECT MPI

IMAGING PROTOCOLS AND ACQUISITIONS; PROCESSING AND QUANTIFICATION

Milena J. Henzlova, Sean R. McMahon, and W. Lane Duvall

CASE 1

HISTORY

53-year-old male with hypertension, gastroesophageal reflux, and high cholesterol presents to the emergency department with intermittent chest pain for 36 hours. The chest pain started at rest while watching TV and was associated with nausea. He described it as a pressure and burning in his central chest. This initial episode lasted for 35 to 45 minutes. The pain returned intermittently over the next day, occurring at rest and with activity. He denies any history of heart disease or cardiac testing.

PHYSICAL FINDINGS

BP: 157/85 mmHg; P: 92 bpm; Ht: 6'1"; Wt: 190 lbs; BMI: 25. His jugular venous pressure is normal and there are no carotid bruits. Lungs are clear to auscultation. Regular rate and rhythm with no murmurs, rubs, or gallops. Abdomen is soft with mild epigastric tenderness. There is no peripheral edema and his extremities are warm with palpable pulses. ECG is shown in Figure 6.1.

LABORATORY FINDINGS

CBC normal; Chem 7 normal; Troponin I negative ×2.

STRESS TEST RESULTS

The patient exercised for 8 minutes 45 seconds on a Bruce protocol without any symptoms of chest pain. He reached a peak heart rate of 145 bpm, which is 87% of maximal age predicted heart rate. Peak blood pressure was 185/80 mmHg. There were no ischemic ST changes during exercise or recovery. Exercise was stopped due to patient fatigue. He was injected with 10 mCi of Tc-99m tetrofosmin at 7 minutes 45 seconds of exercise. Raw/rotating images are shown in Figure 6.2. The perfusion images are shown in Figure 6.3 and gated images in Figure 6.4.

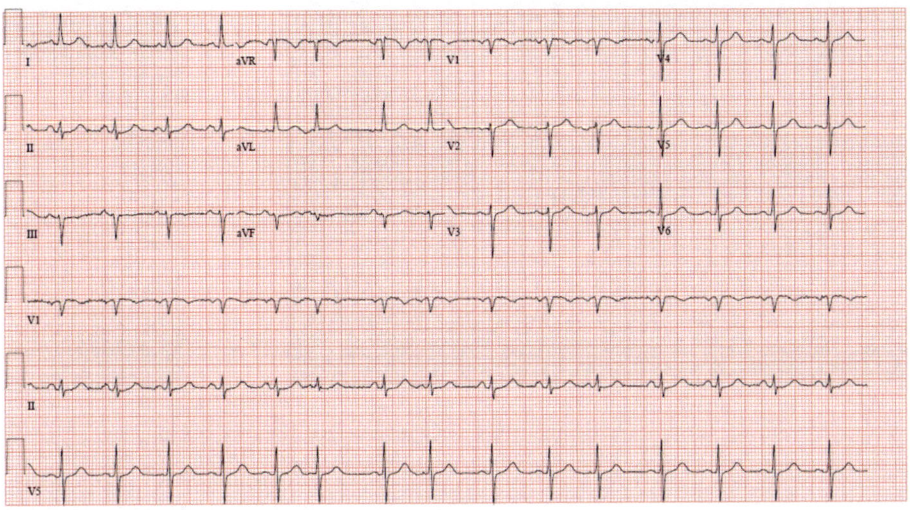

Figure 6.1. Case 1. ECG.

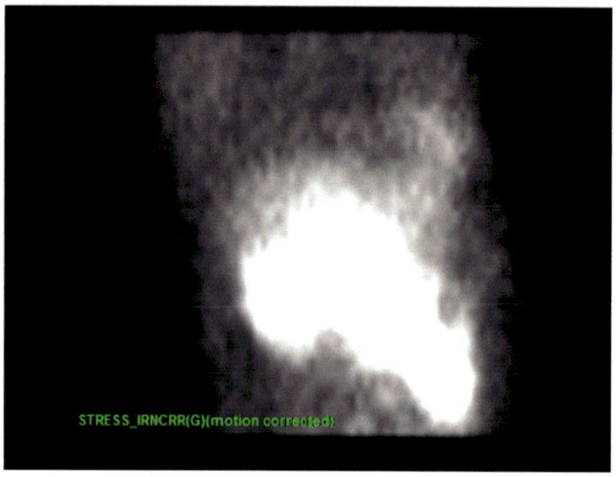

Figure 6.2. Case 1. Raw/rotating images.

The exercise stress portion of the test was unremarkable. Perfusion images show a mild to moderate inferior stress perfusion defect that normalizes with attenuation correction. Regional wall motion is preserved and overall left ventricular systolic function is normal. This is consistent with diaphragmatic attenuation, which can be seen in the rotating images.

LEARNING POINT

Stress-first imaging protocols with SPECT attenuation correction are appropriate for patients at low or intermediate risk of CAD and result in a shorter test with lower radiation exposure to the patient with similar prognostic ability to full rest–stress MPI protocols.

Several studies have investigated appropriate patients for stress-first protocols, with the most simplistic approach dividing patients into those with known or no known CAD.[1,2] Those patients with no known CAD had a high percentage of successful stress-first studies when attenuation correction was used (Figure 6.5). This patient being evaluated in the emergency department has no known CAD, and a stress-first protocol has the potential to evaluate and triage the patient faster than a full rest–stress study.

With a normal stress-only study defined as normal ECG response, normal perfusion, and normal left ventricular function, this patient is at a very low risk for adverse cardiac events. This favorable prognosis of a normal stress-only imaging is comparable to a normal rest–stress study (Figure 6.6).[3,4,5]

CASE 2

HISTORY

A 59-year-old male presents to the office for evaluation of chest pain of 3 months' duration. He reports that the chest pain is a sharp discomfort in the center and left side

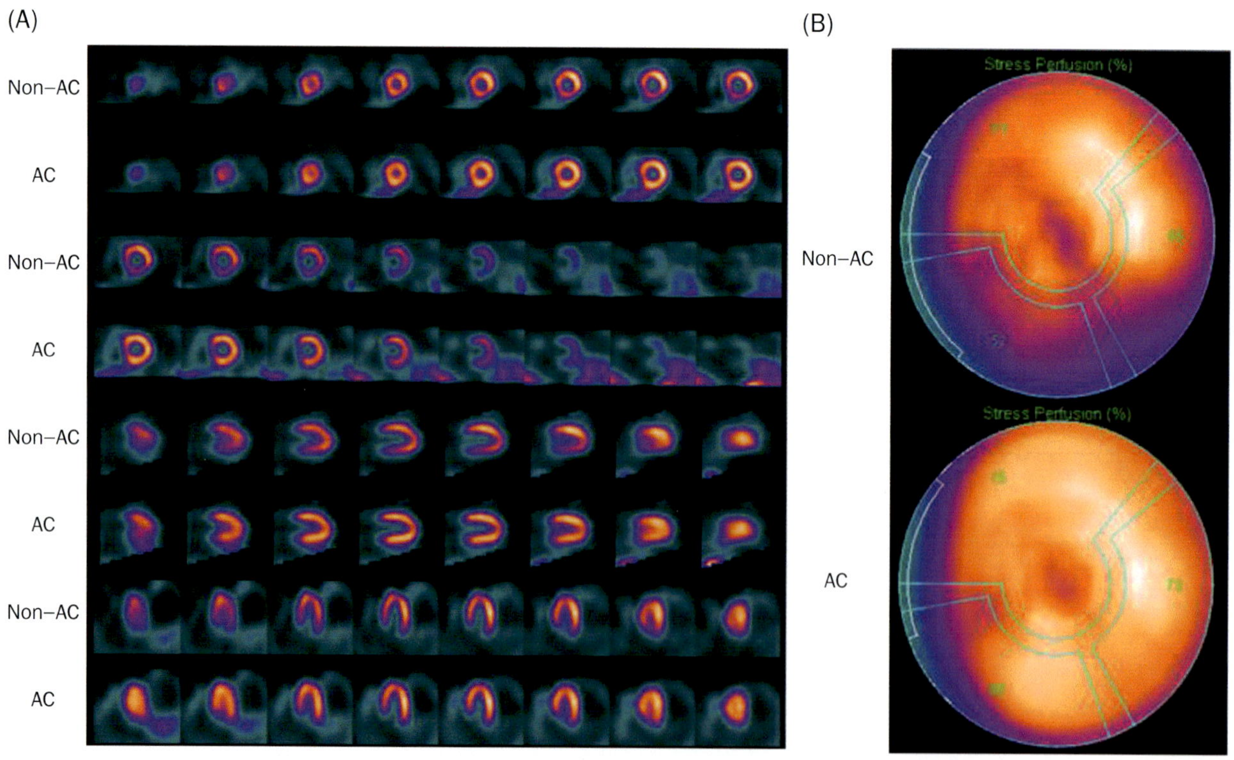

Figure 6.3. Case 1. Non-corrected and Gd-153 scanning line source corrected stress images (A) and polar plot (B).

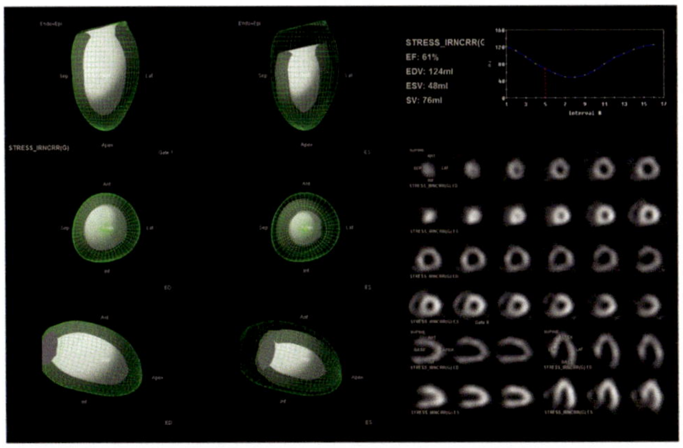

Figure 6.4. Case 1. Gated images.

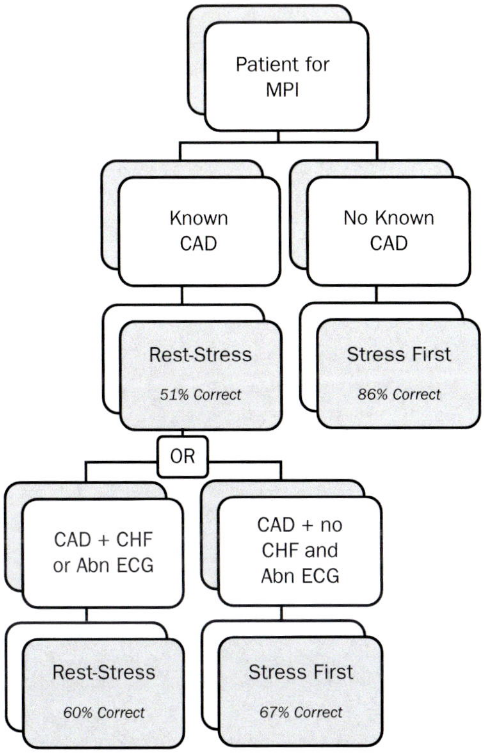

Figure 6.5. In one series, the success rate of stress-first protocols was over 80% in patients with no known CAD and around only 50% with known CAD.[2] From Duvall WL, Baber U, Levine EJ, Croft LB, Henzlova MJ. A model for the prediction of a successful stress-first Tc-99m SPECT MPI. Journal of nuclear cardiology: official publication of the American Society of Nuclear Cardiology 2012;19:1124-34.

of his chest that occurs both at rest and with activity and is sometimes accompanied by shortness of breath and palpitations—a feeling that his heart is going fast. It lasts for several minutes and as long as 30 to 45 minutes. It has usually resolved on its own, but on several occasions he has taken aspirin for relief.

He has a history of high cholesterol, for which he does not take any medications, and is a former smoker. He reports that his blood pressure has been "borderline" at his doctor's office the past few visits. His father had angioplasty in his 70s. He denies any previous cardiac testing.

PHYSICAL FINDINGS

BP: 149/87 mmHg; P: 76 bpm; Ht: 5'11"; Wt: 205 lbs; BMI: 28.6. His jugular venous pressure is normal and there are no carotid bruits. Lungs are clear to auscultation. Regular rate and rhythm with a 1-2/VI systolic murmur at the upper sternal border. Abdomen is soft and overweight. There is no peripheral edema and his extremities are warm with palpable pulses. The ECG is shown in Figure 6.7.

STRESS TEST RESULTS

The patient exercised for 7 minutes 30 seconds on a Bruce protocol with shortness of breath during exercise but without any symptoms of chest pain. He reached a

Meta Analysis of Studies Comparing Prognosis of Normal Stress-only to Normal Stress–Rest MPI

	Study name	Statistics for each study			
Rate ratio		Lower limit	Upper limit	Z-Value	p-Value
1.139	Change 2010	1.047	1.239	3.018	0.003
1.337	Duvall 2010	0.951	1.879	1.673	0.094
0.886	Ueyama 2012	0.512	1.534	-0.431	0.667
2.431	Edenbrandt 2013	1.816	3.255	5.964	0.000
1.206		1.116	1.304	4.708	0.000

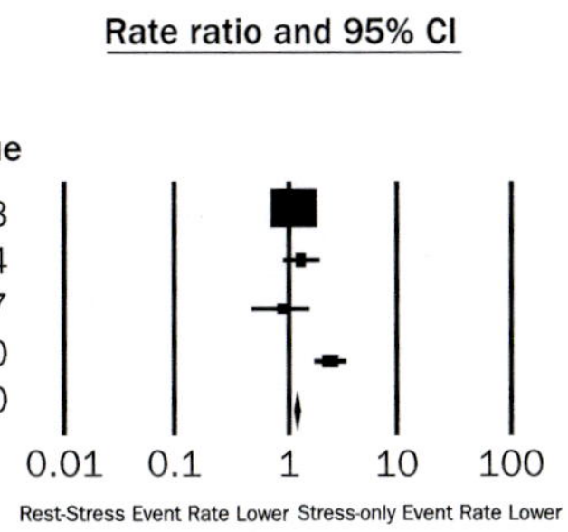

Figure 6.6. Four studies assessed the prognostication of normal stress-only myocardial perfusion imaging compared to a normal full rest–stress protocol. As a whole, the event rate of normal stress-only studies was slightly better than a full rest–stress study.[5] From Hussain N, Parker MW, Henzlova MJ, Duvall WL. Stress-first Myocardial Perfusion Imaging. Cardiology clinics 2016;34:59-67.

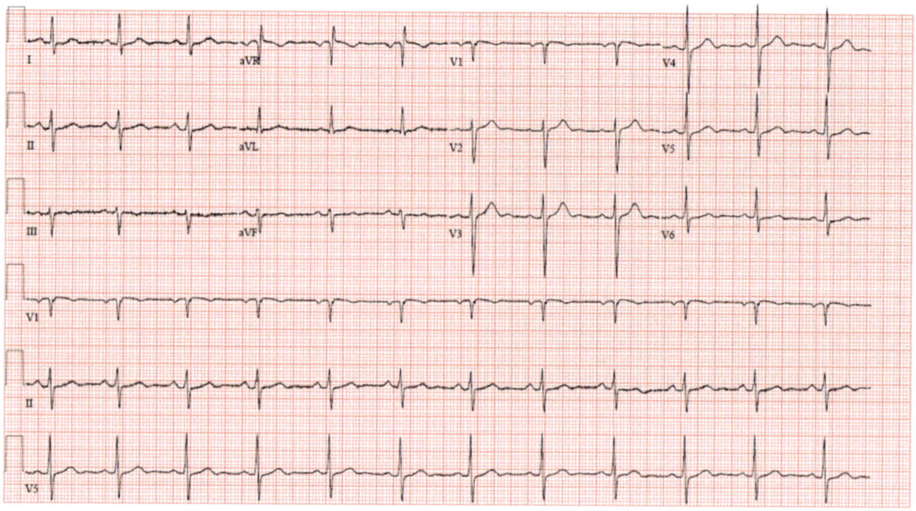

Figure 6.7. Case 2. ECG.

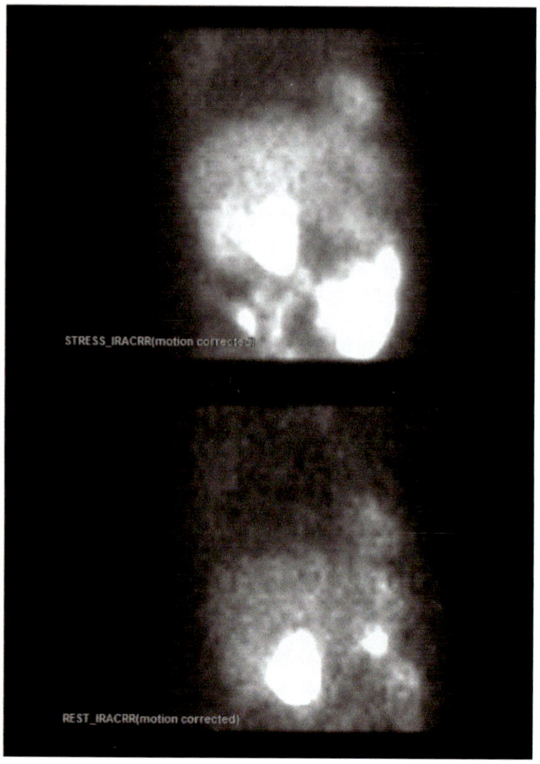

Figure 6.8. Case 2. Raw/rotating images.

peak heart rate of 140 bpm, which is 87% of maximal age predicted heart rate. Peak blood pressure was 180/80 mmHg. Exercise was stopped due to patient fatigue and shortness of breath. There were no ischemic ST changes during exercise or recovery. He was injected with 10 mCi of Tc-99m sestamibi at rest and 30 mCi during exercise.

Raw/rotating images are shown in Figure 6.8. The perfusion images are shown in Figure 6.9 and gated images in Figure 6.10.

The CT attenuation images of a slice showing coronary artery calcification are shown in Figure 6.11.

Perfusion images find a mild reversible anterior perfusion defect. The CT attenuation-correction scan shows a significant amount of coronary calcification localized in the LAD territory. At coronary angiography this patient had LAD 80% mid stenosis, LCx 50% proximal stenosis, and RCA 20% to 30% proximal stenosis.

LEARNING POINT

Assessment of coronary artery calcium burden through the use of SPECT/CT cameras can provide substantial benefit in regards to improved interpretation of perfusion images and patient risk stratification.

In a study by Mouden et al.[6] SPECT MPI interpretation was changed in 37% of patients when perfusion images were interpreted with knowledge of the coronary artery calcium score (Figure 6.12). Overall interpretation was felt to be improved and equivocal studies decreased from 21% to 9%.

The addition of coronary artery calcium burden, even if it is qualitative not quantitative, to the SPECT perfusion results has been shown to improve risk stratification. In a study of 1,047 patients assessed for the presence of coronary calcification visible or not on attenuation-correction CT scans, a worse prognosis was found when coronary calcium was present.[7] This simple visual assessment for coronary calcification provided additional prognostic information for both ischemic and non-ischemic studies (Figure 6.13).

Formal coronary calcium scores can also effectively provide risk stratification that is additive and independent of the SPECT perfusion results in predicting MACE, which

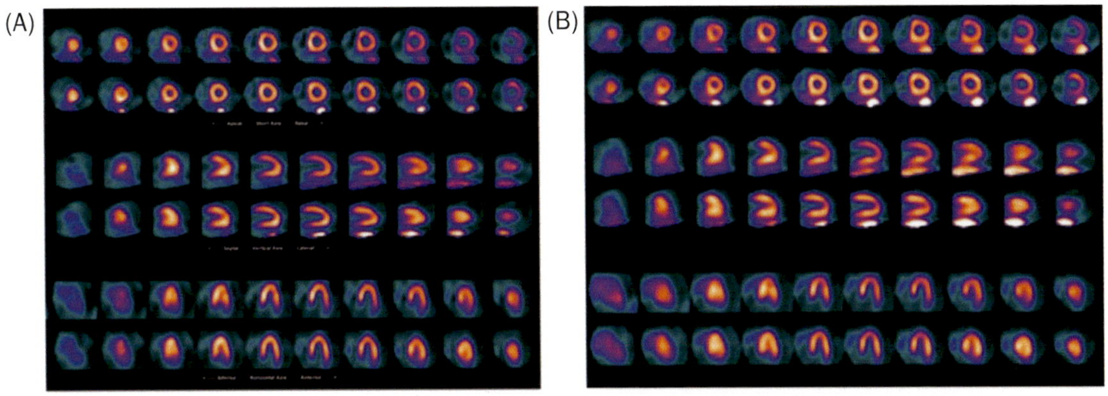

Figure 6.9. Case 2. Non-corrected stress over rest images (A) and CT attenuation-corrected stress over rest images (B).

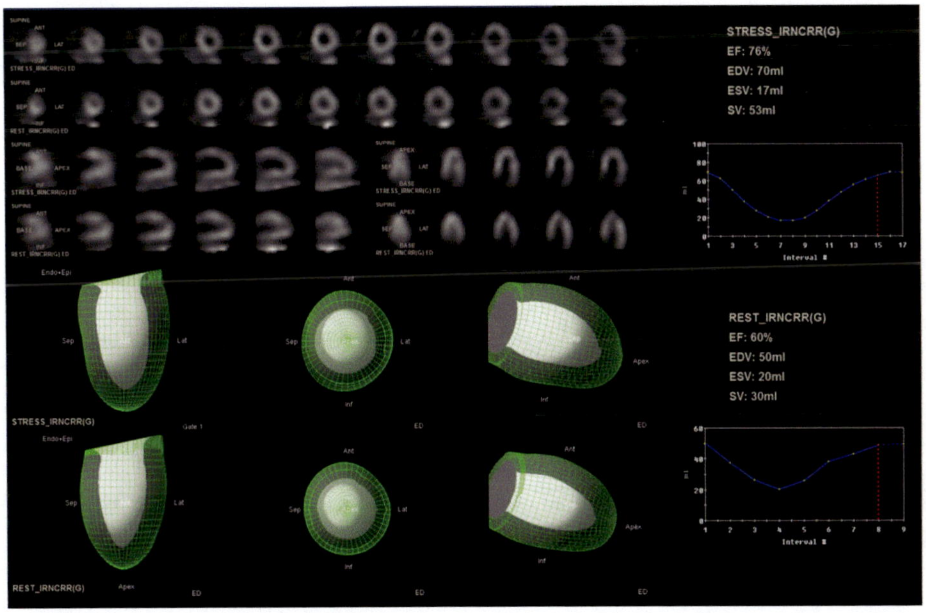

Figure 6.10. Case 2. Gated images.

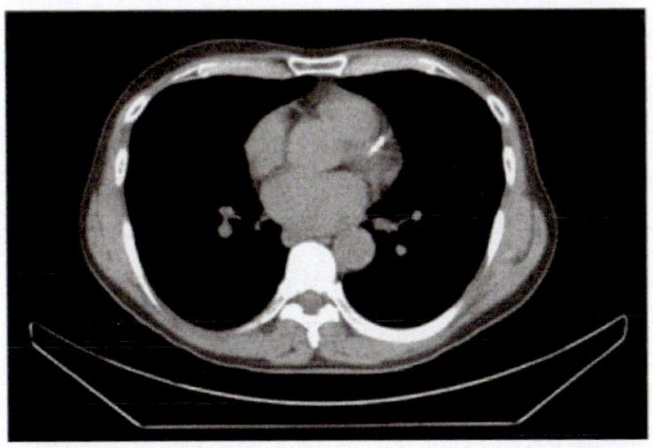

Figure 6.11. Case 2. Attenuation-correction CT scan, illustrative slice.

was nicely shown in a study by Engbers et al. (Figure 6.14).[8] This was shown to hold true not only for abnormal perfusion results, but also within those patients with normal perfusion (Figure 6.15).

With such a high percentage of SPECT myocardial perfusion imaging studies being normal, a study by Berman et al. of over 1,100 patients showed that even with the normal perfusion results, 78% had evidence of coronary atherosclerosis with a coronary artery calcium score above 0.[9] Remarkably, over 30% of patients with normal perfusion had calcium scores above 400 (Figure 6.16).

CASE 3

HISTORY

A 52-year-old male with chronic kidney disease, hypertension, diabetes, ischemic cardiomyopathy, and known coronary artery disease with prior percutaneous coronary intervention

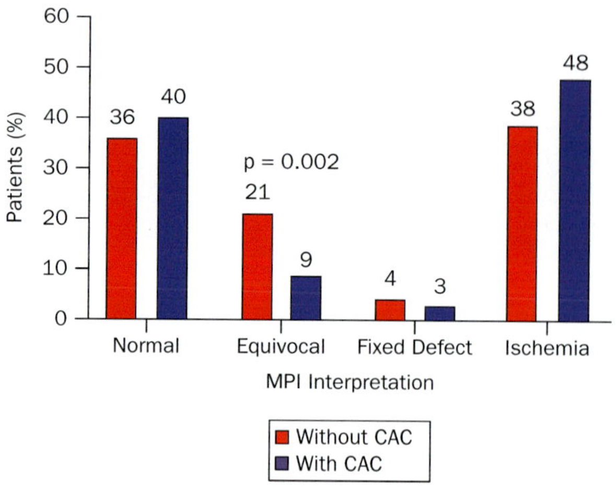

Figure 6.12. Change in MPI interpretation with and without knowledge of coronary artery calcium score. Adapted from Mouden M, Ottervanger JP, Timmer JR, et al. The influence of coronary calcium score on the interpretation of myocardial perfusion imaging. Journal of nuclear cardiology: official publication of the American Society of Nuclear Cardiology 2014;21:368-74.

to the left anterior descending artery 2 years prior presents for evaluation of recently decreased left ventricular ejection fraction (previously 45%, now 35%) with new inferior wall motion abnormalities on echocardiography. He is relatively sedentary and denies symptoms other than fatigue with

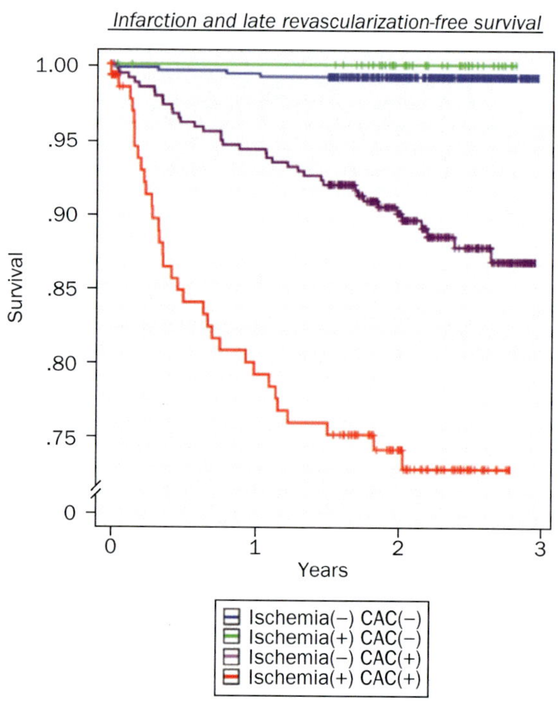

Figure 6.13. Interaction of ischemia and visually assessed presence of coronary calcium on attenuation-correction CT scans on patient prognosis. From Patchett ND, Pawar S, Miller EJ. Visual identification of coronary calcifications on attenuation correction CT improves diagnostic accuracy of SPECT/CT myocardial perfusion imaging. Journal of nuclear cardiology: official publication of the American Society of Nuclear Cardiology 2017;24:711-720; with permission from Springer Nature BV.

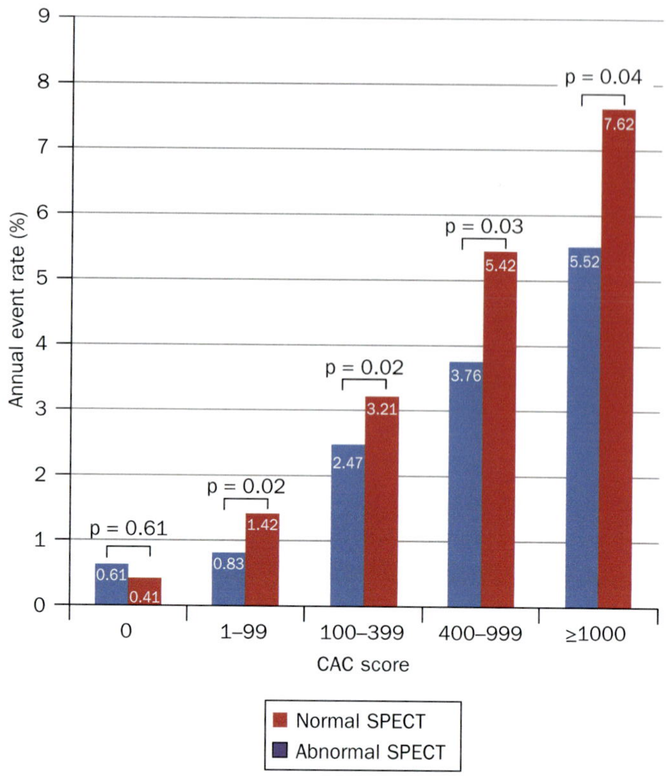

Figure 6.14. Adverse cardiac events are effectively predicted by both coronary artery calcium score and SPECT MPI results. From Engbers EM, Timmer JR, Ottervanger JP, Mouden M, Knollema S, Jager PL. Prognostic Value of Coronary Artery Calcium Scoring in Addition to Single-Photon Emission Computed Tomographic Myocardial Perfusion Imaging in Symptomatic Patients. Circulation Cardiovascular imaging 2016;9.

exertion. He has exercise-limiting knee pain, and therefore vasodilator PET MPI was pursued for evaluation.

PHYSICAL FINDINGS

BP: 95/67 mmHg; P: 88 bpm; Ht: 5'7"; Wt: 165 lbs; BMI: 26. His jugular venous pressure is normal and he has no carotid bruits. He has a regular rate and rhythm with an early peaking systolic ejection murmur heard at the right upper sternal border. Pulmonary auscultation is without wheezing or rales. His abdomen is soft and non-tender. There is no peripheral edema and his peripheral pulses are equal and symmetrical. ECG is shown in Figure 6.17, along with representative images from the echocardiogram (Figure 6.18).

VASODILATOR STRESS FINDINGS

There were no ischemic ECG changes or symptoms after administration of 0.4 mg regadenoson. He had an appropriate heart rate response and became slightly hypotensive to 85/55 with vasodilator stress. He remained asymptomatic and his blood pressure recovered to baseline without intervention. 8.8 mCi of Tc-99m tetrofosmin was injected

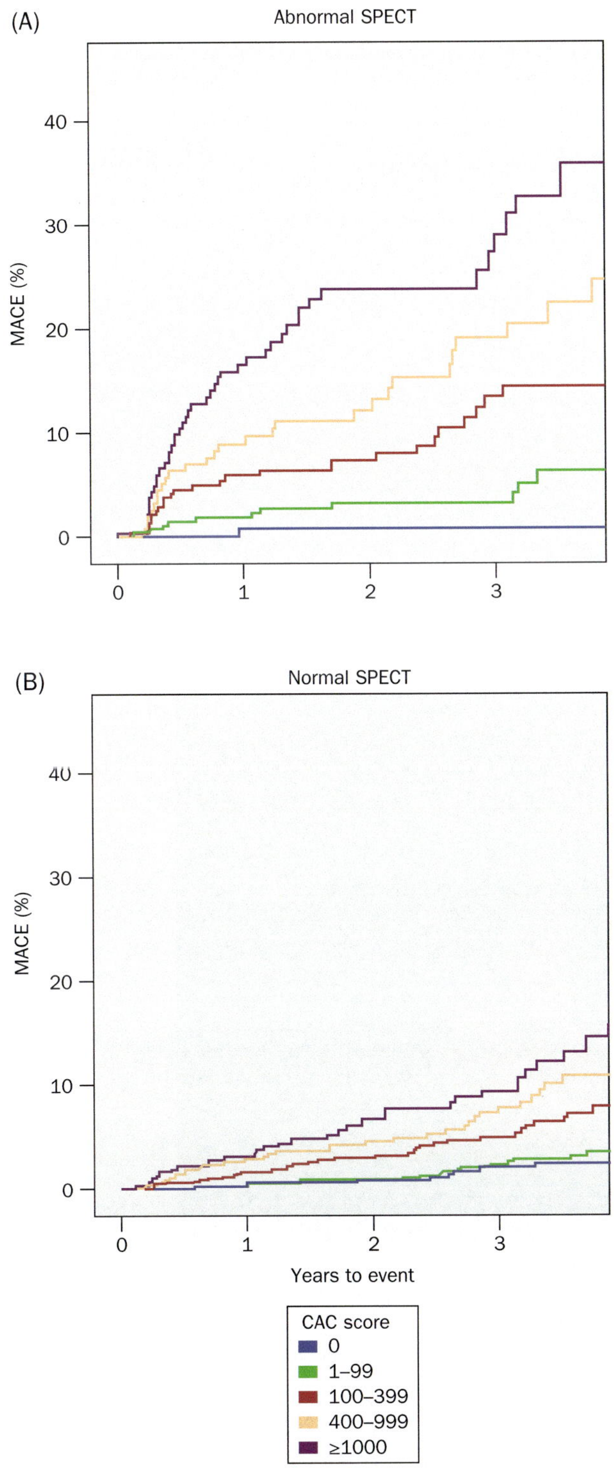

Figure 6.15. Increasing coronary artery calcium scores predicts worsening cardiac event rates in patients with both abnormal (A) and normal (B) SPECT imaging. From Engbers EM, Timmer JR, Ottervanger JP, Mouden M, Knollema S, Jager PL. Prognostic Value of Coronary Artery Calcium Scoring in Addition to Single-Photon Emission Computed Tomographic Myocardial Perfusion Imaging in Symptomatic Patients. Circulation Cardiovascular imaging 2016;9.

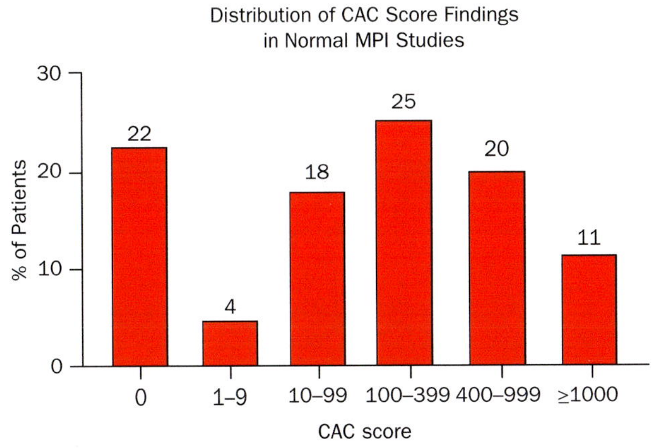

Figure 6.16. Distribution of coronary calcium scores in patients with normal SPECT perfusion. Adapted from Berman DS, Wong ND, Gransar H, et al. Relationship between stress-induced myocardial ischemia and atherosclerosis measured by coronary calcium tomography. Journal of the American College of Cardiology 2004;44:923-30, with permission from Elsevier Science and Technology Journals.

at rest with rest imaging obtained 35 minutes later. At peak stress the patient received 30.1 mCi of Tc-99m tetrofosmin followed by stress imaging 20 minutes later.

The perfusion images are shown in Figure 6.19 and gated images in Figure 6.20. Invasive coronary angiography can be seen in Figure 6.21.

The stress portion of the test was remarkable for mild transient hypotension. Perfusion images demonstrate a large area of moderate to severe ischemia in the anterior, anterolateral, apical, inferior, inferoseptal, and inferolateral segments with mild to moderate concomitant scar in the inferior, apical, and mid antero/inferolateral segments. In addition, there were further high-risk features, including stress-induced decline in ejection fraction and transient ischemic dilation (TID). Left heart catheterization revealed severe triple-vessel coronary artery disease, including severe distal left main artery stenosis with extension into the ostial left anterior descending and left circumflex arteries. The right coronary artery was occluded, filling distally with left to right collaterals. The patient went on to have successful coronary bypass surgery.

LEARNING POINT

The summed difference score (SDS = summed stress score [SSS] – summed rest score [SRS]) and SSS correlate with risk of death or myocardial infarction.[10] In this patient the SDS of 22 and the SSS of 28 indicate extensive ischemia and high risk for major cardiac events. Furthermore, this patient demonstrates several other non-perfusion markers of elevated risk.[11] TID is a specific marker for multivessel or left main coronary disease (88% specific) but lacks sensitivity (44%) for detection of multivessel or left main disease. Similarly, TID has been shown to have a prognostic ability in correlating with

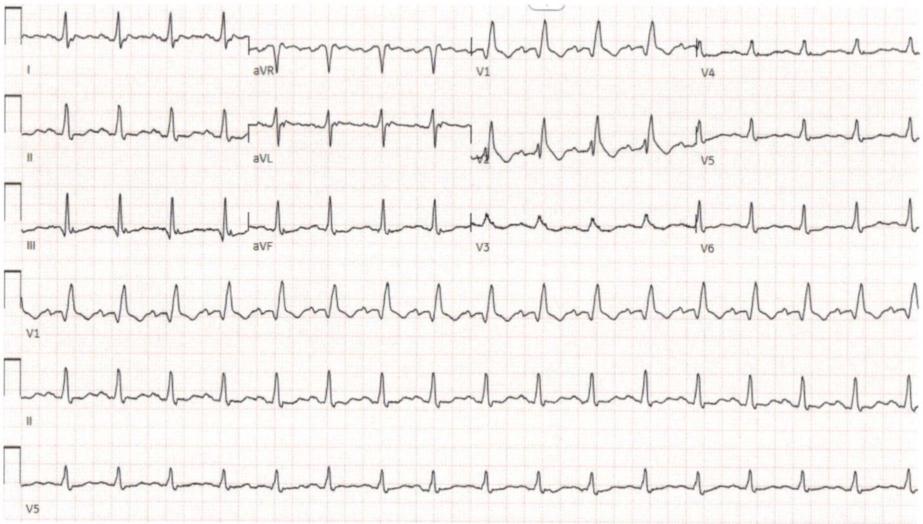

Figure 6.17. Case 3. ECG.

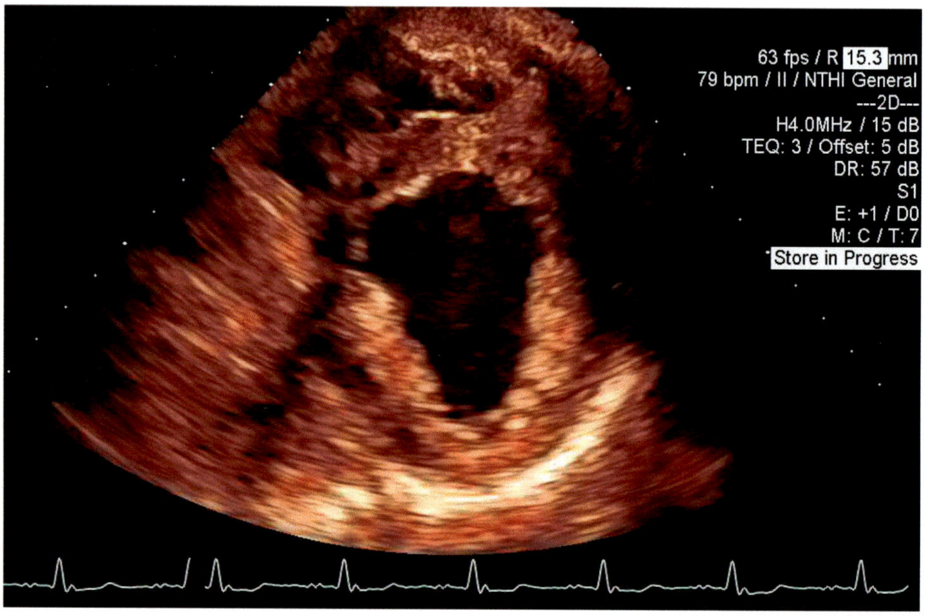

Figure 6.18. Case 3. Echocardiogram.

(A)

(B)

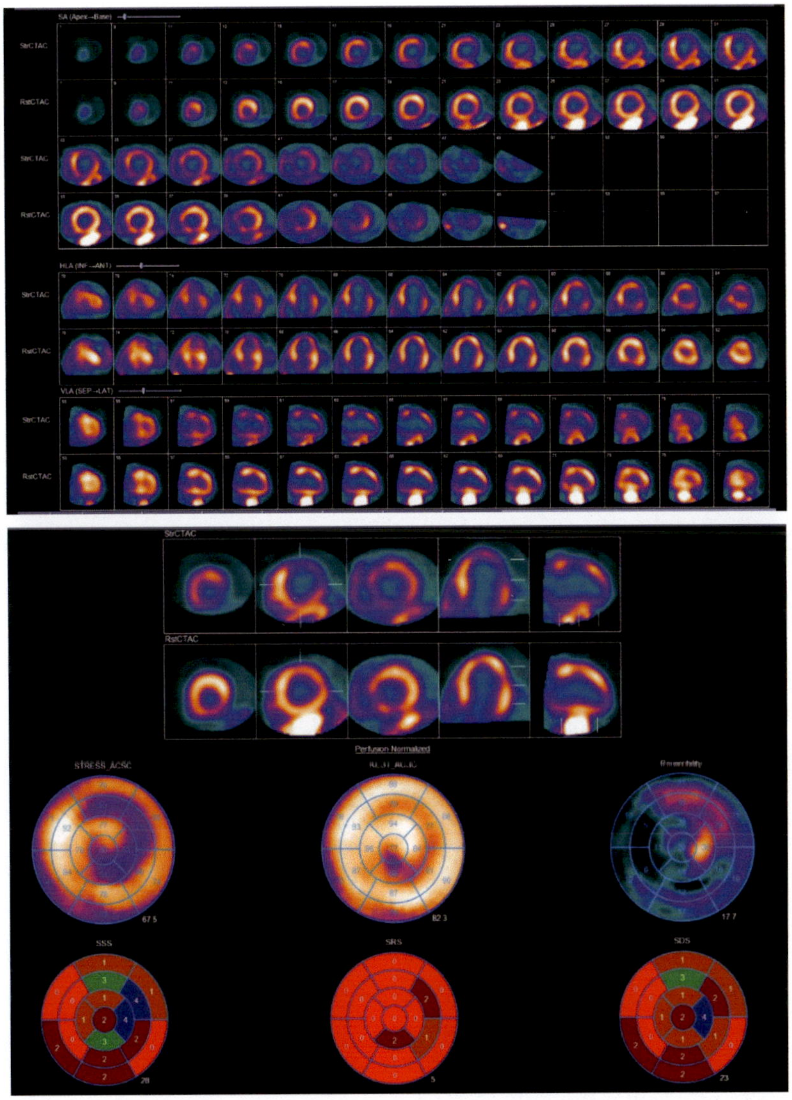

Figure 6.19. Case 3. PET/CT myocardial perfusion images (stress over rest images displayed) (A) and polar plots with automated quantification (B).

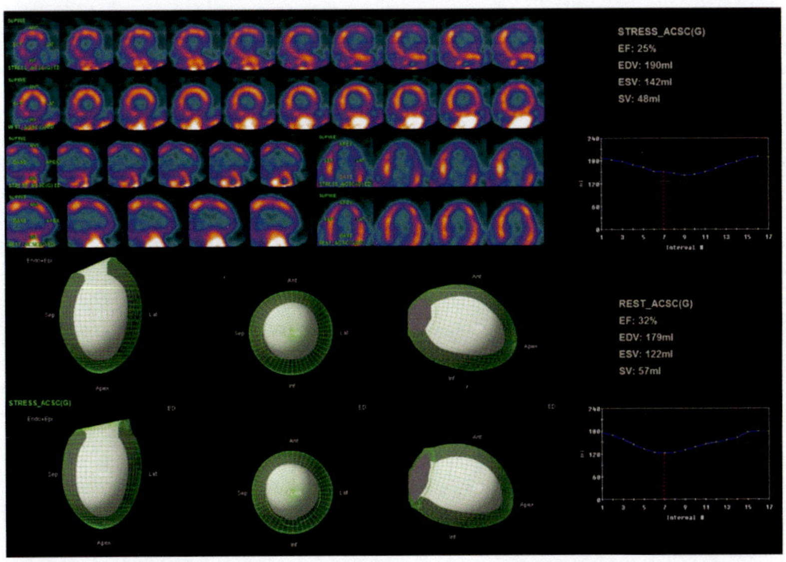

Figure 6.20. Case 3. Gated images (stress and rest).

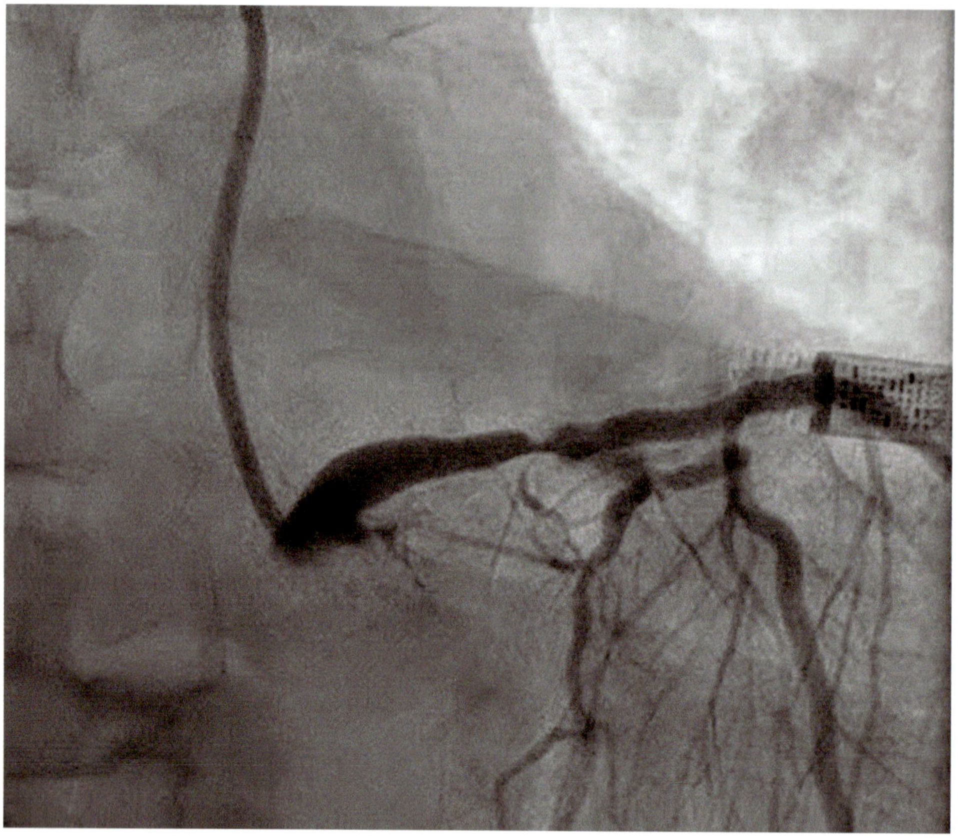

Figure 6.21. Case 3. Invasive coronary angiogram.

cardiac events, particularly in the presence of abnormal perfusion and cardiac risk factors.[12,13] While a depressed ejection fraction on myocardial perfusion imaging has been shown to be an independent predictor of risk,[14] stress-induced decreases in ventricular function in particular are understood to be accompanied by a high risk of cardiac events.[15,16]

REFERENCES

1. Duvall WL, Baber U, Levine EJ, et al. A model for the prediction of a successful stress-first Tc-99m SPECT MPI. *J Nucl Cardiol.* 2012;19:1124–1134.
2. Gowdar S, Chaudhry W, Ahlberg AW, et al. Triage of patients for attenuation-corrected stress-first Tc-99m SPECT MPI using a simplified clinical pre-test scoring model. *J Nucl Cardiol.* 2018;25:1178–1187.
3. Chang SM, Nabi F, Xu J, et al. Normal stress-only versus standard stress/rest myocardial perfusion imaging: similar patient mortality with reduced radiation exposure. *J Am Coll Cardiol.* 2010;55:221–230.
4. Duvall WL, Wijetunga MN, Klein TM, et al. The prognosis of a normal stress-only Tc-99m myocardial perfusion imaging study. *J Nucl Cardiol.* 2010;17:370–377.
5. Hussain N, Parker MW, Henzlova MJ, Duvall WL. Stress-first myocardial perfusion imaging. *Cardiol Clin.* 2016;34:59–67.
6. Mouden M, Ottervanger JP, Timmer JR, et al. The influence of coronary calcium score on the interpretation of myocardial perfusion imaging. *J Nucl Cardiol.* 2014;21:368–374.
7. Patchett ND, Pawar S, Miller EJ. Visual identification of coronary calcifications on attenuation correction CT improves diagnostic accuracy of SPECT/CT myocardial perfusion imaging. *J Nucl Cardiol.* 2017;24:711–720.
8. Engbers EM, Timmer JR, Ottervanger JP, et al. Prognostic value of coronary artery calcium scoring in addition to single-photon emission computed tomographic myocardial perfusion imaging in symptomatic patients. *Circ Cardiovasc Imaging.* 2016;9(5):e003966.
9. Berman DS, Wong ND, Gransar H, et al. Relationship between stress-induced myocardial ischemia and atherosclerosis measured by coronary calcium tomography. *J Am Coll Cardiol.* 2004;44:923–930.
10. Leslie WD, Tully SA, Yogendran MS, et al. Prognostic value of automated quantification of 99mTc-sestamibi myocardial perfusion imaging. *J Nucl Med.* 2005;46:204–211.
11. Bajaj NS, Singh S, Farag A, et al. The prognostic value of non-perfusion variables obtained during vasodilator stress myocardial perfusion imaging. *J Nucl Cardiol.* 2016;23:390–413.
12. Petretta M, Acampa W, Daniele S, et al. Transient ischemic dilation in patients with diabetes mellitus: Prognostic value and effect on clinical outcome after coronary revascularization. *Circ Cardiovasc Imaging.* 2013;6:908–915.
13. Alama M, Labos C, Emery H, et al. Diagnostic and prognostic significance of transient ischemic dilation (TID) in myocardial perfusion imaging: A systematic review and meta-analysis. *J Nucl Cardiol.* 2018;25:724–737.
14. Travin MI, Heller GV, Johnson LL, et al. The prognostic value of ECG-gated SPECT imaging in patients undergoing stress

Tc-99m sestamibi myocardial perfusion imaging. *J Nucl Cardiol.* 2004;11:253–262.
15. Ferro A, Petretta M, Acampa W, et al. Post-stress left ventricular ejection fraction drop in patients with diabetes: A gated myocardial perfusion imaging study. *BMC Cardiovasc Disord.* 2013;13:99.
16. Van Tosh A, Votaw JR, Reichek N, et al. The relationship between ischemia-induced left ventricular dysfunction, coronary flow reserve, and coronary steal on regadenoson stress-gated (82)Rb PET myocardial perfusion imaging. *J Nucl Cardiol.* 2013;20:1060–1068.

7.

ARTIFACTS

William A. Van Decker

CASE 1

HISTORY AND IMAGING FINDINGS

A 58-year-old woman with diabetes, hypertension, abnormal rest ECG "cannot exclude anterior wall myocardial infarction, age indeterminate," is able to walk less than one flight of stairs due to dyspnea. She is 5-foot-2 and 195 lbs. She was referred for a stress pharmacologic technetium 99m sestamibi myocardial perfusion study because of chest discomfort that lasts 5 to 10 minutes at rest or activity but with an inconsistent pattern. Her activity is limited by shortness of breath with less than one flight of stairs.

She underwent same-day rest–stress protocol using a standard SPECT Anger camera. The images are shown in Figure 7.1. The raw planar (rotating) images are shown in Figure 7.2 and ▶ Video 7.1. The gated images are shown in Figure 7.3 and ▶ Video 7.2. The imaging physician recommends repeating the stress images on the new SPECT/CT camera. The attenuation-corrected images are shown in Figure 7.4.

QUESTION

The most useful approach to assessing the initial perfusion finding as real or artifact is:

a. Sinogram assessment for motion
b. Raw planar spin assessment for soft tissue attenuation pattern
c. Gated SPECT wall thickening
d. Attenuation-correction imaging

ANSWER

d. No visual motion in raw spin. Raw spin is helpful for attenuation presence but of limited value in a high-risk patient. Wall thickening is helpful to exclude scar (abnormal rest ECG) but is less helpful when ischemia is considered. Robust attenuation correction applies mathematical science in defining attenuation artifact and is the most useful in this situation.

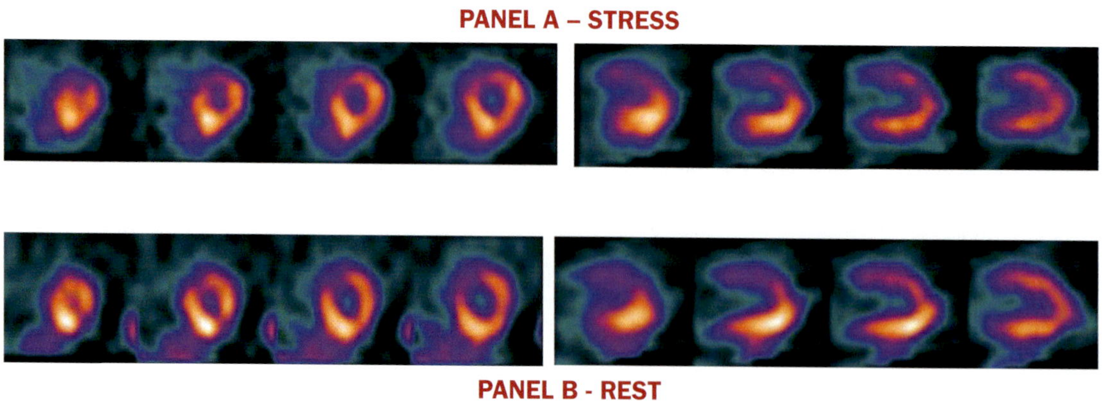

Figure 7.1. Case 1. SPECT image series showing mild fixed anterior defect suggestive of breast attenuation artifact but requires further confirmation in a patient with clinical cardiac risk.

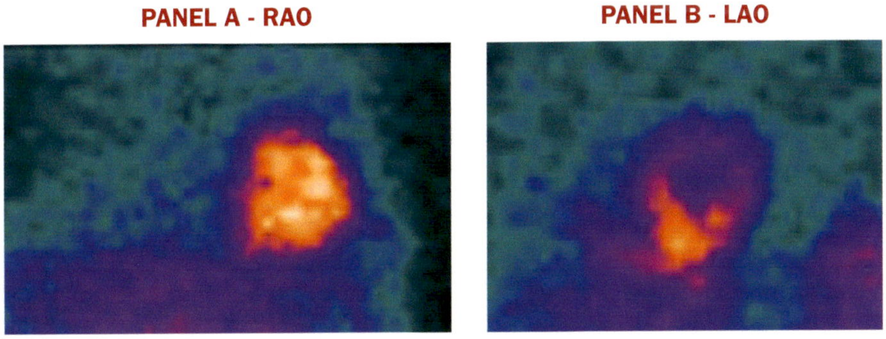

Figure 7.2. Case 1. Traditional raw planar acquisition spin prior to tomographic reconstructions. Shifting curvilinear count attenuating soft tissue as spin moves from RAO to LPO consistent with breast attenuation artifact. The rotating video is shown in Video 7.1.

CASE 2

HISTORY AND IMAGING FINDINGS

A 64-year-old man with atypical angina was referred for a pharmacologic MPI study. He has malignant hypertension and has limited exercise tolerance (less than one block of walking on level ground) due to knee arthritis. His ECG is abnormal with left ventricular hypertrophy and diffuse T-wave inversions.

The images are shown in Figure 7.5. The quality assurance save screen from the initial reconstruction process is shown in Figure 7.6. The repeat reconstructed save screen images are shown in Figure 7.7. The repeat reconstructed tomographic images are shown in Figure 7.8.

QUESTION

What is the best clinical decision based on the image sequences?

a. Send patient to coronary angiography because patient is at high risk (transient ischemic dilatation).

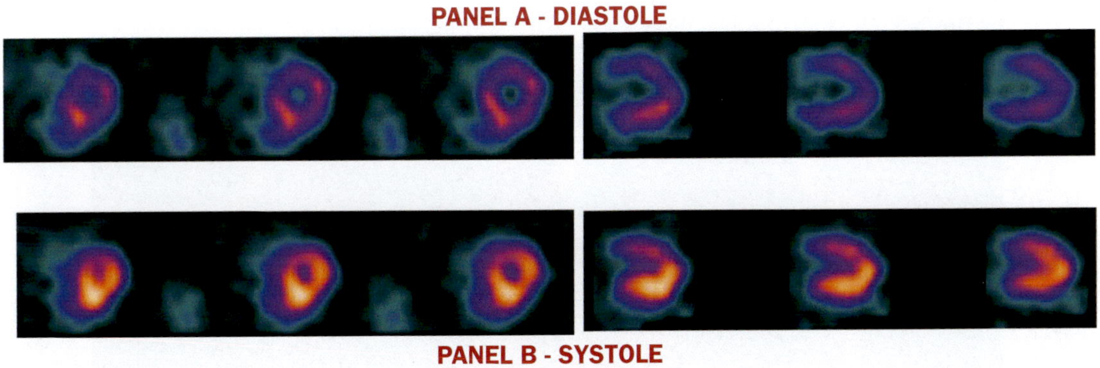

Figure 7.3. Case 1. Gated SPECT images showing normal wall thickening in a region of mild count decrease, making finding more likely to be due to attenuation than myocardial scar (which is usually associated with regional wall motion abnormality and decreased wall thickening). The gated images are shown in Video 7.2.

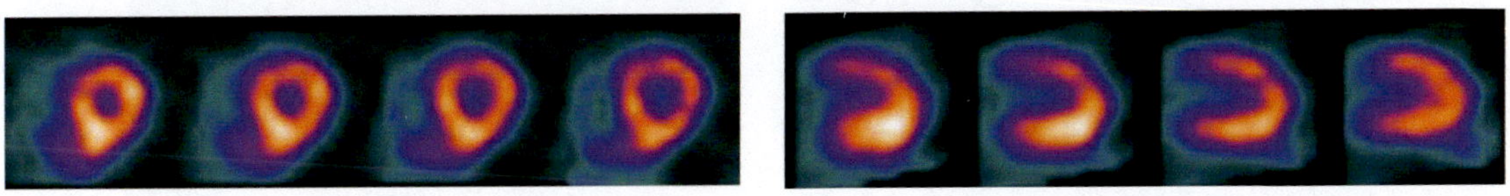

Figure 7.4. Case 1. Attenuation-corrected images showing that attenuation artifact could be normalized utilizing a mathematically fitted attenuation map overlay.

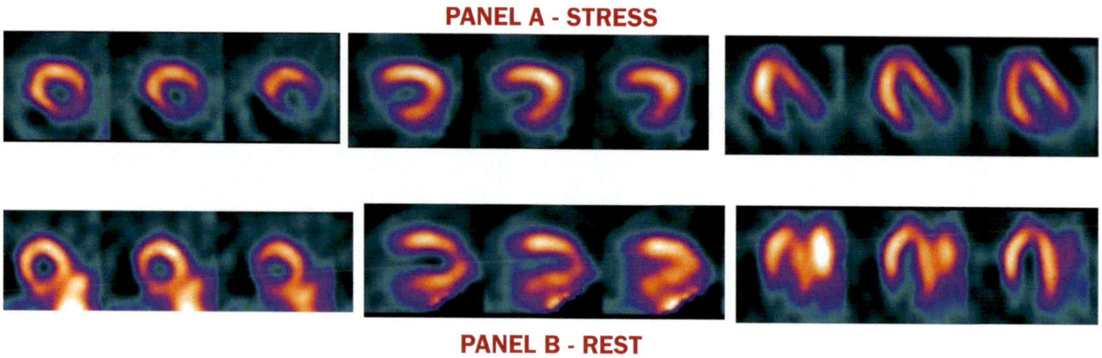

Figure 7.5. Case 2. Tomographic reconstructions images highly suspicious for a variation in the angles of reconstruction between stress and rest acquisitions, with different orientation of the apex and different LV cavity shapes.

b. Send patient home for goal-directed medical therapy, as the scan is low risk.
c. Send patient to coronary angiography based on perfusion pattern (high risk).
d. Send patient to coronary CTA to increase assurance.

ANSWER

b. The initial axes of reconstruction for stress and rest images were very dissimilar (sometimes a result of doing reconstructions after each separate acquisition temporally

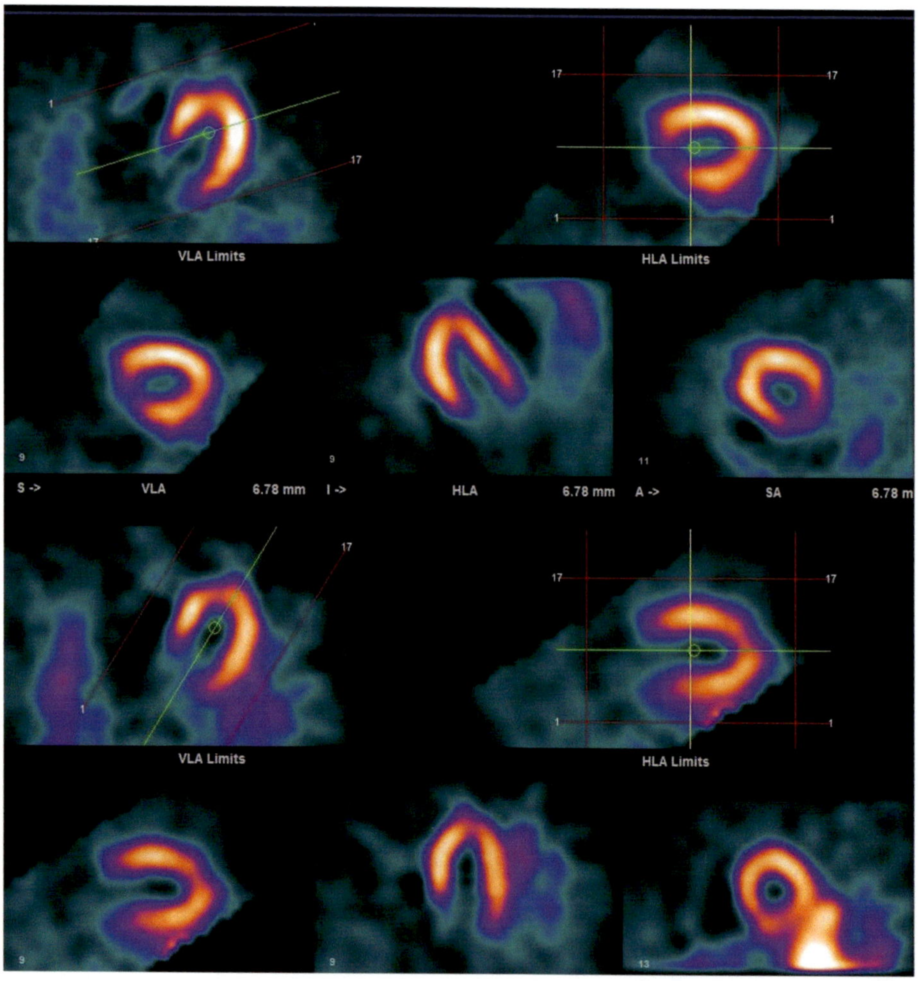

Figure 7.6. Case 2. Reconstruction quality assurance save screen documenting widely different axes of used for stress versus rest reconstruction.

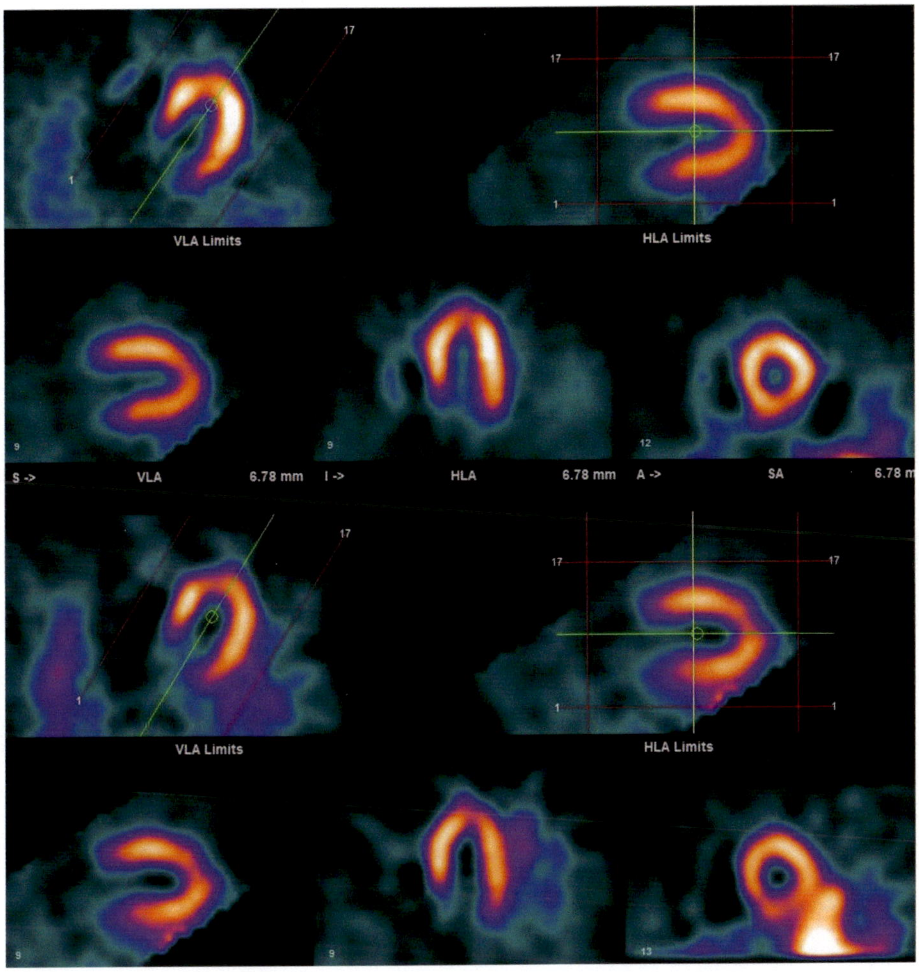

Figure 7.7. Case 2. Reconstruction quality assurance save screen documenting correct angles of reconstruction between stress and rest.

apart, rather than both reconstructions at some time when the study is fully completed, making matching axes easier). These different axes cause different perceptions of cavity size and shape and perfusion. When similar appropriate axes are chosen for reconstruction, both stress and rest appear similar without a large perfusion defect. In this patient with intermediate clinical risk and where hypertension may explain the ECG abnormality, and in the presence of normal perfusion, normal LV size, and normal LVEF, medical therapy is appropriate.

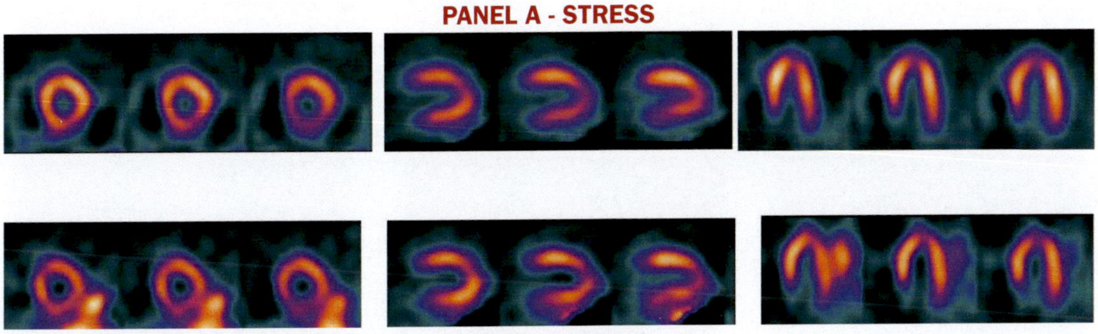

Figure 7.8. Case 2. Same tomographic image set as Figure 7.5, but now both stress and rest images have correct axes of reconstruction; the apex is now at similar position on each series and LV cavity shape is normal.

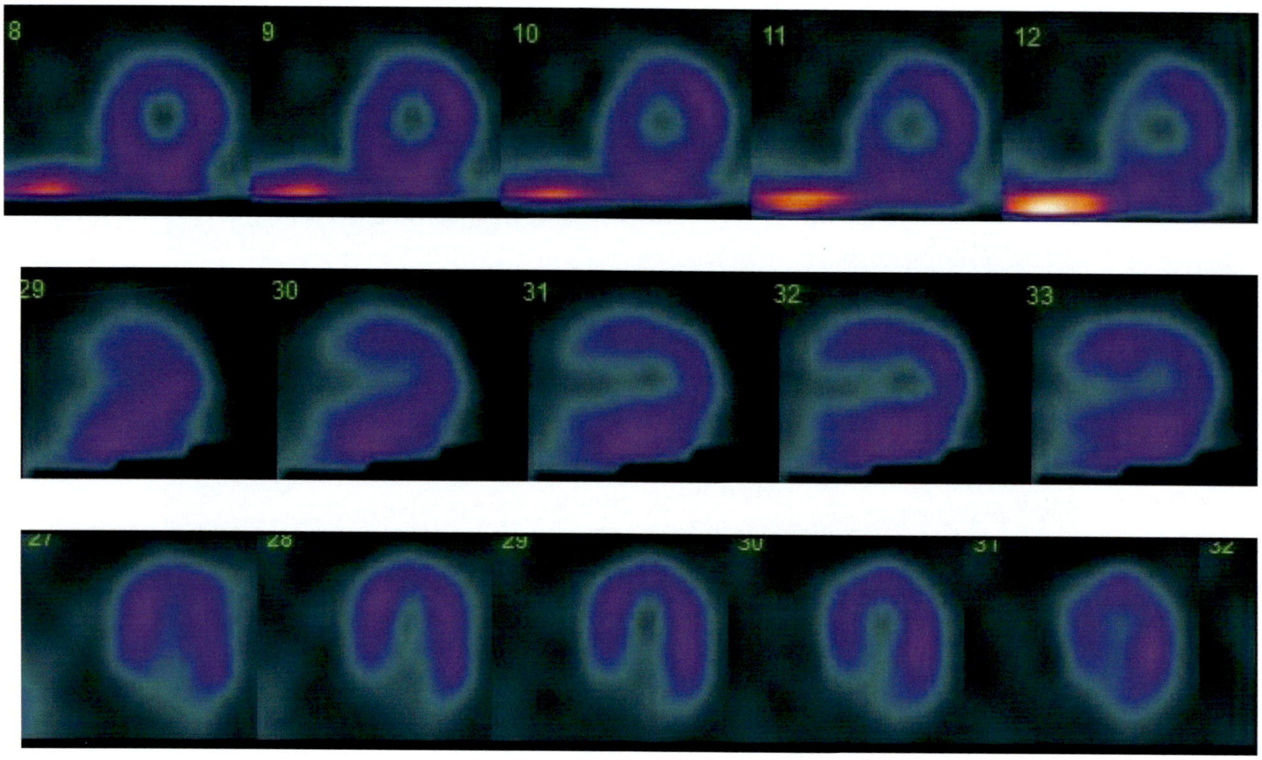

Figure 7.9. Case 3. SPECT tomographic series showing intense extracardiac signal that results in marked downscaling of the cardiac activity.

CASE 3

HISTORY AND IMAGING FINDINGS

A 70-year-old man presents with atypical angina. He has hypertension, hyperlipidemia, and a family history of CAD. The resting ECG showed nonspecific ST-T wave abnormalities. He can walk less than one block due to back pain. He underwent pharmacologic rest–stress MPI.

The technologist reconstructs the tomograms and has difficulty identifying the heart. There is concern for "global hypoperfusion" or dose infiltration (Figure 7.9). After further processing, the images are shown in Figure 7.10. After manual image display manipulation, the images are shown in Figure 7.11. The patient was asked to eat lunch and was re-imaged 2 hours later (Figure 7.12).

QUESTION

What other technique may help clarify this study?

a. Schedule for repeat study with rubidium-82 PET.
b. Repeat SPECT acquisition in 24 hours.
c. Repeat imaging in prone position.
d. Acquire repeat images on different energy level.

ANSWER

a. Very little technetium signal will be left at 24 hours after four half-lives, and therefore a repeat SPECT acquisition in 24 hours is not advisable. A repeat study with thallium-201 could be considered as another option. Prone imaging

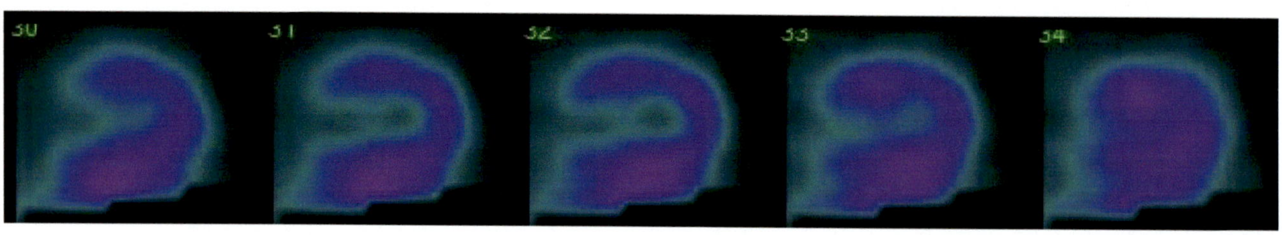

Figure 7.10. Case 3. Attempt to mask the extracardiac activity creates a problem of losing true cardiac activity as well.

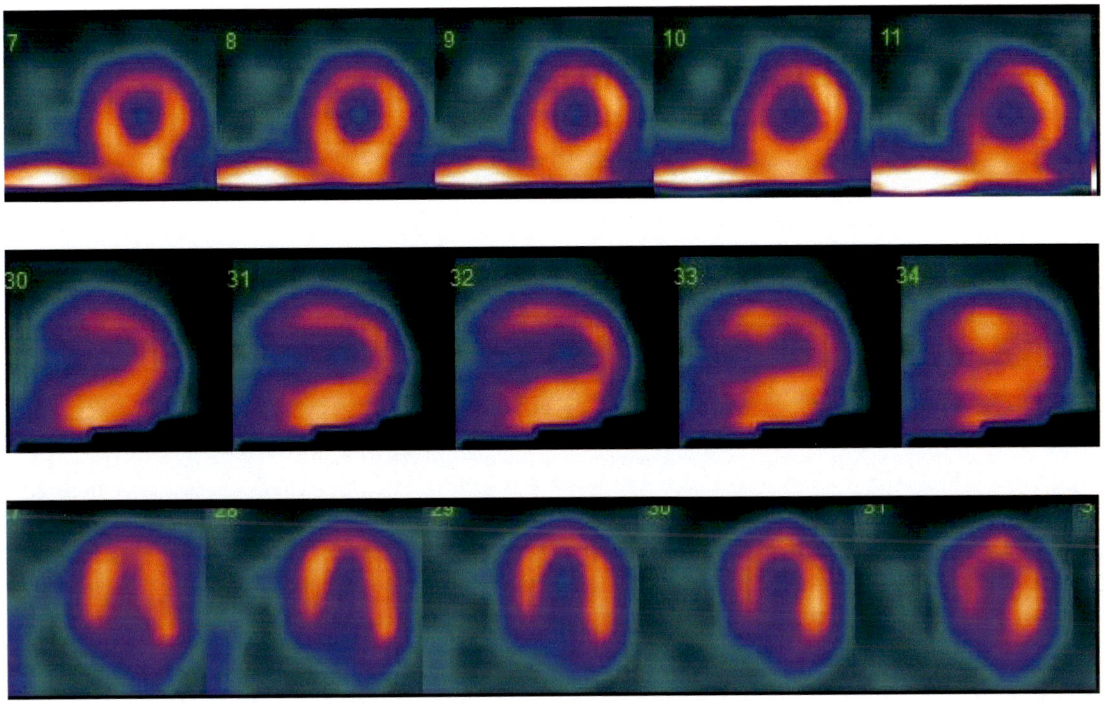

Figure 7.11. Case 3. Manual normalization by adjusting scales may be helpful at times, but the "blooming oversaturation" of the extracardiac activity often remains a problem in precise interpretation.

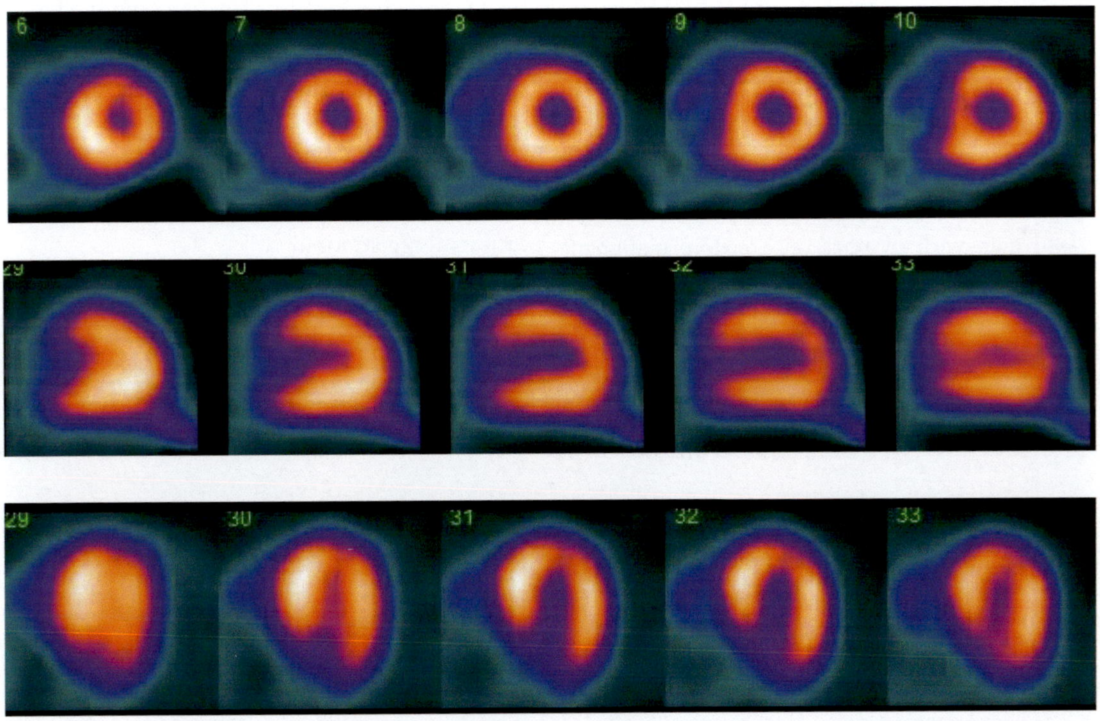

Figure 7.12. Case 3. Technetium-99m perfusion agents are excreted by the hepatobiliary system. Allowing time plus food/water intake (to clear hepatic/transverse colon activity) will create a better normalized image. More often than not, loops of small bowel or transverse colon (rather than the liver activity) butting against the heart create these downscaling problems.

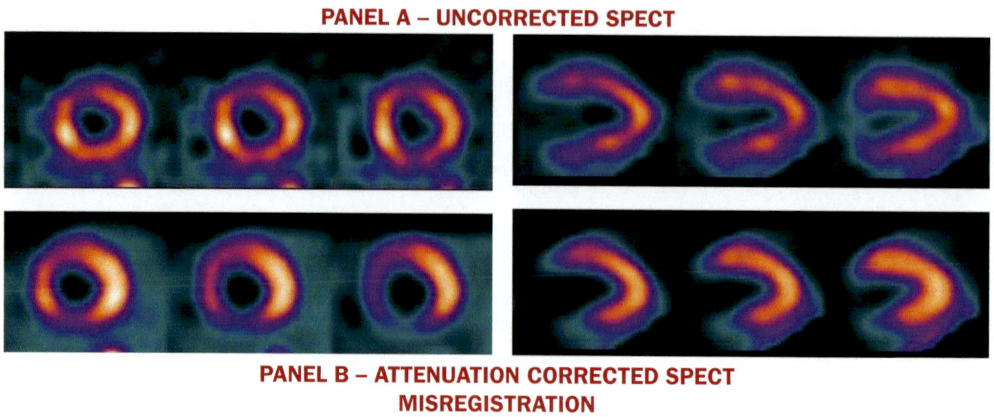

Figure 7.13. Case 4. Odd-appearing perfusion defects on attenuation-correction tomograms in SPECT CT should raise a question about the quality assurance of the CT or the fusion co-registration image (especially if the defect is worse on attenuation-correction images than non-corrected images). Quality assurance checklist should be considered.

does not consistently remove adjacent extracardiac bowel activity. Technetium, whether in gut or heart, is emitting at 140 KeV; changing the energy acquisition level will only decrease global signal but not distinguish site. Rubidium is less likely to have such intense bowel interference (technetium 99m perfusion agents are excreted by the hepatobiliary system; waiting short periods of time after more food frequently moves the hepatic/transverse colon extracardiac activity away from the heart into the descending colon.

CASE 4

HISTORY AND IMAGING FINDINGS

A 50-year-old man with dyspnea on exertion, malignant hypertension, end-stage renal disease on dialysis, and abnormal rest ECG was referred for pharmacologic stress myocardial perfusion imaging. The study was acquired on a SPECT/CT camera. The images are shown in Figure 7.13. The CT equipment quality control save screen and the quality assurance save screen from the SPECT and the CT fusion co-registration for attention correction images are shown in Figure 7.14 and Figure 7.15. The images were then reprocessed and are shown in Figure 7.16.

QUESTION

What is the best method to avoid SPECT-CT image fusion misregistration?

a. Acquire SPECT and CT simultaneously

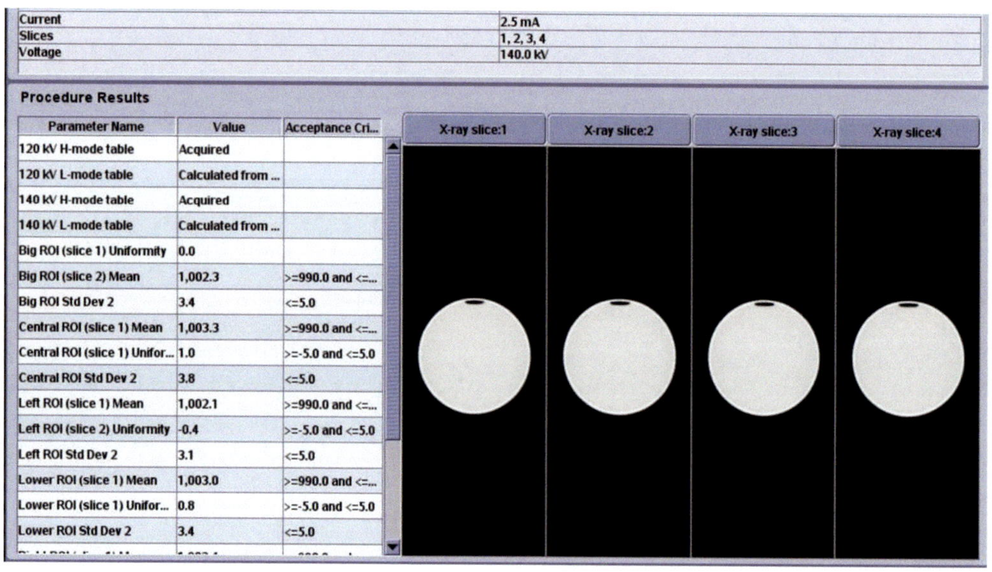

Figure 7.14. Case 4. CT scanners can lose adjustment of their zero Hounsfield unit to water and the last phantom should be checked. CT scan detectors can have problems like nuclear detectors and quality assurance for ring artifacts should be checked.

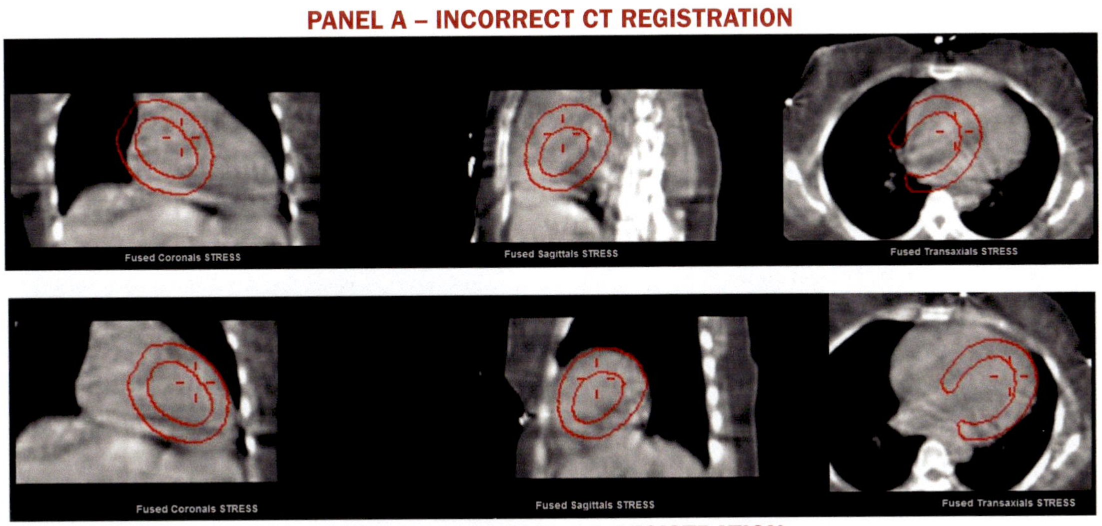

Figure 7.15. Case 4. Attenuation correction relies on near-perfect overlay of the CT attenuation map on the SPECT image, and the co-registration needs to be visually checked to make such co-registration is adequate. If not, the images need to be manually co-registered again.

b. Increase dose of radionuclide
c. Quality control every fusion image visually and save screen for documentation
d. Increase KeV of CT unit

ANSWER

c. Nuclear detectors are mounted in front of the CT ring and the patient table is pushed from the nuclear detectors into the CT ring at the end of the nuclear acquisition sequentially. Simultaneous acquisition is not possible. Neither changing the SPECT tracer dose nor the CT imaging dose affects fusion overlay. Overlay of SPECT and CT must be visually assessed for appropriateness. PET images are always attenuation corrected. With SPECT, a clue of misregistration is lack of perfusion defects on uncorrected images but severe defects on corrected images.

ACKNOWLEDGMENTS

Special thanks to Mathew Mathai, CNMT, Michael Gall, CNMT, and Syed Muhammad Zaidi, MD, for assistance on the image files.

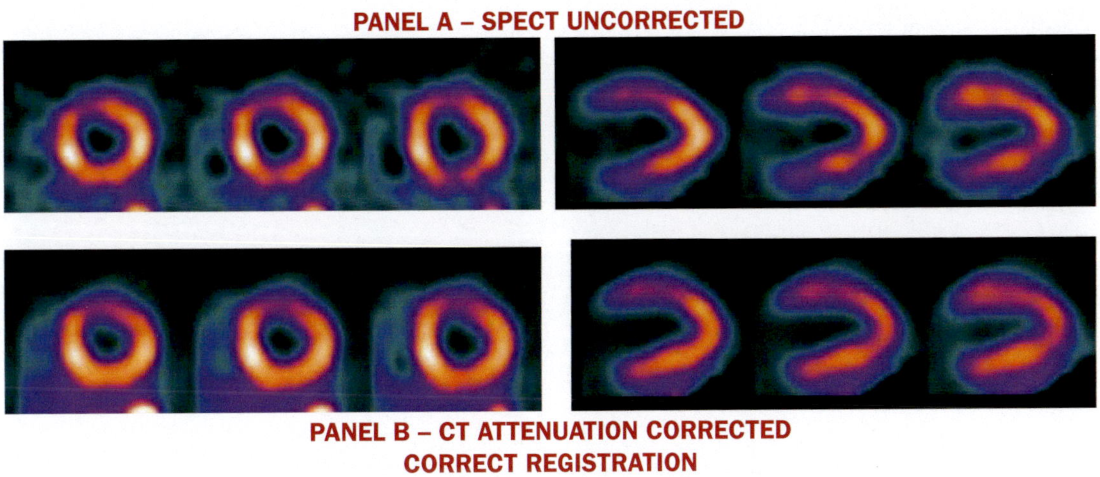

Figure 7.16. Case 4. Same SPECT series as Figure 7.13 but now with SPECT and CT correctly fused co- registered.

BIBLIOGRAPHY

Abreu C, Frade AG. Artefacts and pitfalls in myocardial imaging (SPECT, SPECT/CT, and PET/CT). In *Myocardial Perfusion Imaging*. European Association of Nuclear Medicine (EANM). 2014;109–123.

Burrell S, McDonald A. Artifacts and pitfalls in myocardial perfusion imaging. *J Nucl Med Technol*. 2006;34:193–211.

Case J, Bateman T. Taking the perfect nuclear image: Quality control, acquisition, and processing techniques for cardiac SPECT, PET, and hybrid imaging. *J Nucl Cardiol*. 2013;9:891–907.

DePuey E, Rozanski A. Using gated technetium sestamibi SPECT to characterize fixed myocardial defects as infarct or artifact. *J Nucl Med*. 1995;36:952–955.

Dvorak R, Brown R, Corbett J. Interpretation of SPECT/CT myocardial perfusion images: Common artifacts and quality control techniques. *Radiographics*. 2011;31(7):2041–2057. doi.org// 10.1148/rg.317115090.

Hansen C. The role of the translation table in cardiac imaging display. *J Nucl Cardiol*. 2006;13:571–575.

Piekarski E, Manrique A, Rouzet, et al. Current status of MPI with new SPECT/CT cameras. *Semin Nucl Med*. 2020;50(3):219–226.

8.

REGULATION OF MYOCARDIAL BLOOD FLOW

Henry Gewirtz

QUESTIONS

1. Which of the following principal components of myocardial oxygen demand is a component of two others?
   a. LV contractile state (End-systolic elastance; Ees)
   b. Coronary venous oxygen saturation
   c. Mean left atrial pressure
   d. LV dP/dt
2. The fact that the normal rest endocardial:epicardial (EN:EP) blood flow ratio is greater than one reflects the fact that:
   a. LV forces of contraction are greatest in the epicardial layer
   b. LV forces of contraction are greatest in the endocardial layer
   c. Density of the microvasculature is greater in epicardial layers
   d. Endocardial vasodilator reserve is greater than that of epicardial layers
3. Considering FFR, MFR, iFR, and dP@50 as metrics of myocardial flow reserve, which of the following is *not* correct?
   a. Like FFR and MFR, both iFR and dP@50 require infusion of adenosine (IV preferred) to be clinically useful.
   b. Like FFR, both iFR and dP@50 employ full cardiac cycle pressure measurements for computation of each parameter.
   c. Unlike FFR and MFR, both iFR and dP@50 are independent of the level of mean aortic pressure.
   d. Like FFR and MFR, both iFR and dP@50 are dependent of the level of mean aortic pressure.

ANSWERS

1c. Mean left atrial pressure contributes to both preload and afterload (Laplace equation) and so is a component of two major determinants of myocardial oxygen demand. LV contractile state defined by Ees is an independent determinant as is LV dP/dt, which is sometimes used but is load-dependent and not strictly correct. Coronary venous oxygen saturation is an indirect measure of myocardial oxygen consumption and so reflects the combined effects of all four determinants (heart rate, contractility, preload, and afterload).

2b. Forces of contraction are greatest in endocardial not epicardial layers of the heart (law of Laplace; wall thickness term). Accordingly, the endocardium is rendered transiently ischemic with each systole and dilates more in diastole than epicardium, which has some blood flow in systole (Figure 8.1), and thus endocardium is preferentially perfused (ischemic overshoot) such that the EN:EP ratio is more than 1. The residual vasodilator reserve of the endocardium, however, is less as a result and so it is

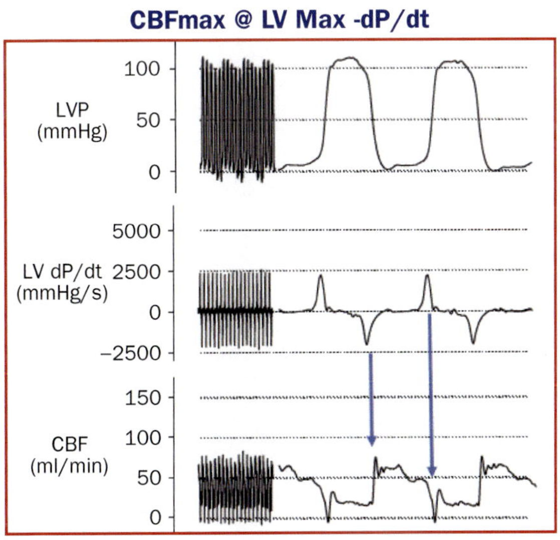

Figure 8.1. Relationship between instantaneous coronary blood flow (CBF) and left ventricular dP/dt. Note that peak coronary inflow occurs in early diastole at the time of maximum negative dP/dt; this is an indication that LV relaxation plays an important role in coronary filling. Similarly, LV pressure peak positive dP/dt coincides with cessation of CBF; this observation indicates that LV contraction all but terminates CBF in systole. (Courtesy of Dirk D. J. Duncker, MD, PhD, Erasmus University, Rotterdam, NE)

rendered more vulnerable to ischemia. The epicardial layers have some systolic flow and lesser compressive forces both in systole and diastole. Thus, they are not ischemic with each systole and do not dip into any of their residual vasodilator reserve. Increased microvasculature in endocardial, not epicardial layers, also may contribute to EN:EP > 1.

3d. Each of these metrics is sensitive to the level of mean aortic pressure (see Equation 4 in Chapter 8 in the main text) since it reflects the driving pressure available in diastole to overcome combined resistance to flow at stenosis, small vessel, and microcirculatory levels. Adenosine is not required for measurements of iFR and dP@50 even though both metrics are indicative of maximal myocardial blood flow, notwithstanding assessment in selected periods of diastole and without need for adenosine.

9.

MEASUREMENT OF MYOCARDIAL BLOOD FLOW BY PET

Heinrich R. Schelbert

QUESTIONS

1. Tracer kinetic models are important for deriving quantitative flows from the arterial radiotracer input function and the myocardial response to it. Which of the following statements is *false*?
   a. They describe the exchange of radiotracer from blood into myocardium and the biochemical fate of the radiolabel in tissue.
   b. They correct for the flow-dependent decline in the radiotracer first-pass extraction fraction.
   c. They employ first-order rate constants for describing the exchange of radiotracer between functional pools.
   d. They are identical for each of the different PET radiotracers of flow.

2. Errors in estimating myocardial blood flow with PET may be caused by (of the statements below, select the one that is *false*):
   a. High spillover of activity from myocardium into the blood pool region of interest
   b. Incomplete sampling of the arterial radiotracer input function when image acquisition is delayed
   c. Adequate correction of cardiac motion during the initial transit of the radiotracer through the central circulation
   d. Misalignment of PET emission and CT transmission images

3. Which of the following statements regarding the test-retest variability is *false*?
   a. The radiotracer should be administered in a consistent fashion.
   b. Measurements of myocardial blood flow should be performed in a quiet ambience.
   c. Fully automated corrections for patient motion worsen the test-retest variability.
   d. Biologic factors influence the variability of test-retesting when performed several days apart.

ANSWERS

1d (please see page 191 (Chapter 9) in Book), 2c (Please see page 193 and 198 (Chapter 9) in Book), 3c (Please see page 192, 196, 197, 201 (Chapter 9) in Book).

10.

MEASUREMENT OF MYOCARDIAL BLOOD FLOW BY SPECT

Juliana Brenande de Oliveira Brito, Gary R. Small, Kathryn J. Ascah, R. Glenn Wells, and Terrence D. Ruddy

QUESTIONS

1. SPECT MPI has several limitations compared to PET MPI. Which recent development in SPECT MPI has facilitated the measurement of SPECT MBF?
   a. SPECT radiotracers with better uptake/flow kinetics
   b. SPECT CZT camera systems with improved temporal resolution
   c. SPECT software using OSEM (Ordered Subsets Expectation Maximization) algorithms with improved image quality
   d. SPECT/CT cameras with validated attenuation correction techniques
2. SPECT MBF and MFR measurements have been validated with comparisons to PET MPI. What advantage has been reported for PET MBF measurement?
   a. PET MFR measurement has greater diagnostic accuracy for identifying coronary stenoses with reduced FFR.
   b. PET measurement of MFR has better specificity for diagnosis of significant coronary stenoses.
   c. PET measurement of MBF has better day-to-day repeatability.
   d. PET MBF measurement does not require attenuation correction.
3. CZT SPECT MPI can be used for measurement of MBF and MFR. What step is essential for accurate and precise results?
   a. A syringe pump for radiotracer injection is necessary since results with hand injection are inconsistent.
   b. A small positioning dose and imaging is required before dynamic imaging of the rest injection.
   c. Dynamic imaging must start before radiotracer injection and continues for several minutes.
   d. Imaging for residual activity is optional prior to dynamic imaging of the radiotracer injection.

ANSWERS

1b. Conventional dual-head SPECT Anger cameras need to rotate around the patient and have limited temporal resolution. The new CZT detector camera systems do not rotate and acquire data continuously like a PET camera, resulting in much better temporal resolution. *Incorrect answers*: a. SPECT MBF measurement is performed with conventional radiotracers (^{201}Tl, ^{99m}Tc tetrofosmin and ^{99m}Tc sestamibi), which have poor uptake/flow kinetics compared to PET radiotracers. c. Although image quality is improved with image reconstruction using OSEM software, this benefit has a small effect for MBF measurement. d. Some studies have shown greater accuracy of SPECT MBF measurement with CT attenuation correction, but the effect is small. Few CZT camera systems have CT capability, and MBF measurement without CT attenuation correction has been well validated.

2c. Day-to-day repeatability of MBF with PET is ~20% and better than ~30% reported with SPECT. *Incorrect answers:* a. Several studies have shown similar diagnostic accuracy of reduced SPECT and PET MFR for detection of coronary stenoses with reduced FFR or >70% luminal diameter reduction on visual analysis. b. Specificity of reduced MFR for diagnosis of obstructive CAD may be reduced due to microvascular dysfunction and diffuse CAD in the absence of severe focal obstructive CAD, whether MFR is measured with PET or SPECT. d. PET MPI does require attenuation correction, which is usually performed with CT.

3c. Dynamic imaging starts about 20 to 30 seconds before radiotracer injection to ensure that the entire radiotracer bolus is imaged. Data are recorded in list mode for several minutes and includes imaging of myocardial uptake. A late start of imaging after the onset of radiotracer injection may result in underestimation of the arterial input function and overestimation of MBF. *Incorrect answers:* a. Although a syringe pump for injection may be preferable with less operator radiation exposure, excellent results have been reported with manual injection. b. A positioning dose is not absolutely required before dynamic imaging but may be helpful for laboratories or technologists with limited experience with CZT cameras and the small camera field of view. After experience with ~50 studies, many centers have adequate expertise with patient positioning and can be confident that imaging will include all the necessary cardiac structures. d. Imaging for residual activity and subsequent correction should be performed in patients who have received a positioning radiotracer dose prior to rest injection or have had a rest injection prior to stress injection (or a stress injection prior to rest injection). Otherwise, myocardial uptake and MBF will be overestimated.

BIBLIOGRAPHY

Acampa W, Zampella E, Assante R, et al. Quantification of myocardial perfusion reserve by CZT-SPECT: A head-to-head comparison with ^{82}rubidium PET. *J Nucl Cardiol.* 2021;28(6):2827–2839. doi:10.1007/s12350-020-02129-w.

Agostini D, Roule V, Nganoa C, et al. First validation of myocardial blood flow reserve assessed by dynamic (99m) Tc-sesamibi CZT-SPECT camera: Head to head comparison with (15)0-water PET and fractional flow reserve in patients with suspected coronary artery disease. The WATERDAY study. *Eur J Nucl Med Mol Imaging.* 2018;45(7):1079–1090.

de Souza ACDAH, Gonçalves BKD, Tedeschi AL, Lima RSL. Quantification of myocardial flow reserve using a gamma camera with solid-state cadmium-zinc-telluride detectors: Relation to angiographic coronary artery disease. *J Nucl Cardiol.* 2021;28(3):876–884. doi:10.1007/s12350-019-01775-z.

Kitkungvan D, Johnson NP, Roby AE, et al. Routine clinical quantitative rest stress myocardial perfusion for managing coronary artery disease: Clinical relevance of test-retest variability. *JACC Cardiovasc Imaging.* 2017;10(5):565–577.

Murthy VL, Bateman TM, Beanlands RS, et al. Clinical quantification of myocardial blood flow using PET: Joint position paper of the SNMMI Cardiovascular Council and the ASNC. *J Nucl Med.* 2018;59:273–293; *J Nucl Cardiol.* 2018;25:269–297.

Otaki Y, Manabe O, Miller RJH, et al. Quantification of myocardial blood flow by CZT-SPECT with motion correction and comparison with ^{15}O-water PET. *J Nucl Cardiol.* 2021;28(4):1477–1486. doi:10.1007/s12350-019-01854-1.

Slomka PJ, Miller RJH, Hu LH, et al. Solid state detector SPECT myocardial perfusion imaging. *J Nucl Med.* 2019;60(9):1194–1204.

Wells RG, Radonjic I, Clackdoyle D, et al. Test-retest precision of myocardial blood flow measurements with ^{99m}Tc-tetrofosmin and solid-state detector single photon emission computed tomography. *Circ Cardiovasc Imaging.* 2020:13(2);e009769.

11.

TREADMILL EXERCISE TESTING

Gregory S. Thomas and L. Samuel Wann

CASE 1

An active 80-year-old man was referred for an exercise stress test for increasing exertional dyspnea. Twenty-three years earlier he had undergone coronary angiography, which demonstrated moderate CAD. He was treated medically until he had an inferior myocardial infarction 13 years later. Angiography at that time demonstrated a 95% posterior descending stenosis (PDA) with moderate disease in the body of the dominant right coronary artery (RCA). Stenoses of 40% in the left main and 70% in the proximal left anterior descending (LAD), two 40% diagonal stenoses, 70% and 60% mid circumflex stenoses were also present. Left ventriculography demonstrated severe hypokinesis of the proximal inferior wall with otherwise normal left ventricular (LV) function. He thus underwent four-vessel CABG with a left internal mammary artery (LIMA) to the LAD and separate saphenous vein grafts to the diagonal, obtuse marginal, and PDA.

Periodic exercise stress tests in the 10 years post-CABG were normal or near normal until the current exercise test.

On the current exercise test, he exercised for 9 minutes on the standard Bruce protocol, stopping secondary to dyspnea. Figure 11.1A shows his resting ECG and Figure 11.1B his exercise ECG in immediate recovery. The exercise ECG demonstrates 2 mm of downsloping ST depression in V5–V6 and inferiorly. One mm of ST elevation is seen in aVR.

His Duke Treadmill Score[1] can be calculated as:

Duke Treadmill Score = Exercise time in minutes on the standard Bruce protocol – 5 × ST deviation – 4 × exercise angina index.

In this patient the equation is 9 – 5 (2) – 0 = −1. A score of −1 would place the patient in the moderate prognostic risk category of scores of +4 to −10. (Scores designated lowest risk are those +5 or greater. Scores designated highest risk are −11 or lower.)

At the time of the exercise test, a pharmacologic stress research study of regadenoson was available and prior to coronary angiography he underwent a research regadenoson 2-day Tc^{99m} sestamibi myocardial perfusion study. The rotating raw images demonstrated no vertical or horizontal movement. His gray scale perfusion images are seen in Figure 11.2 and a splash view of his stress/rest gated images are seen in ▶ Video 11.3.

Coronary angiography of the vein graft to his diagonal is seen in Figure 11.4A. This demonstrated two high-grade stenoses in the mid vein graft with TIMI 2 flow distally. His LIMA and the two other vein grafts were patent. His native LAD had an 80% proximal stenosis and a 95% stenosis of the proximal diagonal that was grafted. His native circumflex and RCA were 100% occluded. He underwent placement of three drug-eluting stents in diagonal graft and his post-intervention diagonal image is seen in Figure 11.4B. The patient did well clinically following this intervention.

The gated SPECT images showed mild proximal inferior wall hypokinesis on stress and rest with otherwise normal LV function. Perfusion imaging showed a severe intensity defect of the mid to distal anterior wall sparing the apex and a small fixed proximal inferior wall defect.

As described in the textbook and by Michaelides et al., the exercise ECG findings of the combination of ST elevation in aVR and anterior ST depression are most consistent with LAD or multivessel disease in the LAD.[2] Coronary angiography demonstrated severe native diagonal disease with severe disease of the vein graft to the diagonal. Post-intervention one can see that the diagonal graft supplied a large segment of the LAD territory. It is also possible that distal disease of the native coronaries beyond graft insertion was present given the long duration of his CAD, which would also explain the substantial ECG changes with exercise.

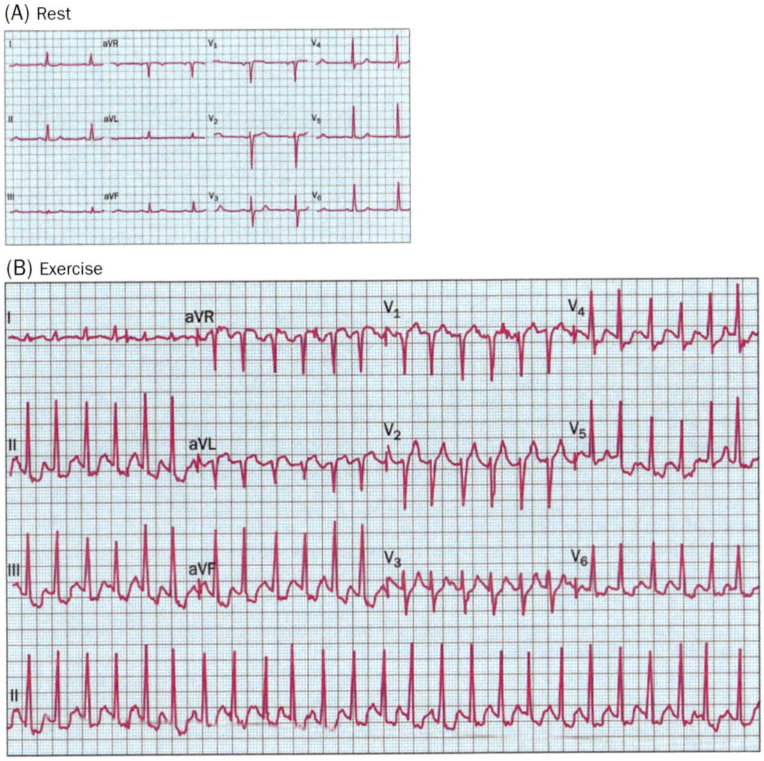

Figure 11.1. Case 1. (A) Normal resting ECG of the patient described in Case 1. (B) The exercise ECG demonstrates 2 mm of downsloping ST depression in V5–V6 and inferiorly. One mm of ST elevation is seen in aVR.

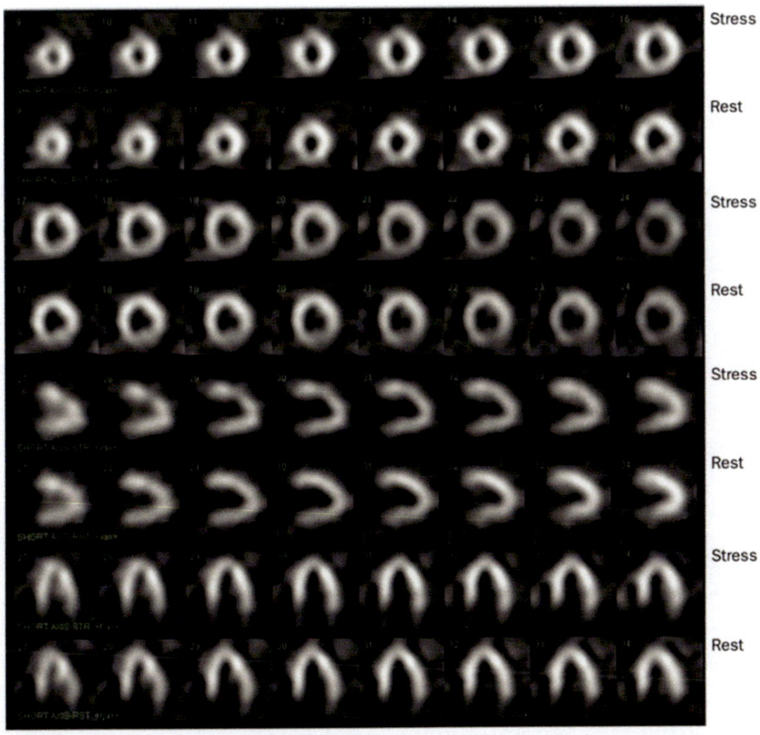

Figure 11.2. Case 1. Gray scale images of the patient's 2-day Tc^{99m} regadenoson stress sestamibi myocardial perfusion study demonstrating a severe intensity defect of the mid to distal anterior wall sparing the apex and a small fixed proximal inferior wall defect.

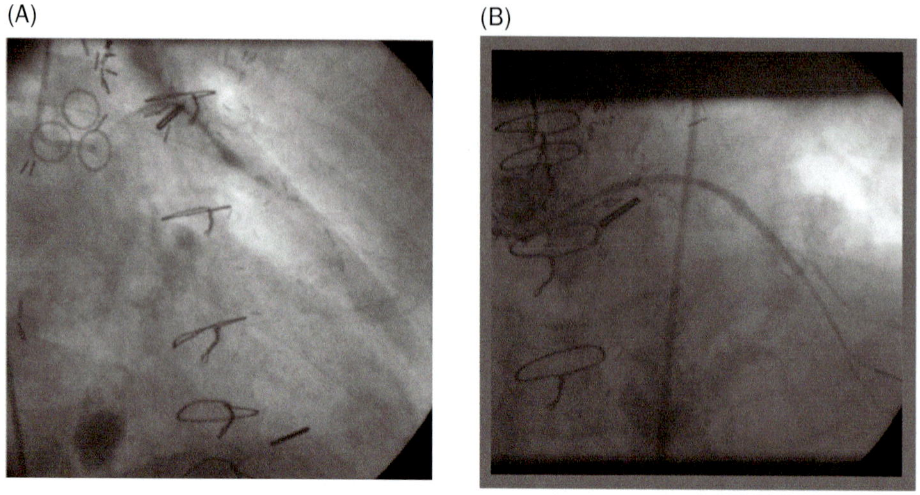

Figure 11.4. Case 1. (A) Coronary angiography of the saphenous vein graft to the diagonal demonstrating two high-grade stenoses with TIMI 2 distal flow. (B) The saphenous vein graft following placement of three drug-eluting stents, now with TIMI 3 flow.

CASE 2

A 58-year-old man with a 6-month history of stable exertional angina was referred for exercise testing with myocardial perfusion imaging. His baseline ECG is normal, though R waves are small in V2–3 (Figure 11.5A). Exercise testing was terminated at 4 minutes of exercise on the Bruce protocol with the ECG changes observed in Figure 11.5B. In this ECG, 2 to 3 mm of ST elevation is present in V2–4 with lesser ST elevation in the contiguous leads of V1 and V5. The inferior leads demonstrated about 1.5 mm of upsloping ST depression.

As described in the textbook, exercise is best terminated if 1 mm or more of ST elevation occurs in an anterior or inferior lead without a Q wave.

The myocardial perfusion study (Figure 11.5C) demonstrates a severe-intensity reversible anterior and anteroseptal reversible defect. As would be expected given the exercise-induced ECG changes and perfusion study, subsequent coronary angiography demonstrated a high-grade LAD stenosis (Figure 11.5D).

Exercise-induced ST elevation in a lead without a Q wave is consistent with transmural ischemia, analogous to the ST elevation that occurs with an ST-elevation MI secondary to an acutely occluded coronary artery. With exercise-induced ST elevation, the coronary stenosis is high grade and the ischemia is transmural because coronary flow is inadequate to supply the full-thickness myocardium during the increased oxygen demand of exercise. As the ischemia is exercise-induced, the ST elevation is transient and resolves during recovery. Unlike exercise-induced ST depression, exercise-induced ST elevation localizes to the area of ischemia.[3] Exercise-induced ST elevation is most common in V2–4, which identifies the LAD as the culprit. ST elevation in leads II, III, and aVF, which is much less common, identifies RCA disease, and the lateral leads of V6, I, and AVL identify circumflex or diagonal branch disease.[4,5]

Exercise-induced ST elevation in a lead with a Q wave typically represents a past LV aneurysm secondary to an MI related to an occluded or high-grade stenosis in the artery subtending that territory and does not indicate ischemia. ST elevation in a lead with a Q wave localizes to the area of the aneurysm.[5,6] As with ST elevation in a lead without a Q wave, ST elevation in a lead with a Q wave is most often seen in LAD territory. As exercise-induced ST elevation adversely impacts the ability of exercise testing to determine if ischemia is present in territories other than that of the ST elevation, MPI represents an option for a more granular ischemic evaluation.

CASE 3

A 45-year-old man had been jogging 5 miles daily until he stopped following the development of knee pain. Two months later, he reported to his primary care physician that he had begun experiencing chest pain at night but not with exercise. He was referred for exercise testing, during which he developed ST elevation in aVR and ST depression in

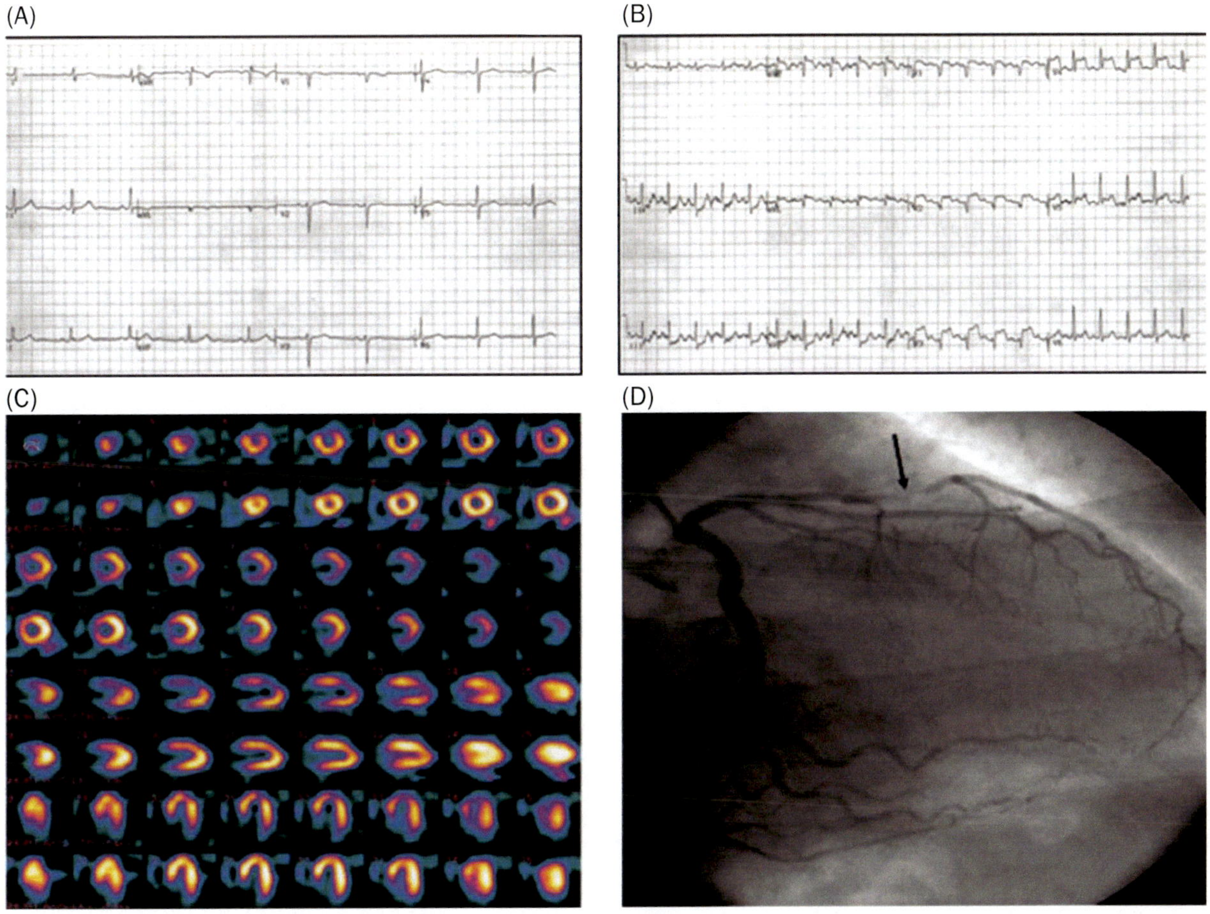

Figure 11.5. Case 2. An example of ST elevation during treadmill exercise testing. A 58-year-old man presented with a 6-month history of stable exertional angina. (A) Baseline ECG is normal. (B) ECG at 4 minutes of exercise shows ST elevation suggesting severe LAD coronary artery disease. (C) Tc-99m-sestamibi SPECT images show severe LAD ischemia. (The stress SPECT images are shown in the first row of each image set and the rest SPECT images in the second row of each image set.) (D) Coronary angiography confirms the presence of a severe mid-LAD stenosis (arrow). Reproduced with permission from Turner J, Brown T. Treadmill Exercise Testing. In: Iskandrian A, Garcia E, editors. Nuclear Cardiac Imaging: Principles and Applications. 5th ed. New York City: Oxford University Press; 2015. p. 225-39.

V4–6, lead I, and inferiorly. ST elevation developed in aVL, and ST elevation increased in V2. He had no chest pain. Figure 11.6A represents his computer-averaged resting ECG and Figure 11.6B his peak exercise ECG.

He was referred to a cardiologist, who recommended an exercise MPI, during which he had cardiac arrest and died.

The lesson in this case is that there was more than enough information to make severe and multivessel CAD likely on his initial standalone exercise test and to proceed with coronary angiography rather than to an exercise test with imaging.

As described in Case 1, exercise-induced ST elevation in aVR with associated anterior ST depression predicts LAD disease or multivessel disease involving the LAD. In the setting of a clinical history of new-onset chest pain, this makes a diagnosis of unstable angina very likely. Another concerning sign is the development of ST elevation in aVL. As described in Case 2, ST elevation in a lead without a Q wave is consistent with transmural ischemia caused by a severe stenosis in the artery subtending the territory. A Q wave was present in aVL but it was small, smaller than one would typically see with an infarction large enough to cause an aneurysm. Thus, transmural ischemia is the most likely cause of the ST elevation. While ST elevation increased with exercise in V2, a Q wave suggestive of a potential past infarction was present in that lead.

Given the combination of an exercise-induced ST elevation in aVR and anterior ST depression suggestive of left main or LAD disease as well as ST elevation in aVL, expeditious coronary angiography was indicated rather than exercise testing with imaging.

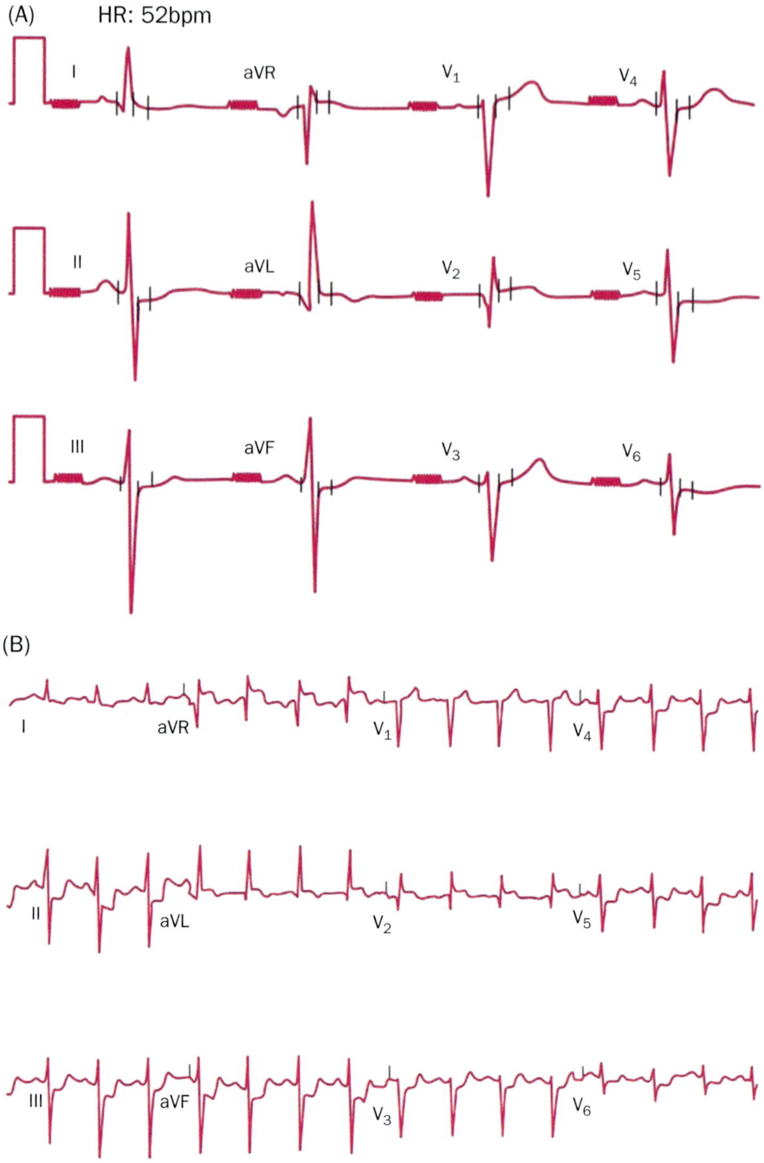

Figure 11.6. Case 3. (A) Averaged resting ECG of a 45-year-old male jogger referred for exercise testing to evaluate new-onset chest pain. One-half to 1 mm of resting ST depression in V4–V6 and inferiorly is present at rest. (B) The 12-lead ECG during treadmill testing demonstrated ST-segment elevation in lead aVR in conjunction with substantial ST depression in the anterior and inferior leads. The patient was asymptomatic during the exercise test. He died during follow-up exercise testing with MPI.

REFERENCES

1. Mark DB, Hlatky MA, Harrell J, et al. Exercise treadmill score for predicting prognosis in coronary artery disease. *Ann Intern Med.* 1987;106:793–800.
2. Michaelides AP, Psomadaki ZD, Aigyptiadou MN, et al. Significance of exercise-induced ST changes in leads aVR, V5, and V1: Discrimination of patients with single- or multivessel coronary artery disease. *Clin Cardiol.* 2003;26(5):226–230.
3. Akil S, Sunnersjo L, Hedeer F, et al. Stress-induced ST elevation with or without concomitant ST depression is predictive of presence, location and amount of myocardial ischemia assessed by myocardial perfusion SPECT, whereas isolated stress-induced ST depression is not. *J Electrocardiol.* 2016;49(3):307–315.
4. Gibbons RJ, Balady GJ, Bricker JT, et al. ACC/AHA 2002 guideline update for exercise testing: Summary article. *J Am Coll Cardiol.* 2002;40(8):1531–1540.
5. Thomas GS, Samtani SR, Ellestad MH. Interpretation of the ECG during exercise and recovery. In: Thomas GS, Wann LS, Ellestad MH, eds. *Ellestad's Stress Testing: Principles and Practice.* 6th ed. Oxford University Press; 2018:160–198.
6. Haines DE, Beller GA, Watson DD, et al. Exercise-induced ST segment elevation 2 weeks after uncomplicated myocardial infarction: Contributing factors and prognostic significance. *J Am Coll Cardiol.* 1987;9(5):996–1003.

12.

PHARMACOLOGIC STRESS TESTING

Efstathia Andrikopoulou, Ami E. Iskandrian, and Fadi G. Hage

CASE 1

A 65-year-old Black woman with prior coronary artery bypass grafting 24 years ago involving implantation of the left internal mammary artery (LIMA) to left anterior descending artery (LAD), hypertension, dyslipidemia, and obesity presents to the cardiology clinic for evaluation of intermittent chest pains. The pains are described as aching in the substernal region with radiation to the left side of the chest, last ~5 minutes of moderate severity, are not consistently related to exertion, and sometimes improve with sublingual nitroglycerin.

Her medications included aspirin 81 mg, atorvastatin 40 mg, amlodipine 10 mg, and hydrochlorothiazide/losartan 12.5 mg/100 mg. She has not tolerated beta-blocker therapy in the past due to bradycardia. She reports quitting smoking several years ago. She drinks alcohol socially and has never used illicit drugs. Her family history is significant for CAD and diabetes in her mother.

On physical examination, her BP is 133/72 mmHg and heart rate is 60 bpm and regular. She weighs 191 pounds with a body mass index of 34 kg/m^2. Her physical exam is otherwise unremarkable. Her resting 12-lead ECG demonstrates sinus rhythm with nonspecific T-wave abnormality (Figure 12.1). Routine laboratory tests were unrevealing.

She was referred for regadenoson MPI using a stress–rest protocol. After receiving 0.4 mg IV regadenoson her heart rate increased from 58 to 109 bpm and BP increased from 117/62 to 139/65 mmHg. She did not experience any discomfort, but her ECG showed ST depression in the inferolateral leads (Figure 12.2).

The stress SPECT MPI images showed normal perfusion pattern at peak stress (Figure 12.3). The gated images showed normal LVEF of 64% and normal wall motion. Since her stress images were normal, rest images were not performed (stress-only protocol).

The referring cardiologist decided to proceed with invasive coronary angiography, which was performed 4 days after the regadenoson MPI. Coronary angiography demonstrated severe ostial and proximal LAD but patent LIMA and no downstream stenoses (Figures 12.4 and 12.5 and ▶ Video 12.1). There was nonobstructive disease in the other vessels. No cardiac intervention was warranted, and the patient was treated with continued medical therapy and lifestyle modification. Over the next 3 years she has done well but continues to experience occasional non-limiting chest pain.

Review of medical records revealed that the patient had discordant results on two prior vasodilator stress tests (ST depression on ECG with normal perfusion on imaging), one with regadenoson 2 years prior and another with adenosine 10 years prior.

MPI has been established to provide a wealth of diagnostic and prognostic data in a wide variety of studies performed in thousands of patients over decades.[1,2] Currently, pharmacologic stress is used in more than half of patients due to their inability to perform a diagnostic exercise stress test. While an exercise stress test provides important data regarding functional capacity and the hemodynamic response to exercise and is generally preferred to pharmacologic stress testing in the majority of patients who can adequately exercise, vasodilator stress also provides significant non-perfusion prognostic data that have been shown to guide clinical management.[3]

As discussed in Chapter 12 in the accompanying book, vasodilator stress testing (with regadenoson or similar agents) induces coronary hyperemia by completely different sets of mechanisms than exercise. Reversible perfusion defects do not always reflect myocardial ischemia but rather heterogeneity of MBF in different vascular territories. The majority of patients with abnormal myocardial perfusion on imaging do not show evidence of ischemia on ECG. Alternatively, when ST depression is seen on ECG with pharmacologic stress (~10%), it is usually accompanied by abnormal myocardial perfusion on imaging. In this setting, the ECG changes indicate the

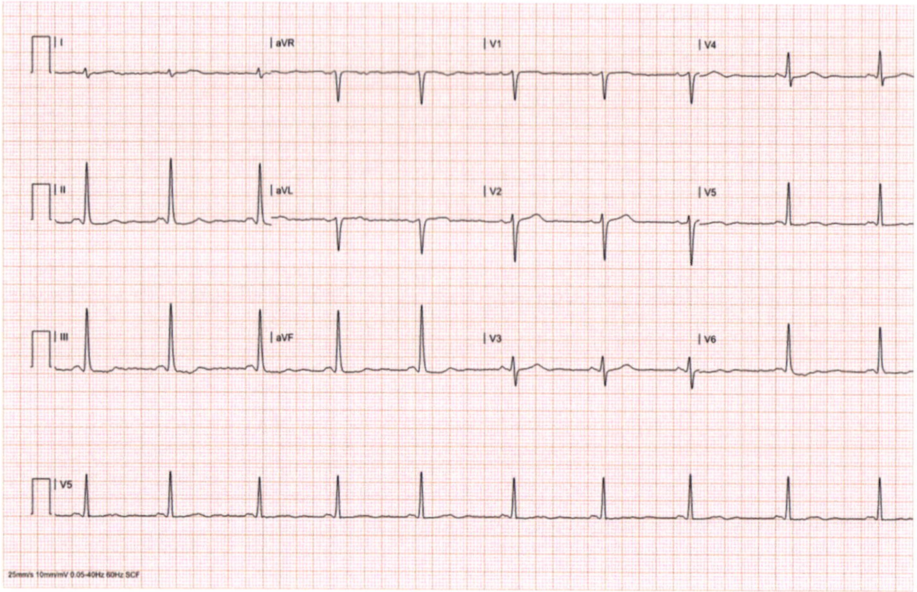

Figure 12.1. Case 1. Baseline ECG demonstrating sinus rhythm with nonspecific T-wave abnormality.

presence of myocardial ischemia (usually due to coronary steal) and correlate with increased risk.

On rare occasions, ST depression with vasodilator stress is seen in patients with normal perfusion on imaging. The diagnostic and prognostic value of the ECG changes in this setting is uncertain, with most studies showing a favorable outcome in these patients over many years of follow-up (see discussion in Chapter 12 of the book and Table 12.11). Importantly, the hypothesis that the ECG changes reflect myocardial ischemia despite a homogeneous MBF due to so-called balanced ischemia is not consistent with the data from the studies provided in Table 12.11. Further, the majority of patients with ST depression on ECG with normal perfusion on imaging with vasodilator stress are women (>80% in most studies), which raises the possibility that the ST segment shift represents an intrinsic gender-related response to vasodilator stress (in a manner similar to the false-positive ECG changes seen in women with exercise) and does not signify myocardial ischemia. In our practice, we have seen many patients (generally women) who show

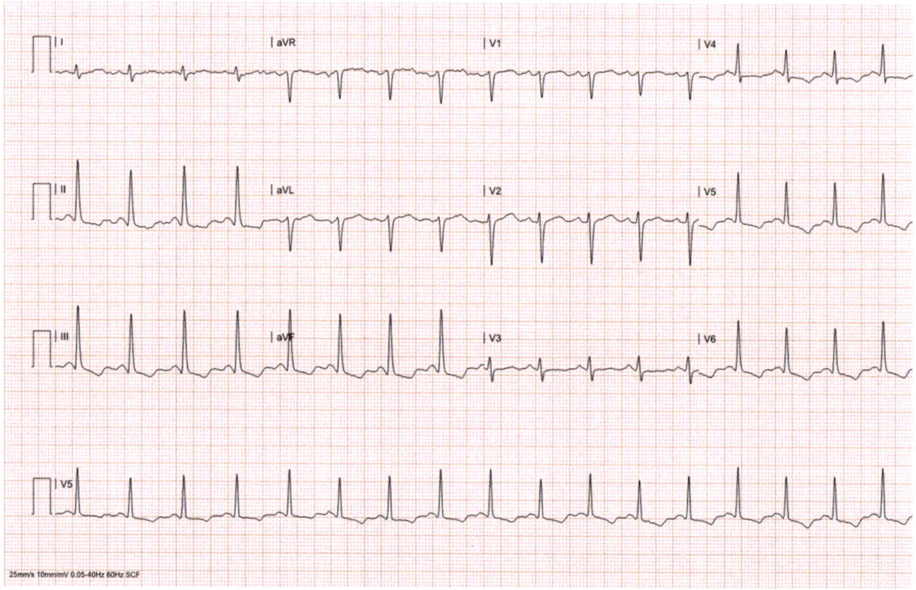

Figure 12.2. Case 1. 12-lead ECG after regadenoson administration showing ST depression in inferolateral leads.

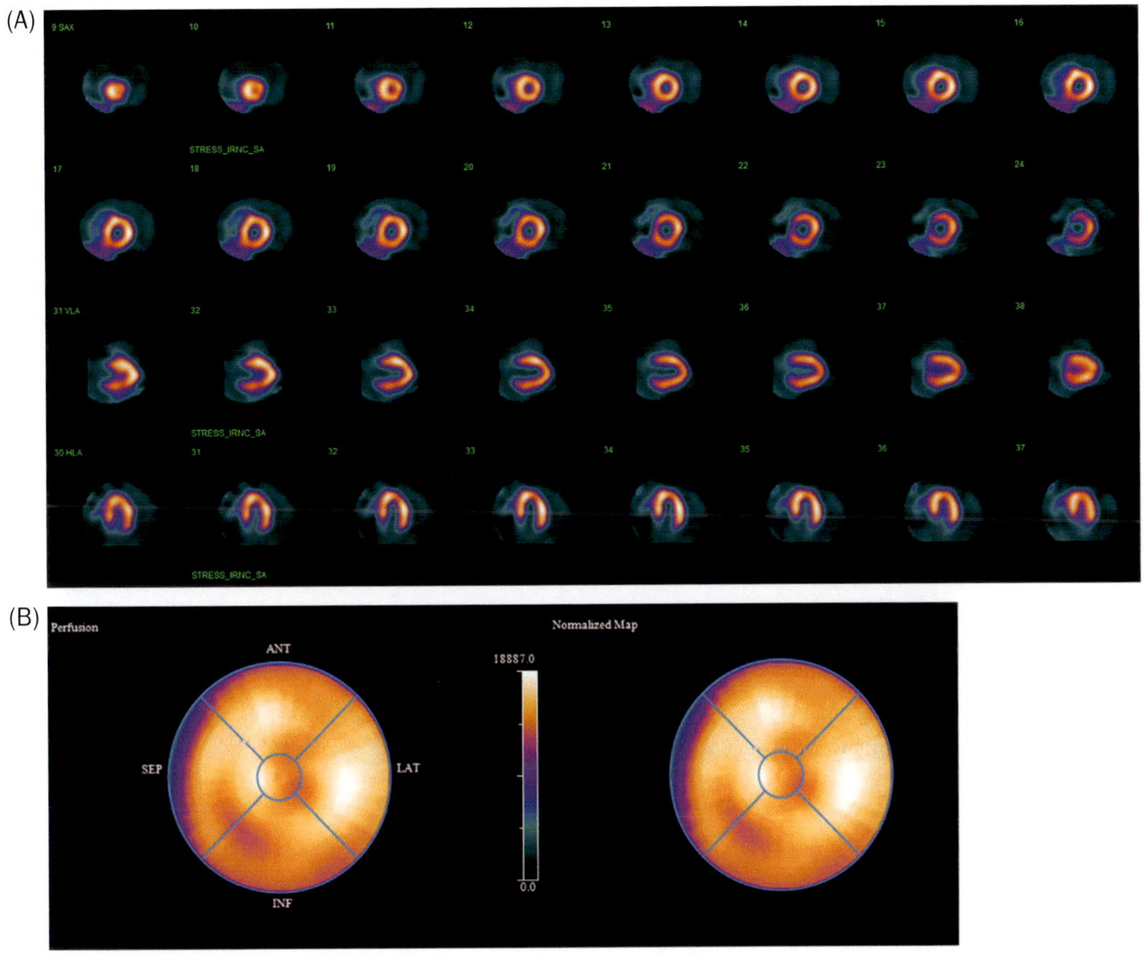

Figure 12.3. Case 1. Regadenoson myocardial perfusion images demonstrating normal perfusion at peak stress (A). The corresponding polar plots are shown in panel B.

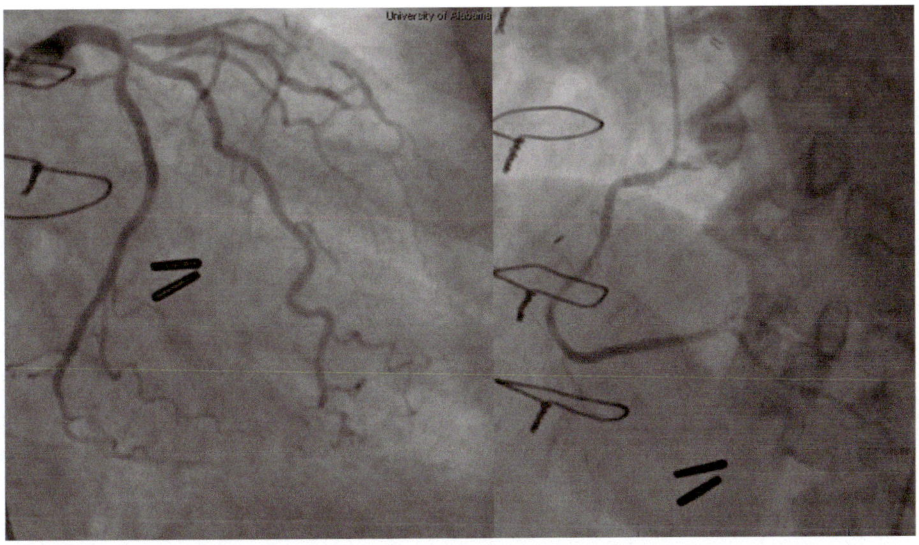

Figure 12.4. Case 1. Coronary angiogram of the left (on the left) and right (on the right) coronary systems. There is severe disease in the ostial and proximal left anterior descending coronary artery but otherwise nonobstructive disease.

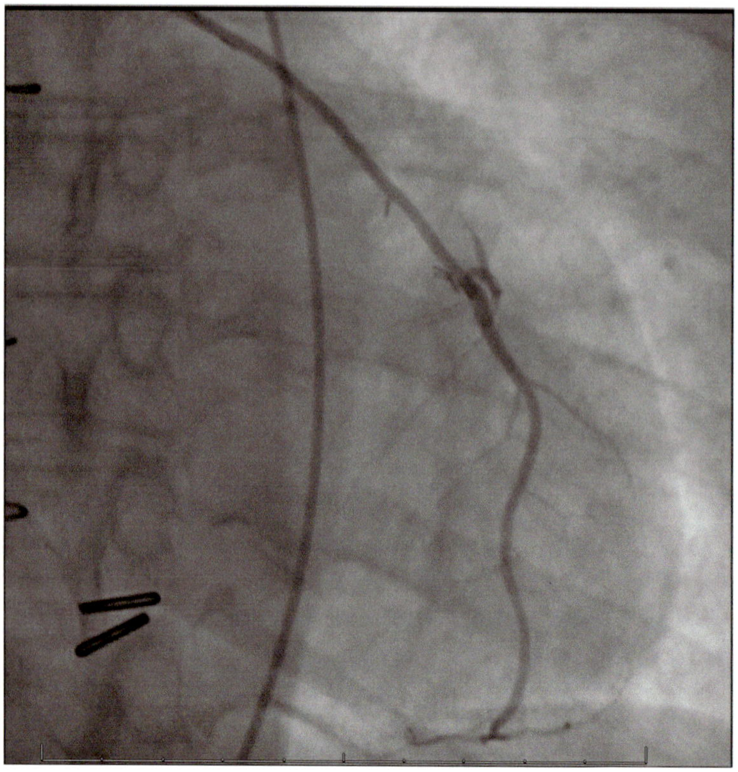

Figure 12.5. Case 1. Angiography of the left internal mammary artery reveals a patent graft to the left anterior descending artery.

this discrepant pattern over multiple stress tests performed several years apart, similar to the patient presented here. This again makes the likelihood that these changes represent ongoing myocardial ischemia in all vascular territories extremely unlikely. It is conceivable, however, that small-vessel disease might be the reason in some of these discordant cases, and measurement of MBF at rest and peak stress might provide useful clues.

In summary, ECG changes during vasodilator stress testing provide complementary data to MPI. The majority of patients with ST-segment depression with vasodilator stress have perfusion abnormalities on imaging. However, when ST depression accompanies normal perfusion, the ECG response is false positive in most patients except when the pretest likelihood for CAD is high. We have seen examples of false-negative MPI that may be related to poor response to vasodilator stress; balanced ischemia is not common or main reason as most patients if they have CAD is in the form of one-vessel disease. For prognostic purposes, the imaging data are more powerful than the ECG data.

CASE 2

A 64-year-old man with obesity, hypertension, dyslipidemia, tobacco use, and known CAD who had prior percutaneous coronary intervention (PCI) with stenting of the right coronary artery (RCA) 1 year prior presents to the cardiology clinic to establish care. He states that the PCI was performed after evaluation of chest pain and shortness of breath with exertion. After his PCI, his shortness of breath worsened, but this was presumed to be secondary to ticagrelor treatment since it resolved when he was switched to clopidogrel. Otherwise, he has been doing well except for the last few weeks, when he started having intermittent sharp substernal chest pain with exertion. These episodes occur several times a week and occasionally are severe enough to have him lie down and stop all activity. He has not tried taking prescribed sublingual nitroglycerin for this pain. He is not physically active.

His current medications include aspirin, clopidogrel, atorvastatin, carvedilol, and isosorbide dinitrate. He has recently stopped taking hydrochlorothiazide, lisinopril, and amlodipine due to concerns for low BP, which causes him to get dizzy when he stands up. On physical exam his heart rate is 59 bpm and BP is 146/79 mmHg. He weighs 231 lbs. and has a body mass index of 35 kg/m^2. His physical examination is otherwise normal. His family history is noncontributory. He endorses smoking a cigar daily but denies using illicit drugs. He lives with his wife.

Review of his records show a coronary angiogram from 1 year ago with severe proximal and mid RCA disease, which was stented. He also had moderate disease in the LAD and left circumflex coronary artery (LCX) (described as 50% diameter stenosis), which were treated medically. An echocardiogram performed 8 months ago was normal, with LVEF of 60%.

He was referred for a stress MPI and, due to his inability to exercise sufficiently, he underwent regadenoson stress. His resting ECG demonstrated sinus bradycardia with nonspecific ST/T-wave changes (Figure 12.6). There were no ECG changes after regadenoson administration.

SPECT MPI images showed a severe perfusion defect of large size in the lateral, inferolateral, inferior walls, and the apex of the LV (Figure 12.7). The rest perfusion pattern was normal. The perfusion abnormality involved 35% of the LV myocardium. There was no TID, but on the gated images there was evidence of stunning, with a drop in LVEF from 52% post-rest to 45% post-stress with regional wall motion abnormality (▶ Video 12.2).

The patient underwent coronary angiography, which demonstrated severe three-vessel disease with 70% stenosis of proximal to mid LAD, 80% ostial stenosis of ramus intermedius, 70% stenosis of proximal LCX with bifurcating obtuse marginal branch showing an ostial complete obstruction with left-to-left and right-to-left collaterals, and 80% in-stent stenosis of a dominant RCA (Figure 12.8).

The patient underwent successful three-vessel arterial coronary artery bypass grafting with LIMA to LAD, right internal mammary to obtuse marginal, and left radial to posterior descending artery (endoscopic vein harvest of the left and right legs had no evidence of usable veins).

The regadenoson MPI in this patient exhibits many high-risk features, including the presence of a large perfusion defect in a multivessel distribution, severe and completely reversible abnormality, and post-stress myocardial stunning. Post-stress stunning is more common with exercise stress but has been described with vasodilator stress, where it is likely mediated by coronary artery steal.[4] It is interesting in this patient that there was no accompanying TID or ST depression on the ECG, features that usually accompany myocardial stunning. Post-stress stunning is more common with PET studies since imaging is done shortly after stress—unlike SPECT, when imaging is delayed 30 to 60 minutes later.[5,6]

CASE 3

A 67-year-old man with diabetes mellitus type 2, hypertension, dyslipidemia, and depression presented to the clinic with exertional retrosternal chest pain that is relieved with rest and associated with dyspnea and diaphoresis of 1 month's duration. The pain was described as tightness

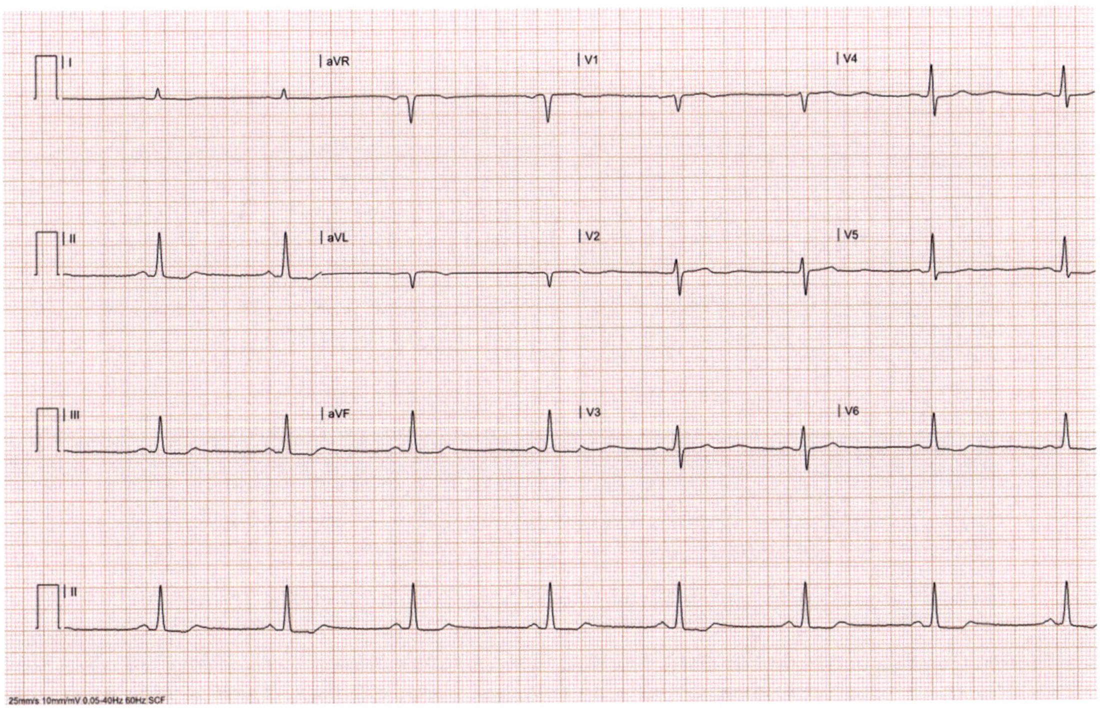

Figure 12.6. Case 2. Baseline ECG demonstrating sinus bradycardia with nonspecific ST/T-wave abnormality.

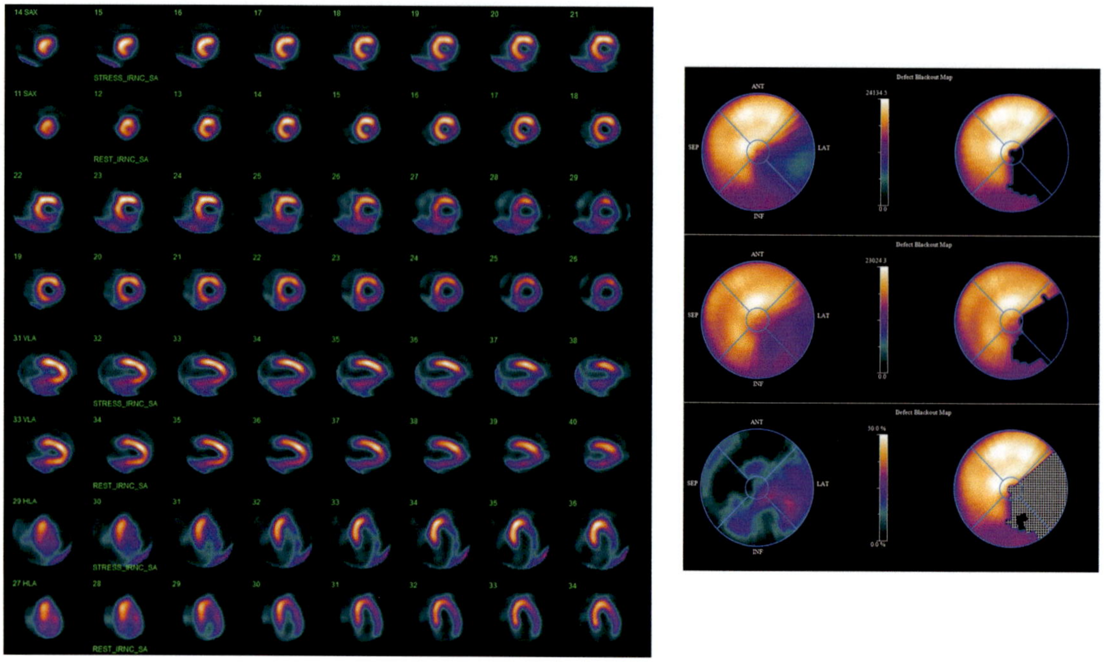

Figure 12.7. Case 2. SPECT MPI images demonstrate a large and severe reversible perfusion defect in the lateral, inferolateral, and inferior walls, and apex of the LV suggestive of ischemia in the distribution of the left circumflex and right coronary arteries. On the polar maps the perfusion abnormality involved 35% of the LV myocardium.

in the chest that reproducibly starts after walking about 300 feet and improves with rest.

His medications included aspirin, metformin, simvastatin, and lisinopril. His family history was significant for CAD in his father. He has never smoked or used illicit drugs.

On physical exam his heart rate was 68 bpm and his BP 110/72 mmHg. He weighed 183 lbs. (body mass index 24 kg/m^2). His resting 12-lead ECG was normal (Figure 12.9). His primary care physician referred him for an exercise stress test. He was able to walk for 6 minutes on the treadmill using a Bruce protocol with no symptoms,

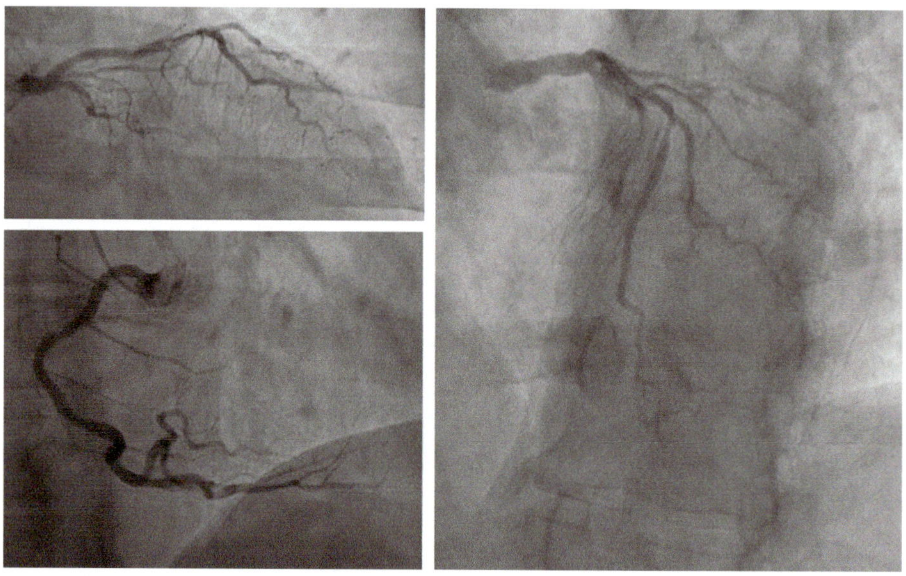

Figure 12.8. Case 2. Coronary angiography demonstrating severe three-vessel disease with 70% stenosis of proximal to mid left anterior descending, 80% ostial stenosis of ramus intermedius, 70% stenosis of proximal left circumflex with bifurcating obtuse marginal branch showing an ostial complete obstruction with left-to-left and right-to-left collaterals, and dominant right coronary artery with mid in-stent restenosis of 80%.

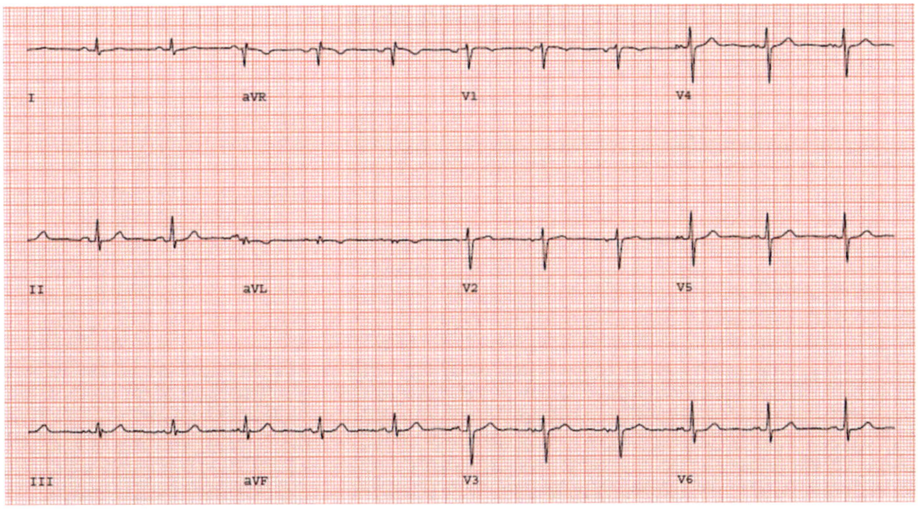

Figure 12.9. Case 3. 12-lead ECG at rest demonstrating normal sinus rhythm with no significant abnormalities.

stopping due to fatigue. The ECG did not show evidence of ischemia. SPECT MPI (Tc-99m sestamibi) showed abnormal perfusion with a large reversible perfusion defect in the distribution of the LAD involving 40% of the LV myocardium (Figure 12.10). The LVEF was normal at 69% with normal wall motion/thickening.

The patient was recruited to the NIH-sponsored ISCHEMIA trial and was randomized to the noninvasive arm. He was started on a beta-blocker and long-acting nitrates, and his angina resolved. On review of the images, the cardiologist was concerned due to the high-risk nature of the test. He recommended to the patient that he undergo coronary angiography, but the patient declined since his symptoms had improved on medical therapy.

After 8 years, a follow-up SPECT MPI was repeated. Since his exercise tolerance has decreased over the years, he underwent regadenoson MPI, which demonstrated a small and mild perfusion defect in the distal anterior wall involving less than 10% of the LV myocardium

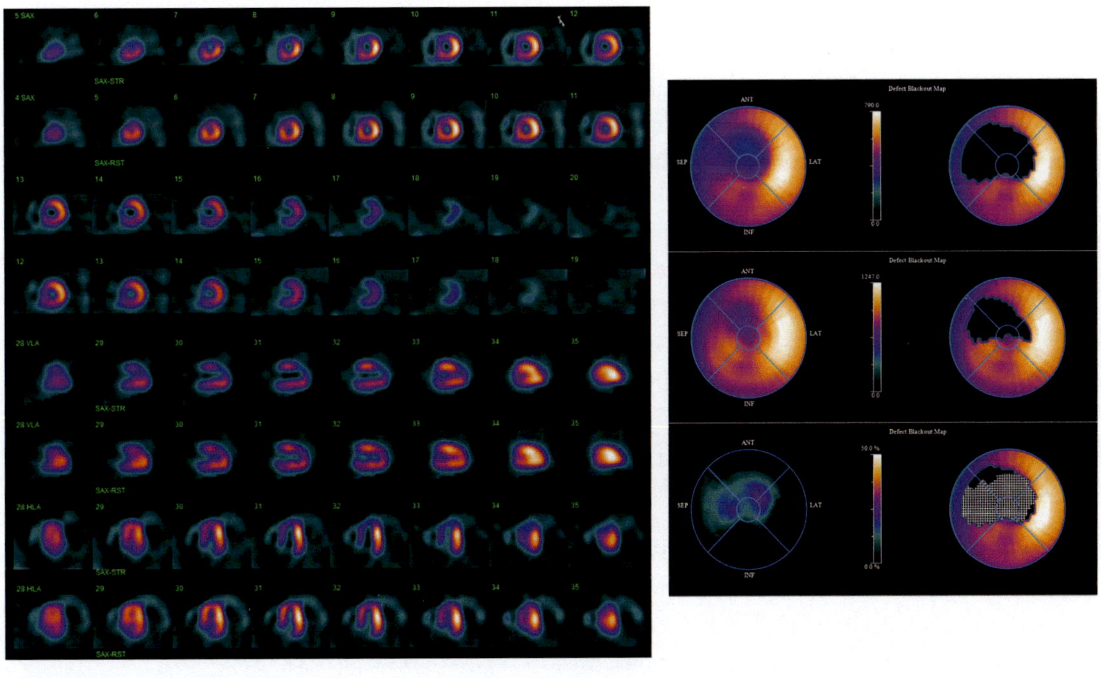

Figure 12.10. Case 3. SPECT MPI images and polar map demonstrating a large reversible perfusion defect in the anterior wall, anterior septum, and apex of the LV involving 40% of the LV myocardium.

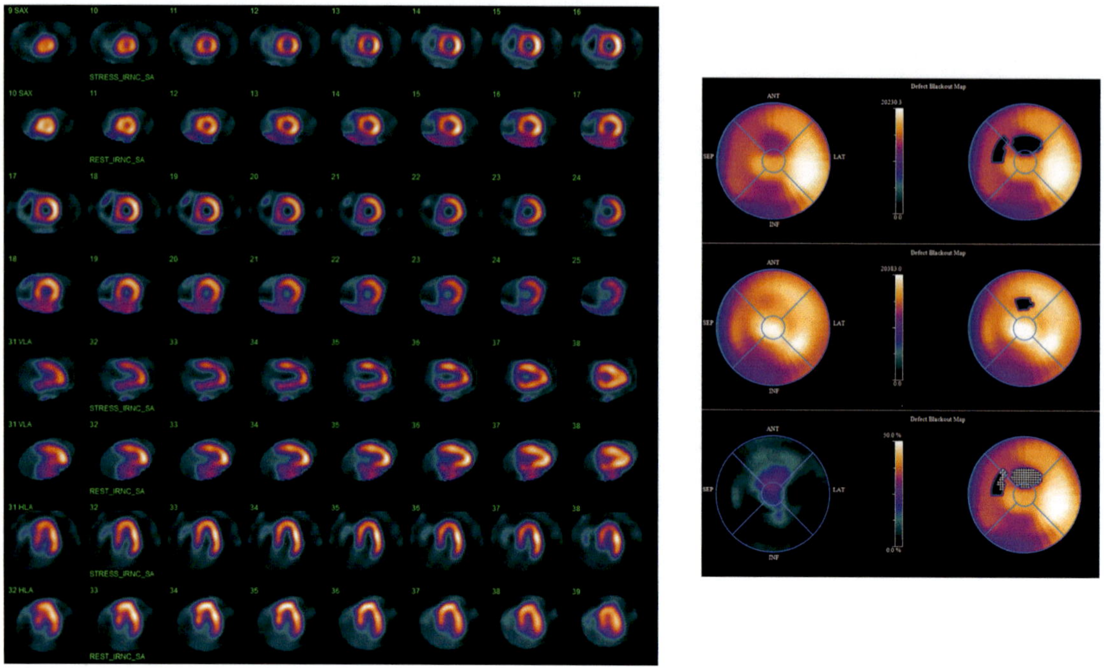

Figure 12.11. Case 3. SPECT MPI images and polar map demonstrating a small reversible perfusion defect in the distal anterior wall of the LV involving <10% of the LV myocardium. Compared to Figure 12.10, the perfusion defect is significantly smaller in size and milder in severity.

(Figure 12.11). Compared to Figure 12.10, the perfusion defect is significantly smaller in size and milder in severity.

The ISCHEMIA trial randomized 5,179 patients with moderate or severe ischemia to an initial invasive strategy (angiography and revascularization when feasible) and medical therapy or to an initial conservative strategy of medical therapy alone and angiography if medical therapy failed.[7] Over a median of 3.2 years there was no significant difference in the primary outcome of death from cardiovascular causes, MI, or hospitalization for unstable angina, heart failure, or resuscitated cardiac arrest between the two arms. One criticism of the trial is that the recruited patients are not representative of patients with moderate to severe ischemia seen in clinical practice. Indeed, most centers had difficulty recruiting patients for this trial since practicing cardiologists did not believe that there is equipoise between the two arms. Although the primary care physician taking care of this patient referred the patient for randomization, the cardiologist felt compelled to try to convince the patient to break protocol and undergo invasive evaluation due to the high-risk findings on MPI. It is informative that although the patient declined and did not undergo invasive evaluation (or coronary revascularization), his symptoms improved, and the perfusion defect size did so as well. Changes in perfusion defect size on serial MPI have been shown to associate with outcomes.[8,9] We note here that these changes are not due to the use of a different stress agent (exercise on the first scan and regadenoson on the second scan). As discussed in Chapter 12 in the accompanying book, MBF with regadenoson is even higher than with exercise, so there is no reason to suspect that using regadenoson resulted in a smaller perfusion defect.

REFERENCES

1. Shaw LJ, Iskandrian AE. Prognostic value of gated myocardial perfusion SPECT. *J Nucl Cardiol.* 2004;11:171–185.
2. Shaw LJ, Hage FG, Berman DS, et al. Prognosis in the era of comparative effectiveness research: Where is nuclear cardiology now and where should it be? *J Nucl Cardiol.* 2012;19:1026–1043.
3. Bajaj NS, Singh S, Farag A, et al. The prognostic value of non-perfusion variables obtained during vasodilator stress myocardial perfusion imaging. *J Nucl Cardiol.* 2016;23:390–413.
4. AlJaroudi WA, Hage FG. Myocardial stunning by gated SPECT: An old tool reinvented in a stunning turn. *J Nucl Cardiol.* 2019;26:841–844.
5. Smith P, Farag A, Bhambhvani P, et al. Prognostic value of absent left ventricular ejection fraction reserve with regadenoson SPECT MPI. *J Nucl Cardiol.* 2022;29(3):978–986.

6 Dorbala S, Vangala D, Sampson U, et al. Value of vasodilator left ventricular ejection fraction reserve in evaluating the magnitude of myocardium at risk and the extent of angiographic coronary artery disease: A 82Rb PET/CT study. *J Nucl Med.* 2007;48:349–358.
7. Maron DJ, Hochman JS, Reynolds HR, et al. Initial invasive or conservative strategy for stable coronary disease. *N Engl J Med.* 2020;382:1395–1407.
8. El-Hajj S, AlJaroudi WA, Farag A, et al. Effect of changes in perfusion defect size during serial regadenoson myocardial perfusion imaging on cardiovascular outcomes in high-risk patients. *J Nucl Cardiol.* 2016;23:101–112.
9. Iskandrian AE, Hage FG, Shaw LJ, et al. Serial myocardial perfusion imaging: defining a significant change and targeting management decisions. *JACC Cardiovasc Imaging.* 2014;7:79–96.

13.

DIAGNOSIS AND RISK ASSESSMENT WITH SPECT MPI

Javier Gomez and Rami Doukky

CASE 1

A 62-year-old man presented to the office for evaluation of a retrosternal, exertional chest pain for 6 months. The pain subsides after resting for approximately 5 minutes. The pain ensues after walking two to three blocks at a fast pace, but he can go up to eight to 10 blocks at a slow pace. He denies other symptoms. His past medical history included diabetes mellitus and hypertension. Three months earlier, his primary care physician started him on metoprolol 50 mg daily and isosorbide mononitrate 30 mg daily, with modest improvement of symptoms. In addition, his medications included metformin 1,000 mg twice daily, ASA 81 mg daily, and lisinopril/hydrochlorothiazide 20 mg/12.5 mg daily. He does not use alcohol, cigarettes, or illicit drugs. He has no family history of CAD.

Physical exam revealed BP 110/72 mmHg, heart rate 56 bpm, and respiratory rate 16 per minute. His body mass index is 35 kg/m^2. He had no jugular venous distension. His chest was clear to auscultation, and the heart sounds were normal. He had no pedal edema. The rest of the exam was unremarkable.

His laboratory workup was notable for hemoglobin A1C 6.6%, total cholesterol 220 mg/dL, high-density lipoprotein 35 mg/dL, triglycerides 150 mg/dL, and low-density lipoprotein 156 mg/dL. He was started on atorvastatin 80 mg daily and referred for 1-day rest/exercise stress ^{99m}Tc sestamibi SPECT MPI for further evaluation. A baseline ECG is shown in Figure 13.1.

He exercised according to the Bruce protocol for 6 minutes and 30 seconds, achieving a peak heart rate 140 bpm (89% of the maximum predicted heart rate). Exercise was limited by fatigue, but he had no chest pain. Stress ECG shown in Figure 13.2 demonstrated upsloping 0.5-mm ST depression, which did not meet ECG criteria for myocardial ischemia.[1] The calculated DTS was 4.5, indicating a moderate-risk category.

The rest and stress SPECT MPI images are shown in (Figure 13.3).

Stress–rest images demonstrated medium to large, moderate to severe, reversible perfusion abnormalities in the septum, apex, and inferior wall. The summed stress score (SSS) was 12 and the summed difference score (SDS) was 9. The calculated ischemic myocardium was 13%. TID was 1.20. LVEF was 56% post-rest and 47% post-stress.

Given the multiple high-risk features on SPECT MPI, the patient was referred for coronary angiography. Coronary angiography images demonstrated a total occlusion of the left anterior descending coronary artery and 80% stenosis in the right coronary artery (Figure 13.4). Based on these findings, the patient was referred for CABG surgery.

This is a case of a 62-year-old man with typical class II stable angina symptoms. He has a high (>90%) pretest likelihood for obstructive CAD based on age, sex, and symptoms according to the Diamond and Forrester estimates.[1] The patient has an interpretable ECG and can exercise. Importantly, he is already on an anti-anginal regimen including a β-blocker, long-acting nitrate, and statin.

Risk stratification based on clinical data alone may have limited value. Diabetes mellitus places this patient in a higher risk category for adverse cardiac events. Observational data suggest that in patients with a high burden of myocardial ischemia, coronary revascularization is associated with improved clinical outcomes, while medical therapy is preferred in patients with low ischemic burden.[2]

Based on available information, this patient has a high pretest likelihood of CAD. Thus, a "negative" noninvasive testing will not rule out CAD, whereas a "positive" test only confirms the high clinical suspicion. Nonetheless, physiologic data derived from stress imaging with MPI, echocardiography, or cardiac magnetic imaging continue to be relevant today, as all these tests are considered appropriate for further risk assessment in patients with a high likelihood of CAD.[3] Another consideration is to proceed directly to invasive coronary angiography. However,

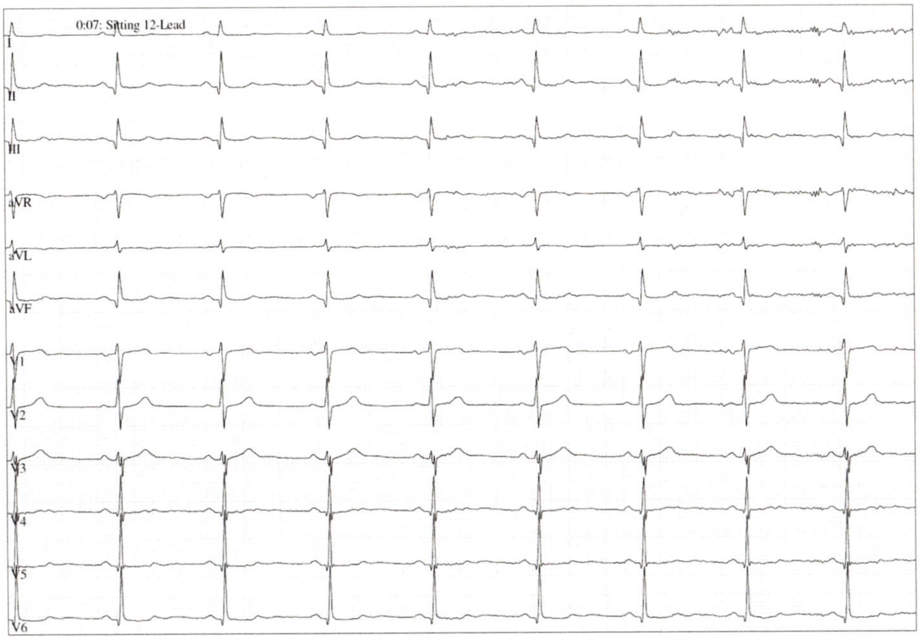

Figure 13.1. Case 1. Baseline 12-lead ECG.

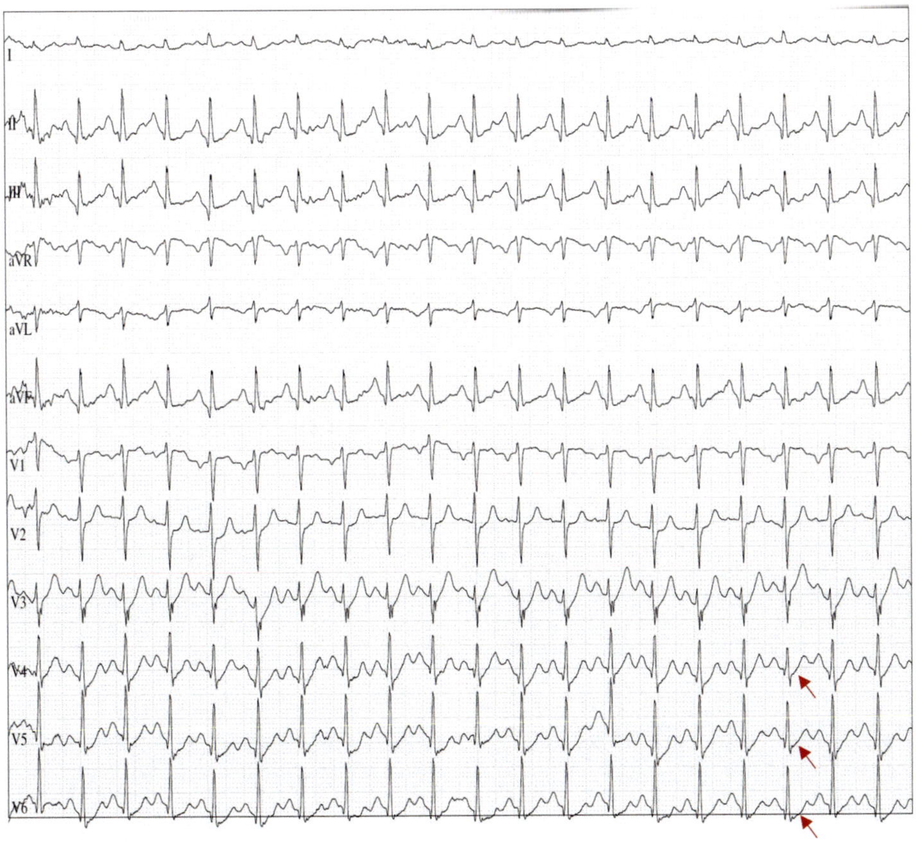

Figure 13.2. Case 1. 12-lead ECG during early recovery after exercise stress.

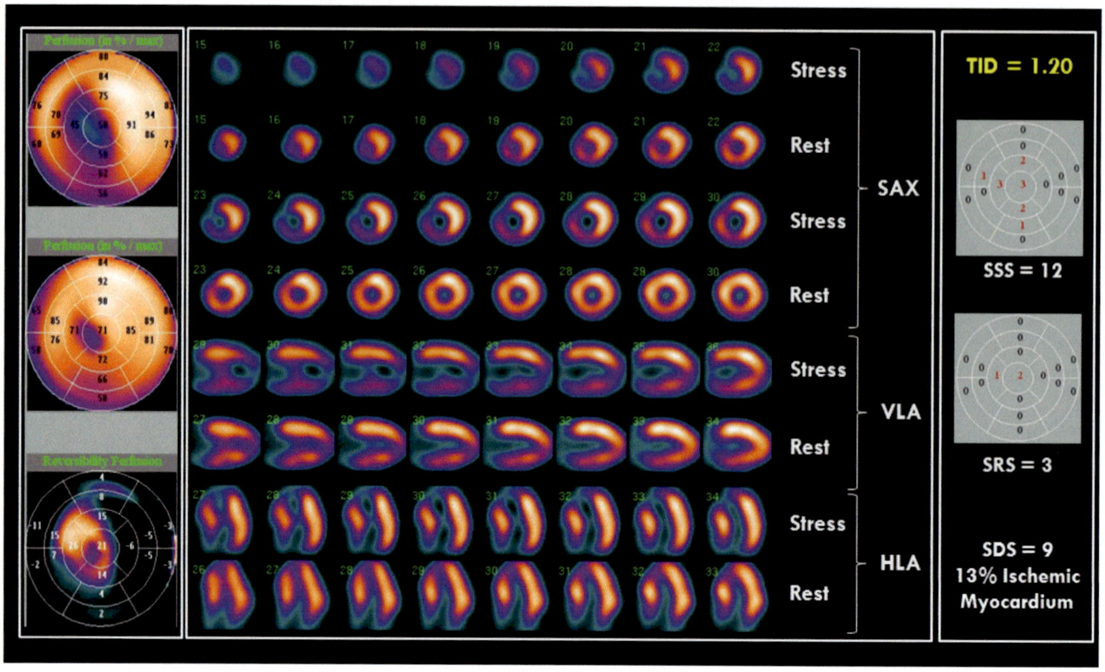

Figure 13.3. Case 1. SPECT MPI. HLA, horizontal long axis; SAX, short axis; SDS, summed difference score; SRS, summed rest score; SSS, summed stress score; TID, transient ischemic dilation VLA vertical long axis.

available data show that functional information derived from SPECT MPI provides incremental prognostic value to clinical data, exercise tolerance test data, and coronary angiography, while angiography data do add prognostic risk prediction to MPI. Nonetheless, coronary angiography and ancillary tools remain the gold standard to confirm epicardial obstructive coronary disease and to plan revascularization, if indicated.

In this case, stress MPI was appropriately selected and provided valuable prognostic information to guide decision-making.[4] The patient exercised for 6 minutes and 30 seconds with a 0.5-mm ST depression on ECG and no reproduction of symptoms, yielding a DTS of 4.5. By exercise parameters alone the patient would be categorized at intermediate risk with expected 1-year mortality rate of 2.9%. MPI data provided additional diagnostic and prognostic information that aided in decision-making. MPI demonstrated perfusion abnormalities involving multivessel distribution with a summed stress score of 12 and a summed difference score of 9. The burden of myocardial ischemia for this patient was 13%, which favors coronary revascularization, especially in a symptomatic patient on medical therapy. Furthermore,

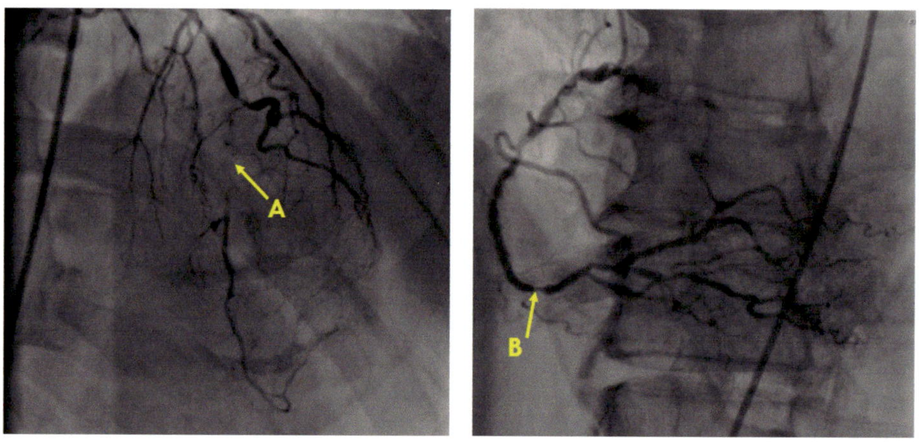

Figure 13.4. Case 1. Invasive coronary angiography. (A) Total occlusion of the left anterior descending coronary artery (arrow). (B) Severe 80% stenosis of the distal right coronary artery (arrow).

the presence of TID above the abnormal threshold of > 1.19 defined for 1-day rest/exercise stress Tc-99m protocol is another marker for multivessel CAD.[5]

The benefit of revascularization in addition to optimal medical therapy versus medical therapy alone in patients with moderate to severe ischemia was recently challenged in the ISCHEMIA trial.[6] However, it is important to consider the limitations of the ISCHEMIA trial. Prior to the publication of the study results, it was generally accepted that coronary revascularization improves outcomes of patients with moderate to severe myocardial ischemia. Therefore, physicians were reluctant to randomize patients with significant ischemia to medical therapy alone. Thus, patients with severe disease who are most in need for coronary revascularization were not commonly enrolled, biasing the trial toward the null. In fact, 14% of patients enrolled in the trial did not meet the ischemia eligibility criteria after review by the core laboratory. Additionally, the investigators allowed patients with a positive ECG treadmill test (without imaging) to be included to increase recruitment. There are limited data to suggest that treadmill testing, without imaging, can accurately identify patients who might benefit from coronary revascularization. Based on current data, functional testing to determine the cause of symptoms, stratify risk, and guide management remains a valuable tool in clinical practice.

CASE 2

A 56-year-old woman was referred to your office for evaluation of a 3-month complaint of an epigastric burning sensation. The symptoms are associated with exertion after walking one block and improve with 3 to 5 minutes of rest. These symptoms did not occur at rest. She has a past medical history of hypertension, type 2 diabetes mellitus, dyslipidemia, knee osteoarthritis, and peripheral vascular disease. Her exercise tolerance is limited to less than two blocks at a slow pace due to knee pain. She takes metformin 1,000 mg twice daily, aspirin 81 mg daily, lisinopril 20 mg daily, and atorvastatin 80 mg daily. She weighs 82 kg, her height is 1.68 m, and her BMI is 29 m^2/kg.

Vital signs showed BP 126/84 mmHg, heart rate 68 bpm, and respiratory rate 14/min. Her oxygen saturation was 98% on room air. The jugular venous pressure was normal, the heart sounds were normal, and there was no gallop or murmur. Lungs were clear to auscultation. Pulses were equal and there was no peripheral edema.

A 12-lead ECG was obtained (Figure 13.5) and demonstrates normal sinus rhythm with right bundle branch block.

Due to the abnormal ECG and exertional nature of symptoms, the patient was referred for a transthoracic echocardiogram and a 1-day rest/regadenoson-stress SPECT MPI. Transthoracic echocardiogram showed normal LV systolic function with LVEF 58%, grade 1 diastolic dysfunction, and no other significant abnormalities. The regadenoson stress ECG portion (Figure 13.6) demonstrated a 1-mm horizontal ST depression in the inferior and lateral leads and was considered positive for myocardial ischemia by ECG criteria.

SPECT MPI (Figure 13.7) demonstrated large defects of moderate severity involving the entire anterior, basal to mid anterolateral, basal to mid inferolateral, and apical lateral segments of the LV, which were completely reversible when compared with resting images. Additionally, TID was present with a value of 1.38. Both the summed stress score and the summed difference score were 12, with a burden of ischemic myocardium of 18%.

Invasive coronary angiography revealed triple-vessel coronary artery disease with 80% stenosis in the mid segment of the left anterior descending coronary artery, 70% stenosis in the proximal left circumflex coronary artery, and

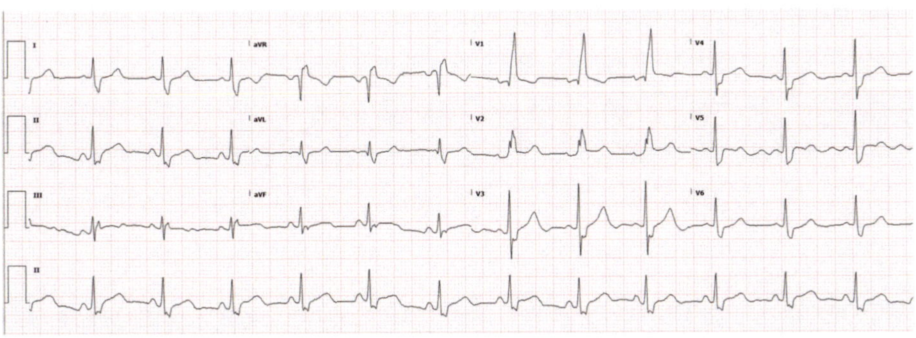

Figure 13.5. Case 2. Baseline 12-lead ECG.

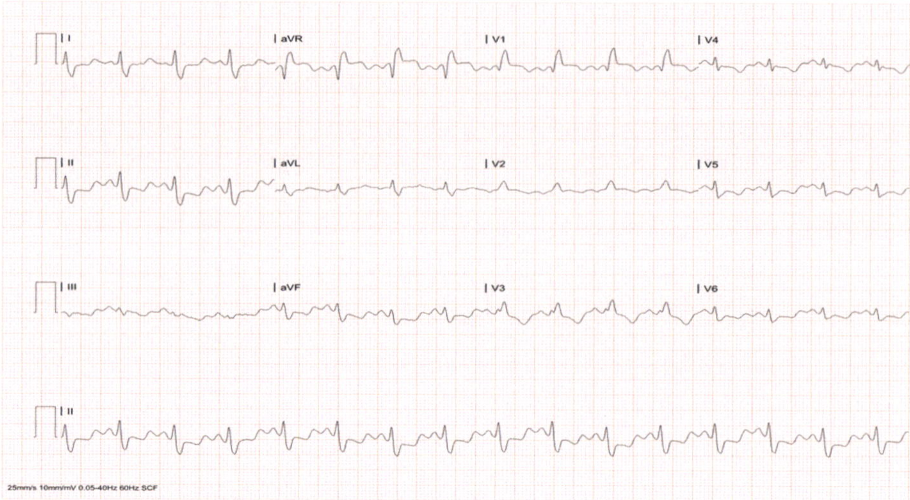

Figure 13.6. Case 2. 12-lead ECG at peak stress after regadenoson injection

80% diffuse stenosis in the proximal right coronary artery. The patient was referred for CABG surgery.

This case illustrates a woman with atypical angina, signifying an intermediate pretest probability of CAD based on the Diamond and Forrester classification. Exercise ECG is recommended in patients with a low pretest probability of CAD and could have been considered despite the patient having an abnormal ECG at baseline. Her ECG demonstrated complete right bundle branch block. Although right bundle branch block can frequently be associated with ST-T changes in leads V1–V3, the test diagnostic performance in the V4–V5 and limb leads is similar to that with normal resting ECG. Thus, her baseline ECG is considered interpretable.

Current stress testing guidelines consider the baseline ECG to be uninterpretable in the presence of left bundle branch block, pre-excitation, ventricular paced rhythm, and >1 mm of ST depression.[7] It has been shown that anginal symptoms can frequently be atypical or subtle in women and patients with diabetes mellitus. Current criteria consider the use of SPECT MPI to be "appropriate" in patients with new symptoms and an intermediate pretest probability. Moreover, given her limited ability to undergo adequate exercise stress, vasodilator stress with SPECT MPI is an appropriate choice of stress testing in this patient.[3]

MPI demonstrated perfusion abnormalities in the territory of the left anterior descending and left circumflex coronary arteries, with a summed difference score of 12

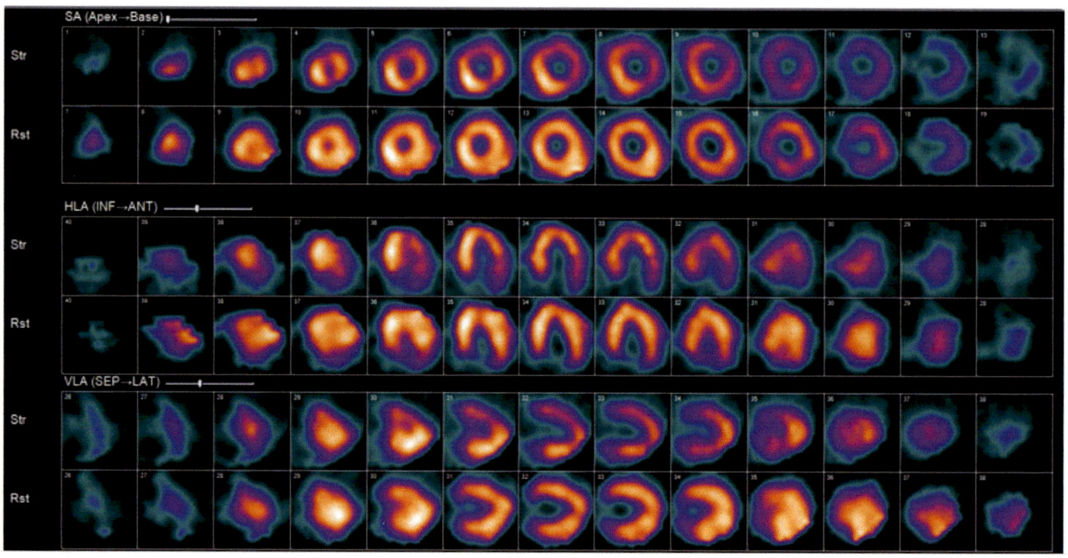

Figure 13.7. Case 2. SPECT MPI. HLA, horizontal long axis; Rst, rest; SA, short axis; Str, stress; VLA vertical long axis.

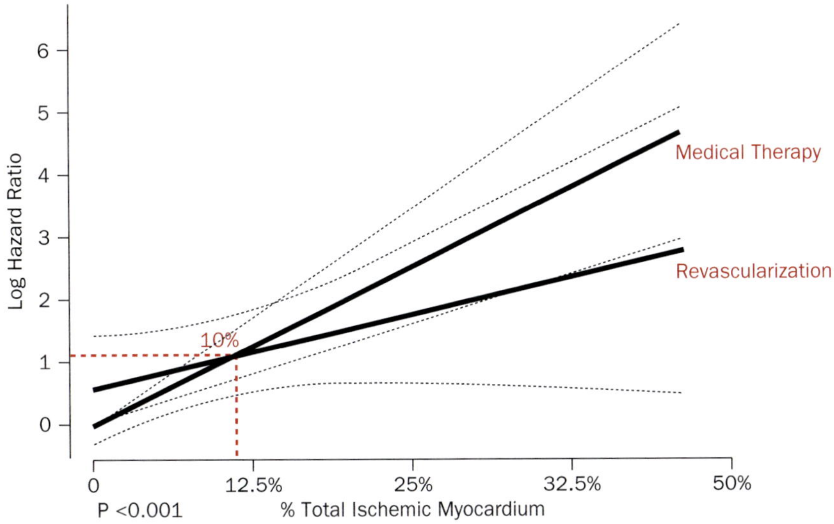

Figure 13.8. Relationship between percent of ischemic myocardium and hazard ratio for revascularization and medical therapy. Modified from Hachamovitch R, Hayes SW, Friedman JD, et al. Comparison of the short-term survival benefit associated with revascularization compared with medical therapy in patients with no prior coronary artery disease undergoing stress myocardial perfusion single photon emission computed tomography. *Circulation*. 2003;107(23):2900–2907, with permission.

and a burden of ischemic myocardium of 18%. Perfusion abnormalities in multivessel territories indicate the high-risk nature of this scan. In addition, a TID ratio of 1.38 is above the abnormal threshold of 1.31 defined for 1-day rest/regadenoson stress Tc-99m protocol.[5] Based on SPECT MPI findings, the patient was referred for invasive coronary angiography, which showed multivessel obstructive CAD, confirming SPECT MPI findings.

Regarding revascularization, the patient had class II to III angina symptoms, and she was not on an optimal anti-anginal regimen. Therefore, an initial trial of optimal medical therapy may seem reasonable. On the other hand, a high burden of ischemia and TID portend a high risk of future cardiac events.

The question is whether this patient would have a better outcome with coronary revascularization plus optimal medical therapy versus optimal medical therapy alone. Hachamovitch et al.[8] demonstrated the benefit of early coronary revascularization compared with medical therapy for patients with moderate to large stress-induced myocardial ischemia. In patients with more than 10% ischemic myocardium, coronary revascularization was associated with a 50% risk-adjusted reduction in cardiac death and all-cause mortality (Figure 13.8). Conversely, a strategy of medical therapy was associated with a lower mortality risk in the setting of no or mild ischemia (<10% ischemic myocardium).

The relationship between percent ischemic myocardium and the benefit from revascularization was present irrespective of LVEF. These findings were supported by the nuclear sub-study of the COURAGE trial that compared outcomes of patients with baseline stress MPI and a repeat stress MPI after 6 to 18 months of treatment.[9] These analyses demonstrated that percutaneous coronary intervention added to optimal medical therapy was more effective in reducing ischemia and improving angina than optimal medical therapy alone, particularly in patients with moderate-to-severe pretreatment ischemia.

CASE 3

A 62-year-old woman presented for an evaluation of intermittent retrosternal chest pain episodes for the last 2 months. The episodes are retrosternal, may happen with or without exertion, and are not always relieved by rest. She has a past medical history of chronic back pain, hypertension, and dyslipidemia, for which she was on chlortalidone 25 mg daily and atorvastatin 40 mg daily. She denied any prior history of CAD. Vital signs demonstrated BP 128/74 mmHg and heart rate 76 bpm. Her height and weight were 93 kg (205 lbs) and 170 cm (5 feet 7 inches), respectively. Physical exam was unremarkable. A baseline ECG (Figure 13.9) was unremarkable.

The patient was referred for a regadenoson-stress-first (only) Tc99m SPECT MPI protocol. Images were obtained using a standard gamma camera with low energy, high resolution collimation (LEHR) without AC. SPECT MPI (Figure 13.10) demonstrated a small defect of mild severity involving the inferior wall. The summed stress score was

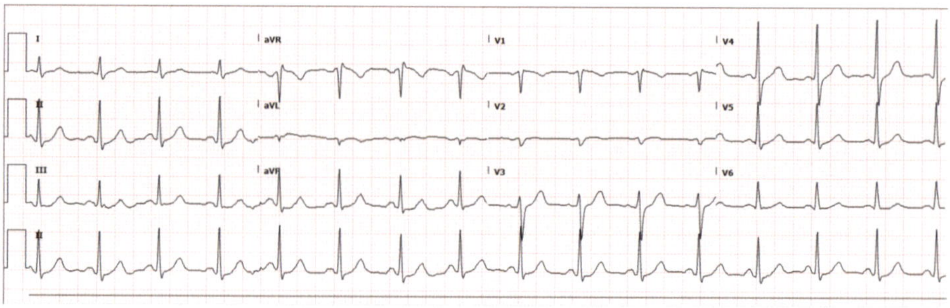

Figure 13.9. Case 3. Baseline 12-lead ECG.

4. Gated stress SPECT images demonstrated normal LVEF of 58% and no regional wall motion abnormalities.

Upon review of the images, the patient underwent repeat imaging using a prone position, which demonstrated resolution of the inferior wall defect (Figure 13.11).

The case illustrates a 62-year-old woman presenting with non-anginal chest pain, placing her at an intermediate pretest probability for CAD by the Diamond and Forrester classification.[1] Current multimodality imaging criteria for detection of coronary artery disease consider the use of SPECT MPI as "appropriate" in this scenario.[3] The patient is selected for a stress-only SPECT MPI protocol. In selected patients, stress-only SPECT imaging has been shown to be a viable alternative to rest–stress SPECT imaging to improve laboratory efficiency and reduce radiation exposure. However, AC or attenuation compensation with multi-position image acquisition is often necessary for confident interpretation of these images. In a cohort of 1,383 patients referred for clinically indicated stress-only Tc-99m AC SPECT, Mathur et al.[10] demonstrated that without AC, less than half of the studies were considered normal, but with AC, a higher percentage of the studies were

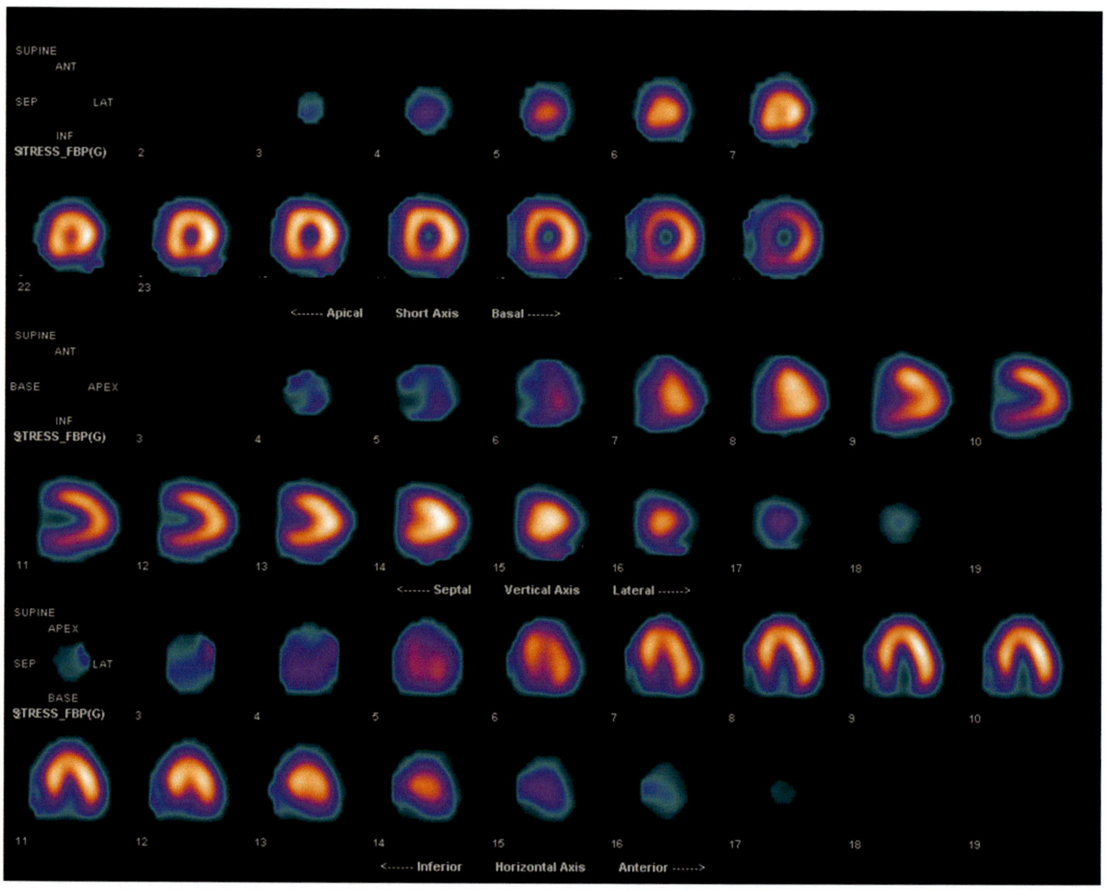

Figure 13.10. Case 3. SPECT MPI.

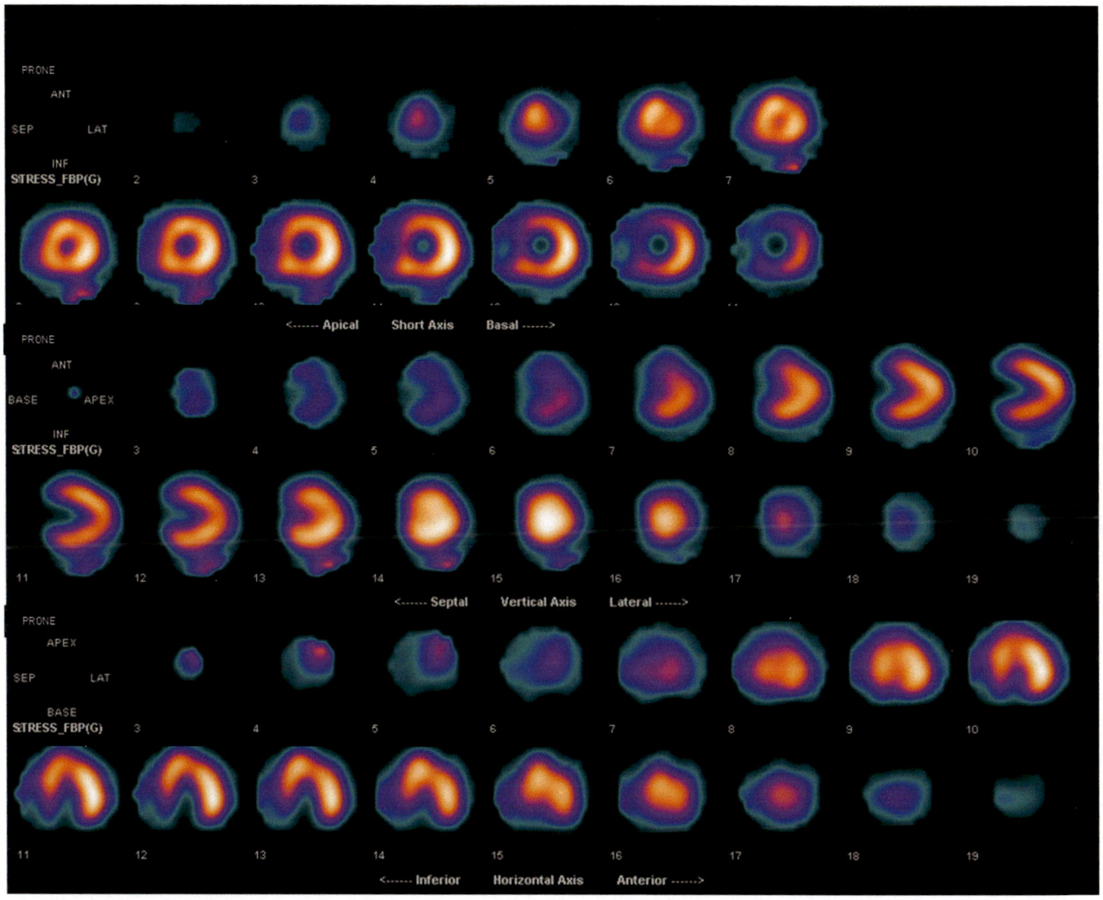

Figure 13.11. Case 3. SPECT MPI in prone position.

interpreted as normal. Moreover, non-AC SPECT image interpretation revealed that 58% (802/1,383) of patients had abnormal stress images. AC image interpretation of the abnormal non-AC images reclassified 83% (666/802) of these as normal. In patients with normal stress-only scans, the annualized event rate of adverse cardiac events was very low (0.7%), as shown in Figure 13.12. Our patient had supine images that demonstrated decreased radiotracer uptake in the inferior segments of the LV. Due to the lack of AC, it could not be determined whether the abnormality

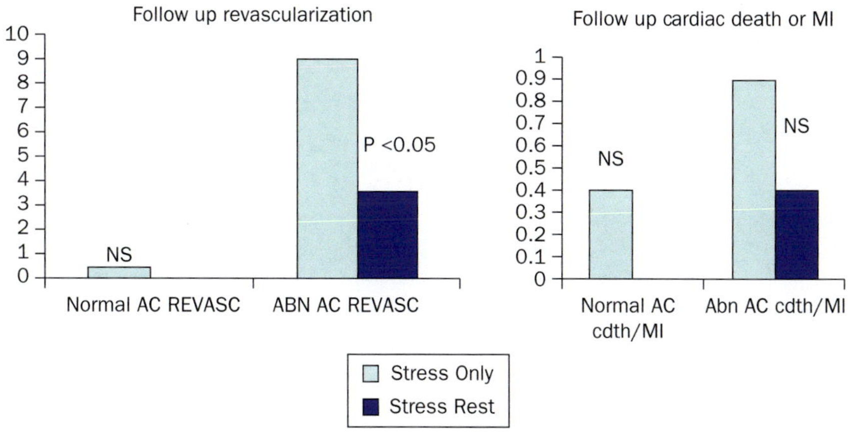

Figure 13.12. Percent of follow-up cardiac events in AC normal and abnormal stress-only studies and stress–rest cohorts. Abn, abnormal; cdth, cardiac death; REVASC, revascularization; NS, nonsignificant. Reproduced from Mathur S, Heller GV, Bateman TM, et al. Clinical value of stress-only Tc-99m SPECT imaging: Importance of attenuation correction. *J Nucl Cardiol*. 2013;20(1):27–37, with permission.

seen corresponds to a true perfusion defect or soft tissue attenuation. In this case, the defect resolved on prone imaging indicating normal myocardial perfusion, highlighting the importance of AC. The patient in this case can be reassured and advised on lifestyle and risk factor modifications.

REFERENCES

1. Diamond GA, Forrester JS. Analysis of probability as an aid in the clinical diagnosis of coronary-artery disease. *N Engl J Med.* 1979;300(24):1350–1358.
2. Hachamovitch R, Hayes SW, Friedman JD, et al. Comparison of the short-term survival benefit associated with revascularization compared with medical therapy in patients with no prior coronary artery disease undergoing stress myocardial perfusion single photon emission computed tomography. *Circulation.* 2003;107(23):2900–2907.
3. Wolk MJ, Bailey SR, Doherty JU, et al. ACCF/AHA/ASE/ASNC/HFSA/HRS/SCAI/SCCT/SCMR/STS 2013 multimodality appropriate use criteria for the detection and risk assessment of stable ischemic heart disease. *J Am Coll Cardiol.* 2014;63(4):380–406.
4. Doukky R, Hayes K, Frogge N, et al. Impact of appropriate use on the prognostic value of single-photon emission computed tomography myocardial perfusion imaging. *Circulation.* 2013;128:1634–1643.
5. Xu Y, Arsanjani R, Clond M, et al. Transient ischemic dilation for coronary artery disease in quantitative analysis of same-day sestamibi myocardial perfusion SPECT. *J Nucl Cardiol.* 2012;19(3):465–473.
6. Maron DJ, Hochman JS, Reynolds HR, et al. Initial invasive or conservative strategy for stable coronary disease. *N Engl J Med.* 2020;382(15):1395–1407.
7. Gibbons RJ, Balady GJ, Bricker JT, et al. ACC/AHA 2002 guideline update for exercise testing: Summary article. *J Am Coll Cardiol.* 2002;40(8):1531–1540.
8. Hachamovitch R, Rozanski A, Shaw LJ, et al. Impact of ischaemia and scar on the therapeutic benefit derived from myocardial revascularization vs. medical therapy among patients undergoing stress-rest myocardial perfusion scintigraphy. *Eur Heart J.* 2011;32(8):1012–1024.
9. Shaw LJ, Heller GV, Casperson P, et al. Gated myocardial perfusion single photon emission computed tomography in the clinical outcomes utilizing revascularization and aggressive drug evaluation (COURAGE) trial, Veterans Administration Cooperative study no. 424. *J Nucl Cardiol.* 2006;13(5):685–698.
10. Mathur S, Heller GV, Bateman TM, et al. Clinical value of stress-only Tc-99m SPECT imaging: Importance of attenuation correction. *J Nucl Cardiol.* 2013;20(1):27–37.

14.

SPECT MPI FOR RISK ASSESSMENT IN SPECIAL GROUPS

DIABETES MELLITUS, KIDNEY TRANSPLANT, LIVER TRANSPLANT, ASYMPTOMATIC, OBESE

Alberto Cuocolo, Emilia Zampella, Valeria Gaudieri, and Roberta Assante

CASE 1

A 56-year-old man with diabetes, hypertension, hypercholesterolemia, family history of CAD, and obesity (BMI 55 kg/m^2) was referred for exercise testing because of atypical angina of 2 months' duration. The physical examination was unremarkable except for massive obesity. He failed to complete exercise testing due to poor exercise tolerance. He underwent pharmacologic stress–rest imaging using a CZT SPECT camera. Stress images were acquired in both the upright and supine positions (Figure 14.1). Figure 14.2 shows stress

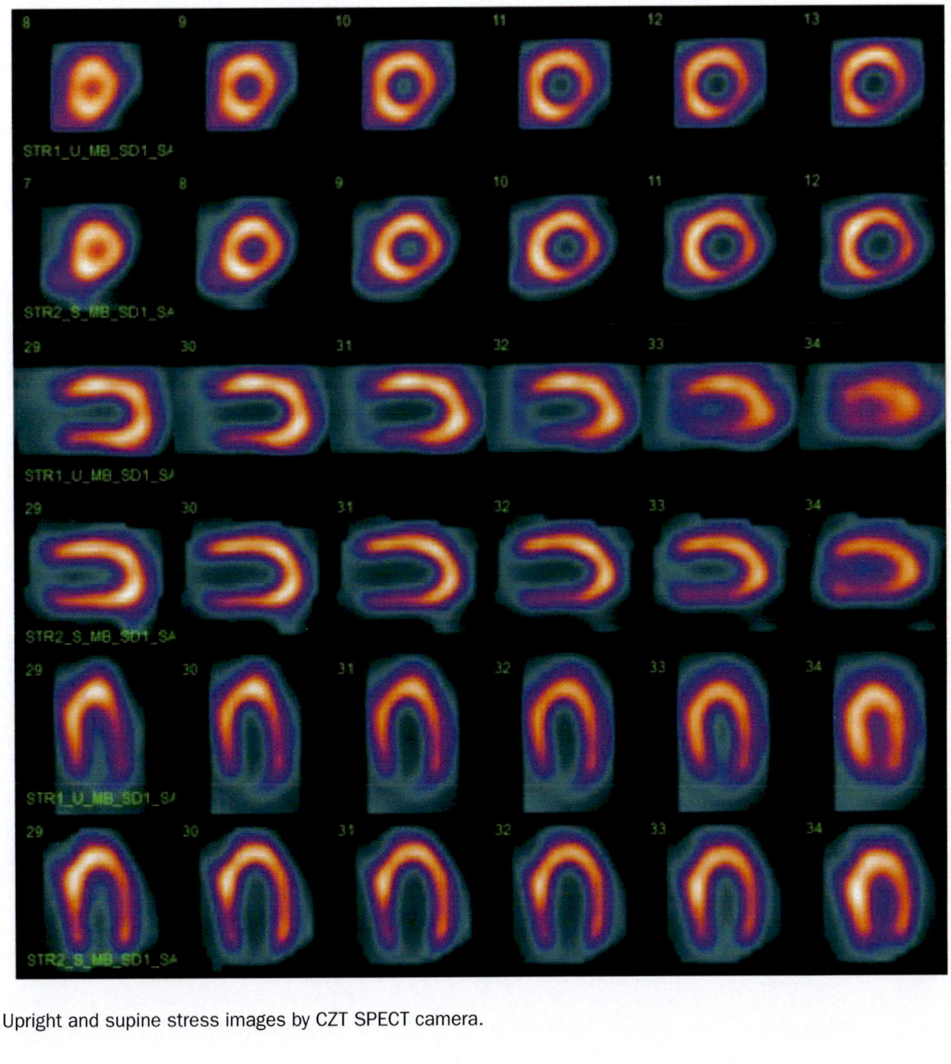

Figure 14.1. Case 1. Upright and supine stress images by CZT SPECT camera.

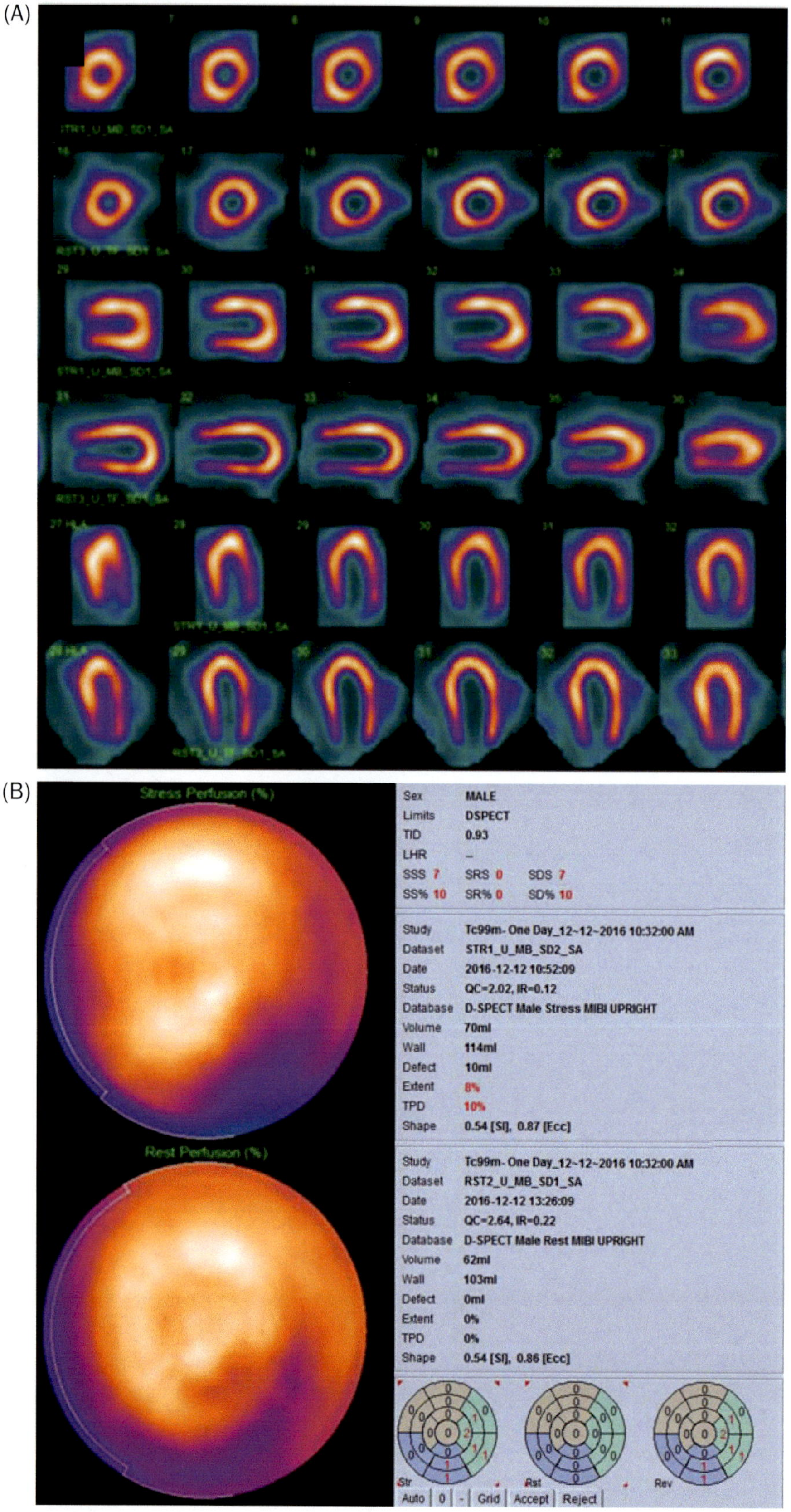

Figure 14.2. Case 1. Dipyridamole stress–rest MPI by CZT SPECT camera (A). Stress and rest semiquantitative perfusion analysis using QPS (Cedars-Sinai Medical Center, Los Angeles, CA) (B).

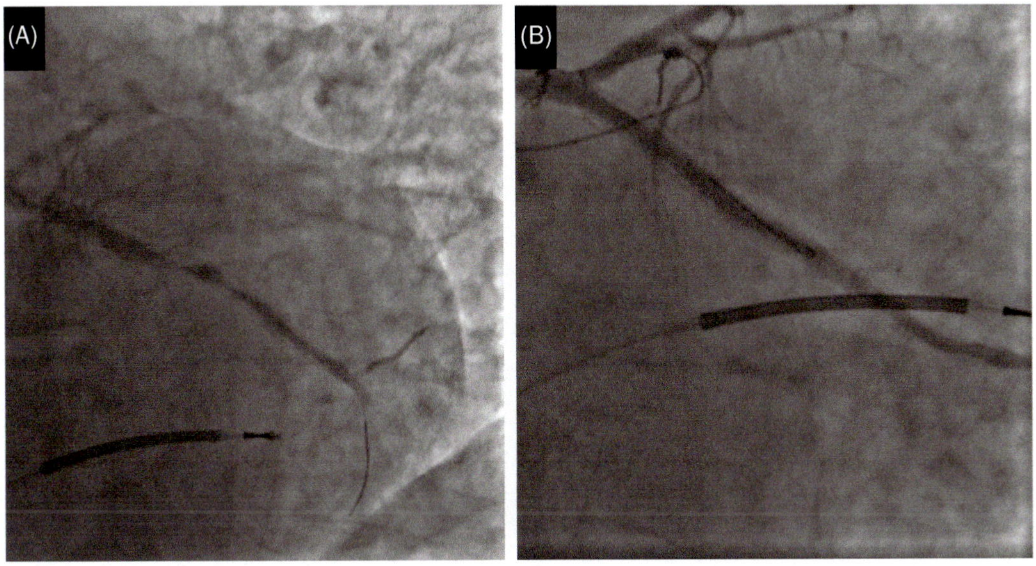

Figure 14.3. Case 1. Coronary angiography performed 1 week after CZT SPECT MPI.

and rest perfusion imaging (A) and semiquantitative analysis (B).

QUESTION

1. The images in Figure 14.2 show:
   a. Normal perfusion
   b. Small apical reversible defect
   c. Large anterior fixed defect
   d. Infero-lateral reversible defect

ANSWER

1d. The CZT SPECT images show a reversible perfusion defect in the infero-lateral wall involving 10% of LV myocardium.

Coronary angiography (Figure 14.3) performed 1 week after CZT SPECT imaging shows a severe stenosis of the left circumflex artery (A) successfully treated (B) with stenting. A repeat stress imaging study 12 months later (Fig. 14.4) showed normal stress myocardial perfusion.

In obese patients, to reduce attenuation-related artifacts, stress images can be acquired in upright and supine positions. In this patient the perfusion defect in the infero-lateral wall did not change in the two acquisitions, suggesting that it was a non-artifactual defect. The imaging findings modified the diagnostic program of the patient, who underwent coronary angiography and coronary revascularization. Serial MPI showed a significant improvement in perfusion between baseline and follow-up studies, demonstrating the effectiveness of the therapeutic approach.

CASE 2

A 51-year-old diabetic man with hypertension, hypercholesterolemia, family history of CAD, and atypical angina was referred for CT coronary angiography (Fig. 14.5). The images showed a <50% stenosis of the left anterior descending artery (LAD; yellow arrow) and a 50% stenosis of the right coronary artery (RCA; red arrow). The patient then underwent dynamic stress–rest MPI using CZT SPECT camera. Images, polar maps, and myocardial perfusion reserve data are shown in Figures 14.6, 14.7 and 14.8.

QUESTION

1. The images in Figures 14.6, 14.7 and 14.8 show:
   a. Normal perfusion and normal reserve
   b. Normal perfusion and abnormal reserve
   c. Abnormal perfusion and abnormal reserve
   d. Abnormal perfusion and normal reserve

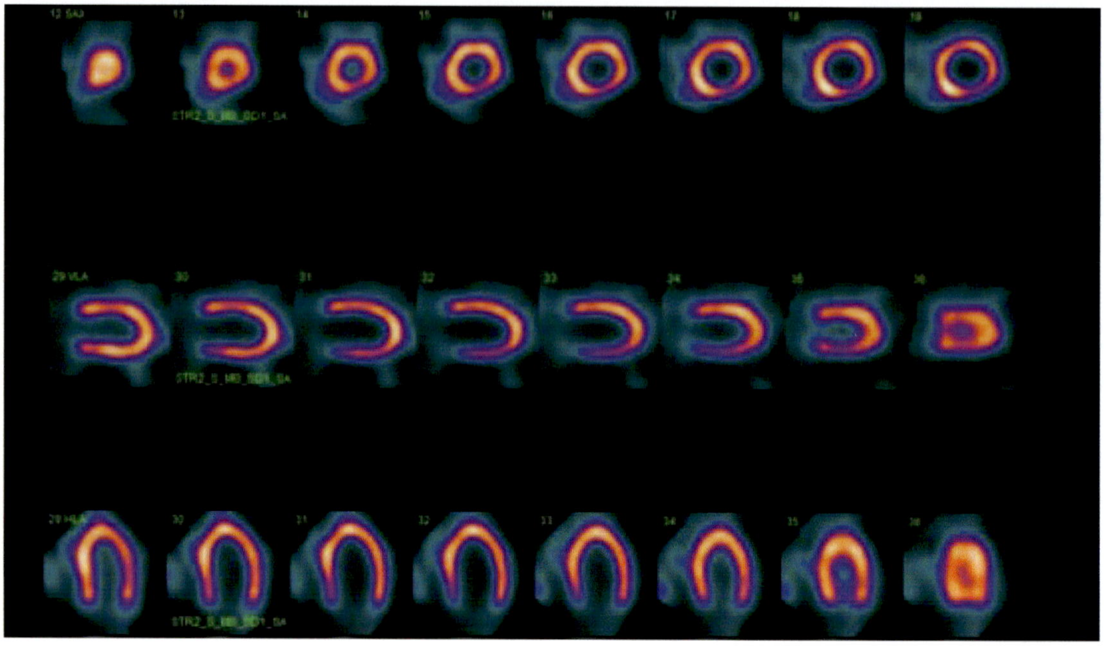

Figure 14.4. Case 1. Dipyridamole stress-only MPI by CZT SPECT camera performed 1 year after coronary revascularization.

ANSWER

1a. The images show normal myocardial perfusion. Flow quantification shows a normal regional and total myocardial perfusion reserve.

Coronary angiography CT is recommended as the initial test to diagnose CAD in symptomatic patients with low-intermediate risk of CAD. Stenoses assessed to be 50% to 90% are not necessarily functionally significant. Therefore, functional imaging for myocardial ischemia is recommended if coronary angiography CT has shown CAD of uncertain functional significance or is not diagnostic.

In this case, MPI excludes the presence of ischemia, avoiding invasive testing. Furthermore, the dynamic acquisition allows the evaluation of MPR both global and regional, showing a preserved vasodilator function.

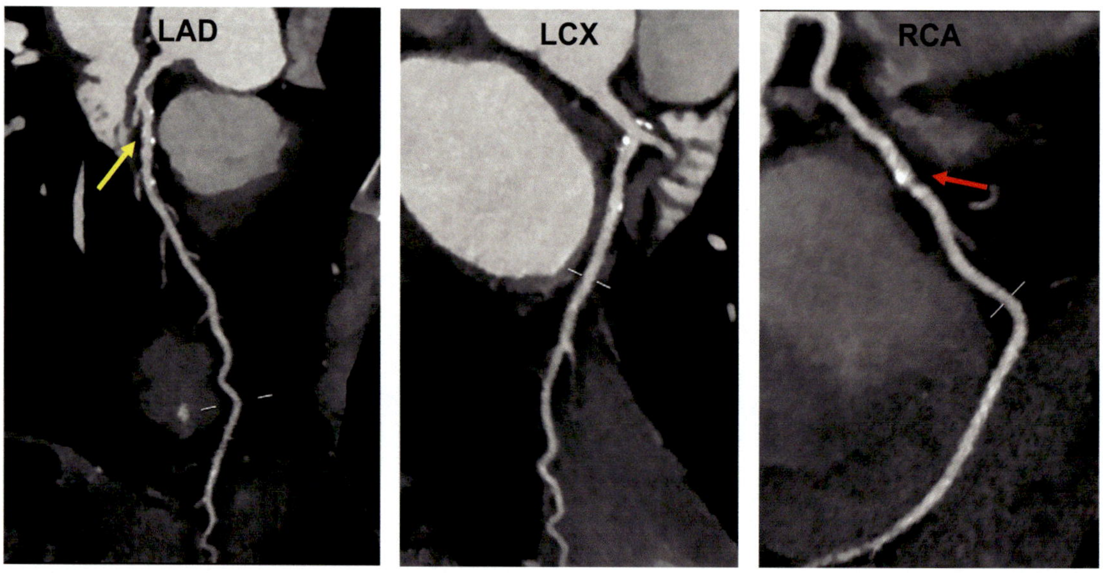

Figure 14.5. Case 2. CT coronary angiography (performed before MPI). LCX, left circumflex.

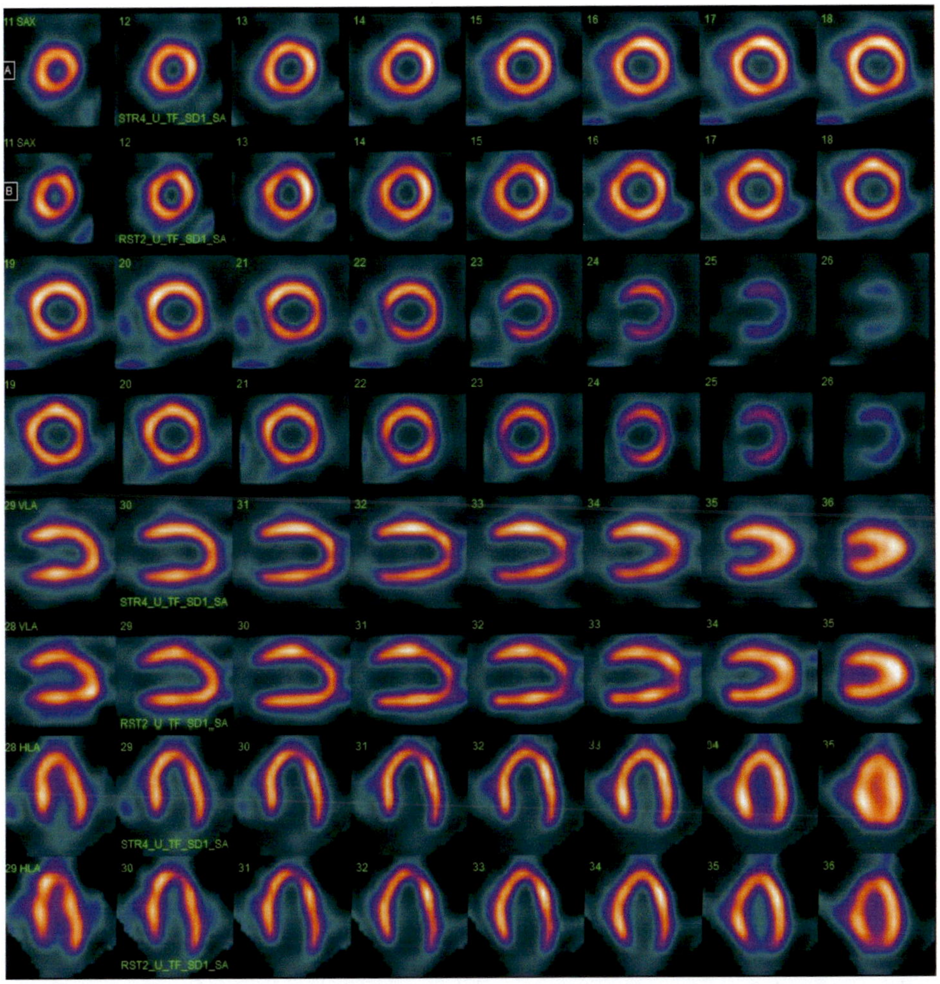

Figure 14.6. Case 2. Dipyridamole stress–rest imaging by CZT SPECT camera.

CASE 3

A 59-year-old male smoker with hypercholesterolemia, obesity, and atypical angina underwent CT coronary angiography (Figure 14.9). CT imaging showed extensive calcifications of the left anterior descending artery (LAD), with 50% stenosis at mid segment (yellow arrow), and 50% stenosis of the right coronary artery (RCA, red arrow). The patient then underwent dynamic stress–rest MPI by CZT SPECT camera. Images, polar maps, and myocardial perfusion reserve data are shown in Figures 14.10, 14.11 and 14.12.

QUESTIONS

1. Images in Figures 14.10 and 14.11 show:
   a. Normal perfusion
   b. One-vessel disease
   c. Two-vessel disease
   d. Three-vessel disease
2. Evaluation of myocardial perfusion reserve in Figure 14.12 shows:
   a. Normal regional and total reserve
   b. Normal regional reserve but reduced total reserve
   c. Reduced regional reserve in all three vascular territories and reduced total reserve
   d. Reduced regional reserve in only one vascular territory and reduced total reserve

ANSWERS

1c. CZT SPECT images show a reversible perfusion defect in the anterior and inferior walls with total perfusion defect size of 12%.

2d. Flow quantification shows a reduced reserve in the territory of the left anterior descending coronary artery and a reduction of total reserve.

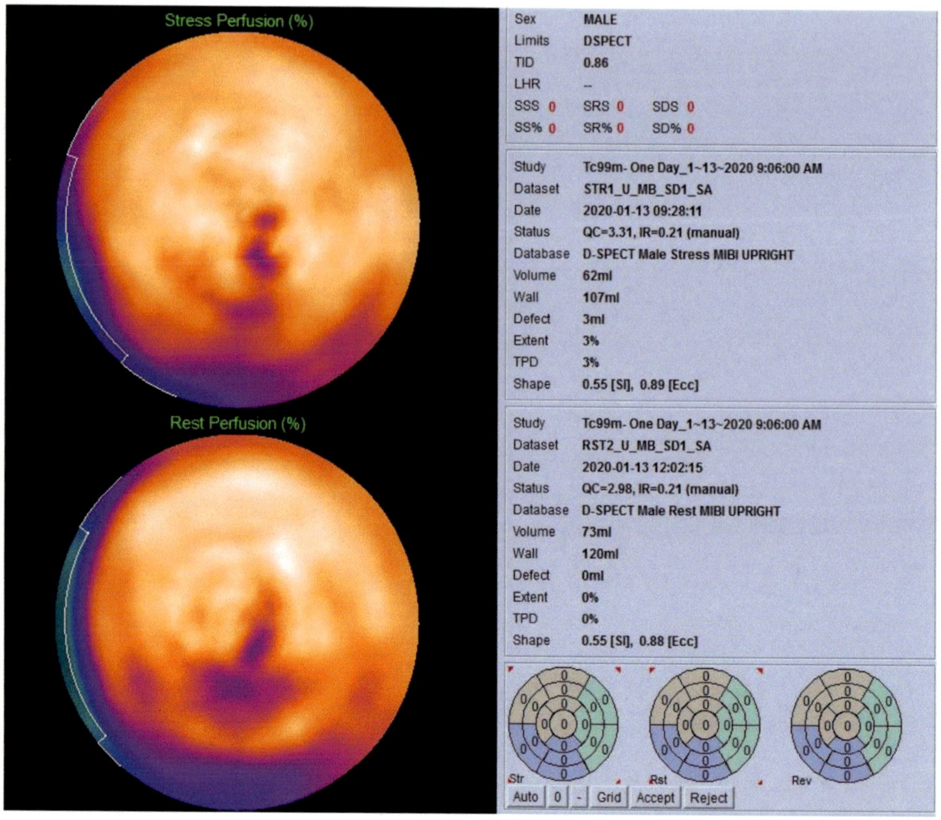

Figure 14.7. Case 2. Stress and rest semiquantitative perfusion analysis using QPS (Cedars-Sinai Medical Center, Los Angeles, CA).

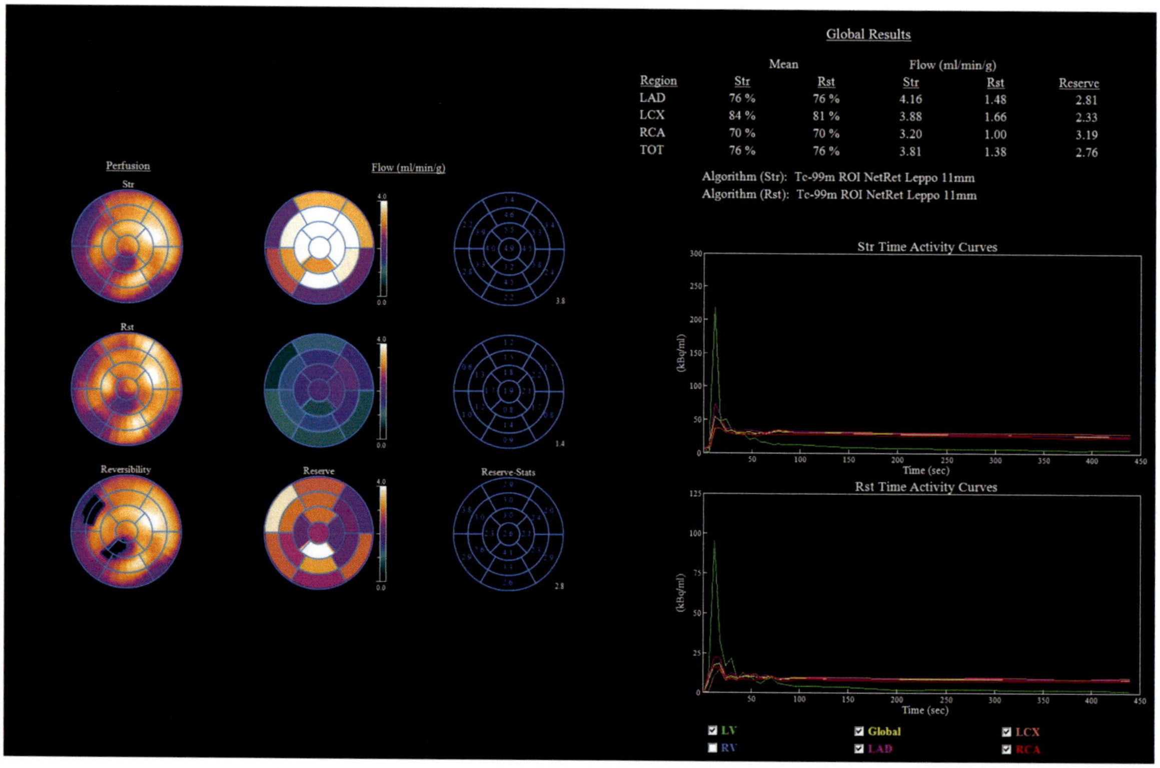

Figure 14.8. Case 2. Myocardial blood flow and myocardial perfusion reserve quantification by dynamic CZT SPECT imaging.

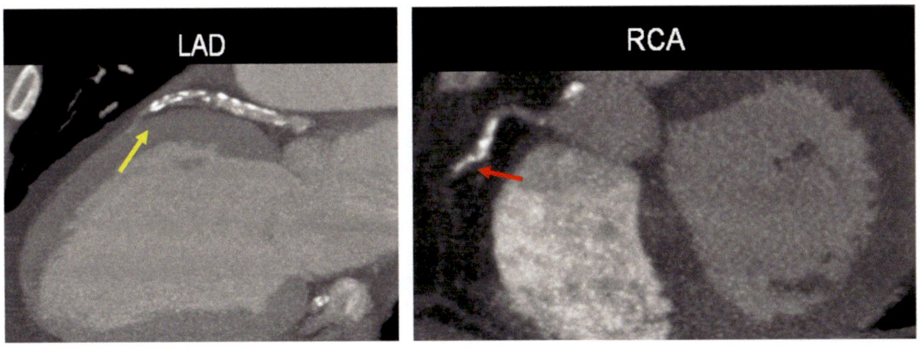

Figure 14.9. Case 3. CT coronary angiography performed before MPI.

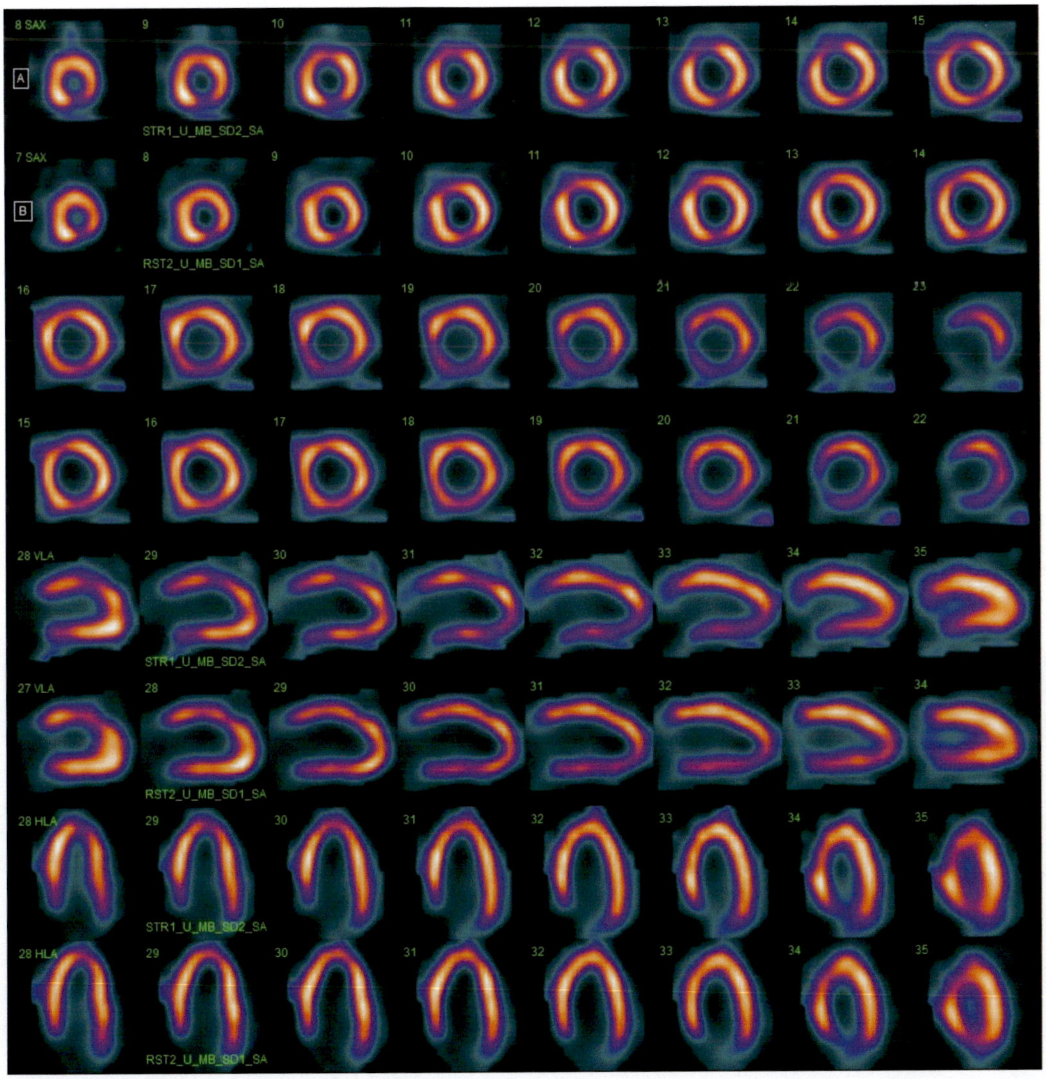

Figure 14.10. Case 3. Dipyridamole stress–rest imaging by CZT SPECT camera.

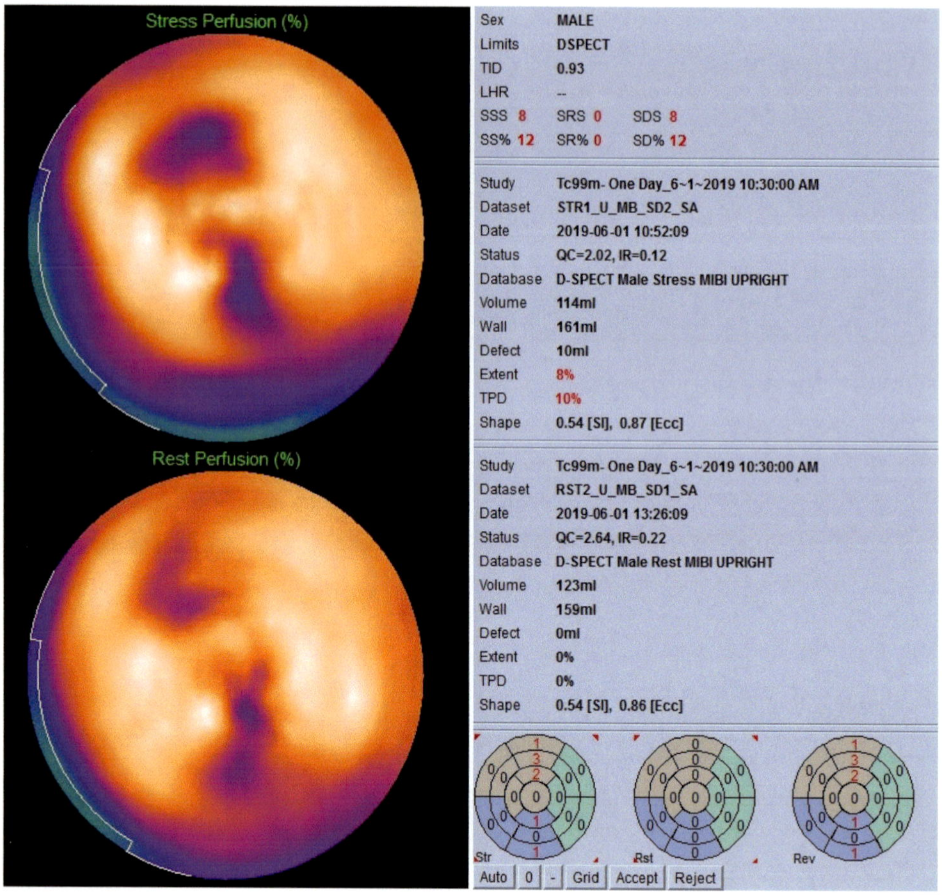

Figure 14.11. Case 3. Stress and rest semiquantitative perfusion analysis using QPS (Cedars-Sinai Medical Center, Los Angeles, CA).

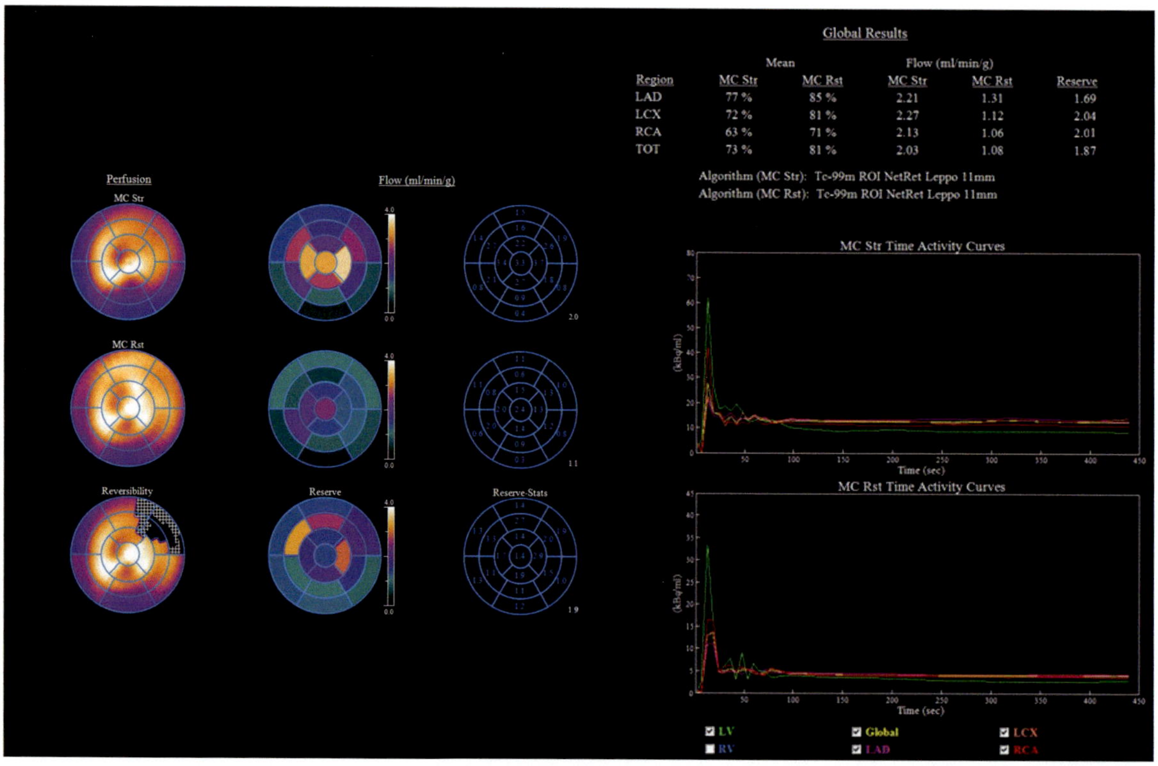

Figure 14.12. Case 3. Myocardial blood flow and myocardial perfusion reserve quantification by dynamic CZT SPECT imaging.

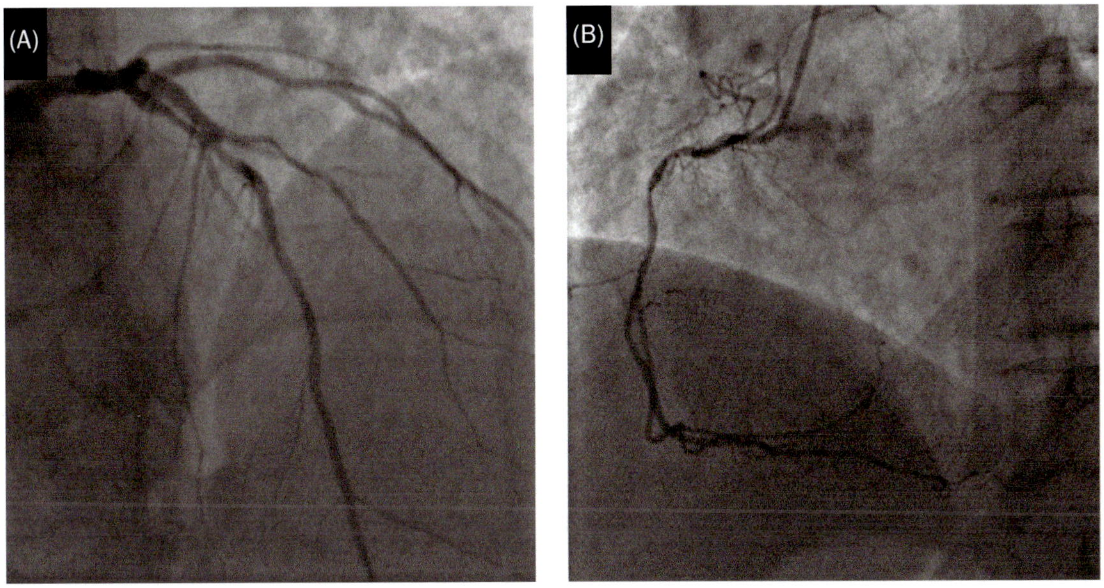

Figure 14.13. Case 3. Coronary angiography performed after CZT SPECT imaging.

Coronary angiography (Fig. 14.13) performed 3 weeks after SPECT shows a severe stenosis of the left anterior descending coronary artery (treated) (A) and an intermediate stenosis of a small right coronary artery (not treated) (B).

In the case of multivessel disease, MPI is able to provide information on the severity and extent of the perfusion defect, guiding the choice of the vessel to be treated. In this case, ischemia mainly involved the anterior wall, in accordance with the reduction of MPR in the LAD territory and the angiographic data that showed severe stenosis. The scintigraphic results also guided the therapeutic choice to treat only one of the two stenotic vessels, since ischemia in the inferior wall was mild and therefore was treated with medical therapy.

15.

SPECT MPI AND RISK ASSESSMENT BEFORE NON-CARDIAC SURGERY

Daniel C. Fisher and Lawrence M. Phillips

CASE 1

You are asked to evaluate a 68-year-old man with multiple risk factors for CAD who presents for preoperative risk assessment prior to lung mass resection. He has hypertension and dyslipidemia and smoked a pack per day for 35 years, quitting 5 years ago. On questioning, he denies chest pain or prior MI, but he has had limited exercise, walking only a block or two and stopping due to dyspnea on exertion. His medications include atorvastatin and amlodipine. On exam, his blood pressure is 124/72 mmHg and his heart rate is 74 bpm. His heart is regular rate and rhythm without significant murmur or gallop. Lungs are clear to auscultation bilaterally. Extremities are without edema. His EKG shows normal sinus rhythm with an intraventricular conduction delay.

QUESTION

1. What is the most appropriate of the following regarding his preoperative evaluation?
   a. Clear him for surgery without hesitation.
   b. Recommend an exercise stress test.
   c. Recommend a pharmacologic stress test.
   d. Proceed to cardiac catheterization.

ANSWER

1c. The preoperative evaluation is an opportunity to assess the patient and the risk of the planned surgery. The planned thoracic surgery has an elevated risk. Given his poor functional status (likely <4 METs), the decision of how to proceed depends on whether further testing will impact decision-making or perioperative patient care. Assuming the surgery is not an emergency, and that an abnormal stress test might alter management perioperatively, it is reasonable to proceed with noninvasive stress testing. Given his limited exercise tolerance, a pharmacologic stress test is likely the best option.

You refer the patient for pharmacologic stress testing with regadenoson. The patient has mild symptoms of dyspnea with infusion, and there are no significant EKG changes during the test. Nuclear images are shown in Figure 15.1.

QUESTIONS

2. What are your recommendations based on the stress test?
   a. Request coronary CTA.
   b. Refer the patient for cardiac catheterization.
   c. Adjust medications prior to surgery.
   d. Proceed with planned surgery without further cardiac evaluation.
3. What findings on nuclear imaging would have lead you to consider cardiac catheterization preoperatively?
   a. Small or mild perfusion defects with stress or rest
   b. Multiple defects of moderate size or a large reversible defect
   c. Transient ischemic dilatation
   d. All of the above
   e. b or c

ANSWERS

2d. The nuclear images are normal, without evidence of ischemia or infarction. There is no evidence of abnormal

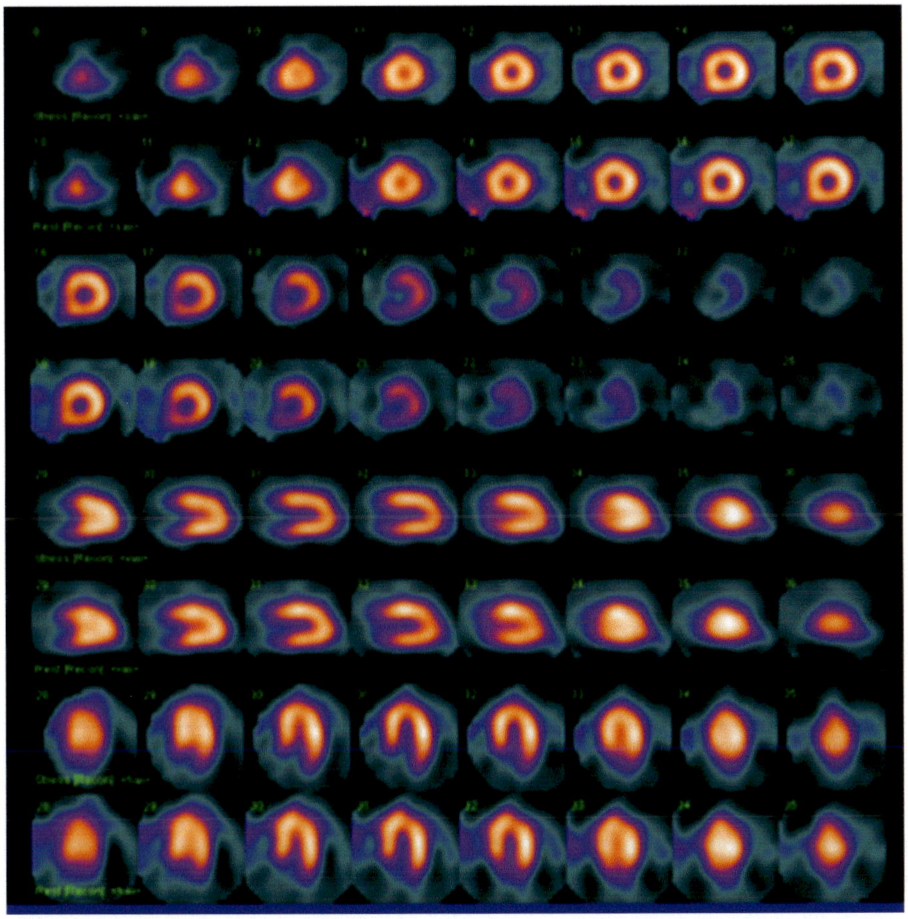

Figure 15.1. Stress and Rest SPECT MPI.

transient ischemic dilatation. Given the absence of ischemia (or infarction) on imaging, there is a no need for further cardiac evaluation prior to surgery.

3e. High-risk findings on nuclear imaging include the presence of a large reversible perfusion defect (particularly anterior) or multiple perfusion defects of moderate size. Transient ischemic dilatation is another high risk feature suggestive of severe coronary disease. Cardiac catheterization should be considered in such cases prior to proceeding with surgery.

CASE 2

A 65-year-old man was referred for preoperative evaluation prior to reversal of colostomy. He was a former smoker with a history of hypertension, gastroesophageal reflux disease, and dyslipidemia. He had known prior coronary artery bypass grafting surgery ×3 vessels 11 years prior. He also had a prior cerebrovascular accident without significant residual. He denied chest pain or dyspnea with exertion, but his exertion was limited to walking about two blocks slowly. Medications included aspirin, carvedilol, enalapril, and rosuvastatin. On exam, his body mass index was 34, his heart sounds were normal, and his lungs were clear. His baseline EKG showed sinus rhythm with Q waves seen in the septal leads and an IVCD. His electrocardiogram was unchanged from prior visits (Figure 15.2).

Given his history of coronary artery bypass surgery with a limited exercise tolerance and plans for an intermediate-risk surgery, he was referred for pharmacologic stress testing with MPI. He was given regadenoson per protocol with mild symptoms of dyspnea during the injection but no notable EKG changes.

The nuclear images (stress sitting and supine and rest sitting) were interpreted as showing a large, moderate-severe severity fixed defect in the left anterior distribution and only minimal ischemia (Figure 15.3). Both rest and post-stress gated analysis showed a normal-sized LV cavity with markedly reduced systolic function (LVEF = 30%).

Based on these results, no additional testing or intervention was deemed necessary prior to the planned surgery.

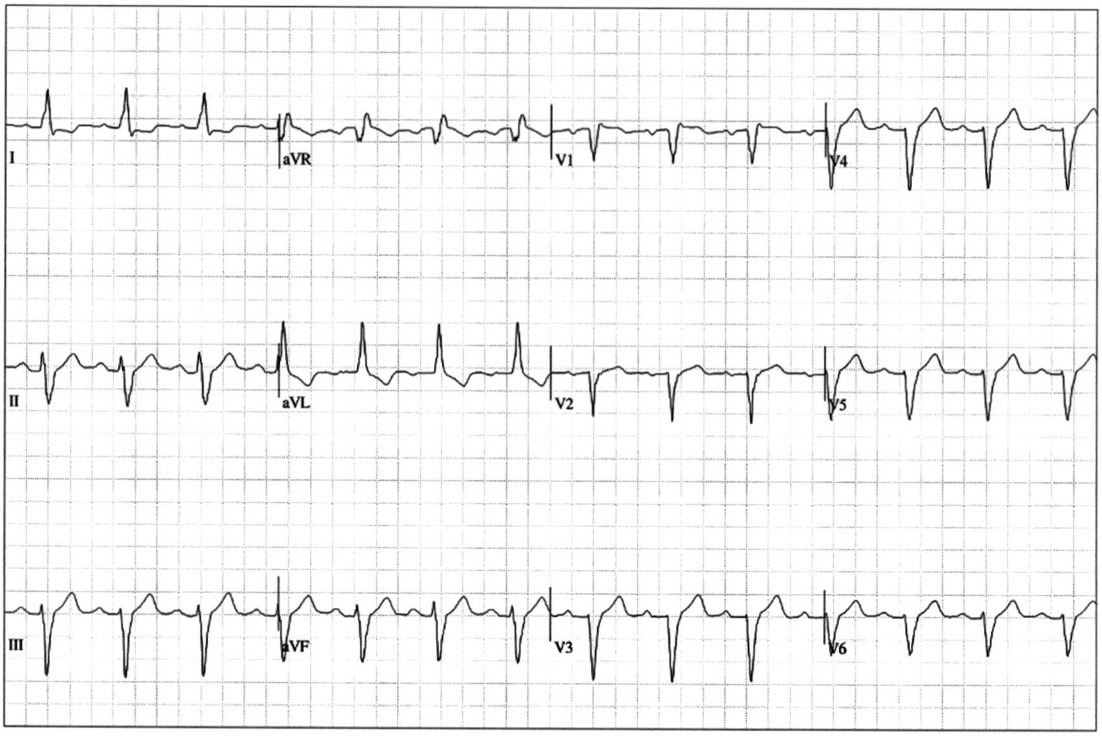

Figure 15.2. Baseline EKG showing sinus rhythm with septal Q waves and IVCD.

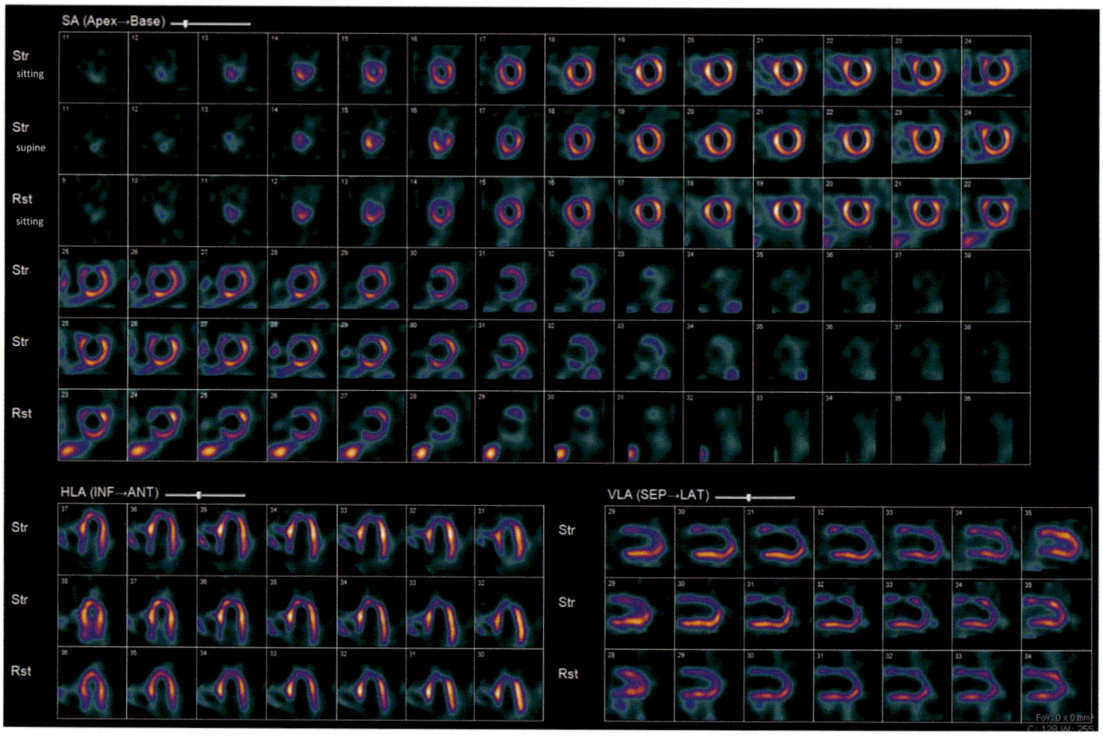

Figure 15.3. SPECT MPI (stress sitting and supine and rest sitting).

Baseline EKG

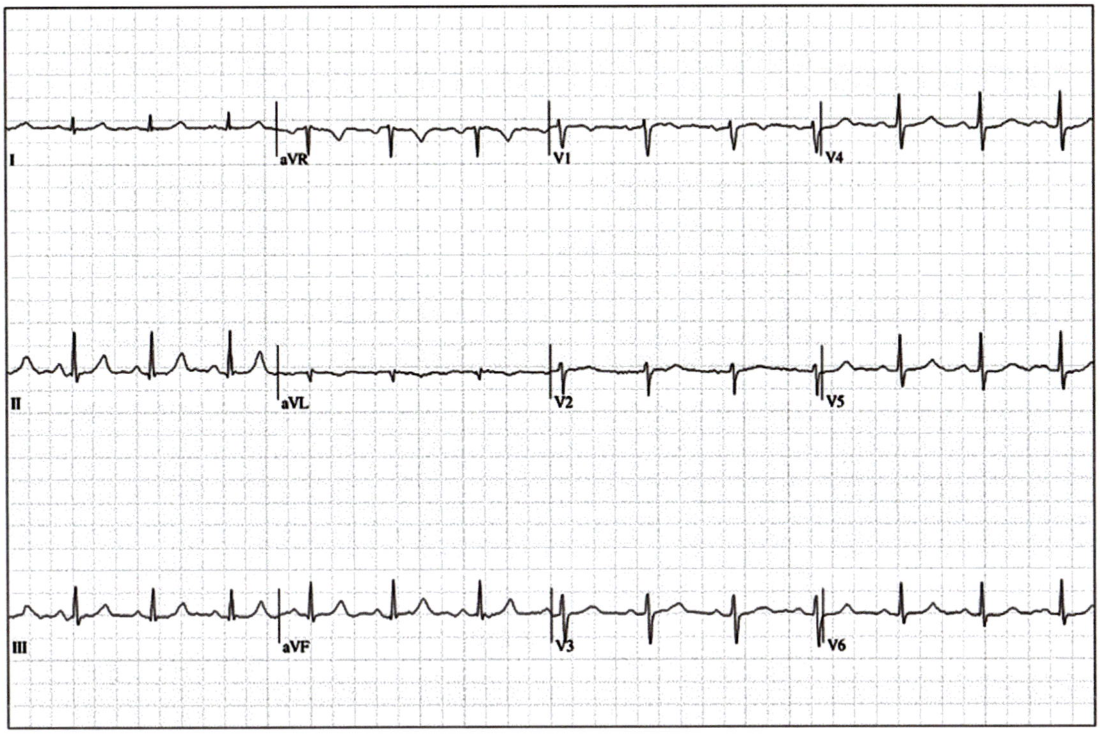

Figure 15.4. Baseline EKG showing normal sinus rhythm with no baseline ST segment deviation.

EKG in Early Recovery

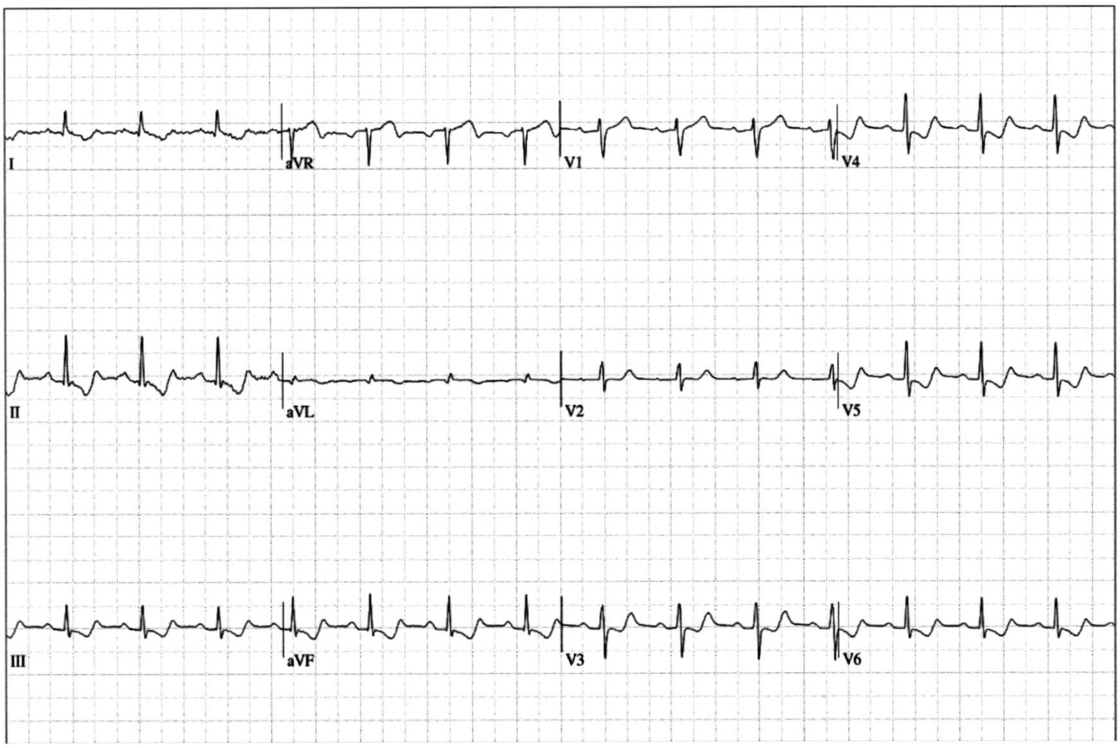

Figure 15.5. Post-Exercise EKG with 2-mm downsloping ST depressions in the inferior and anterolateral leads.

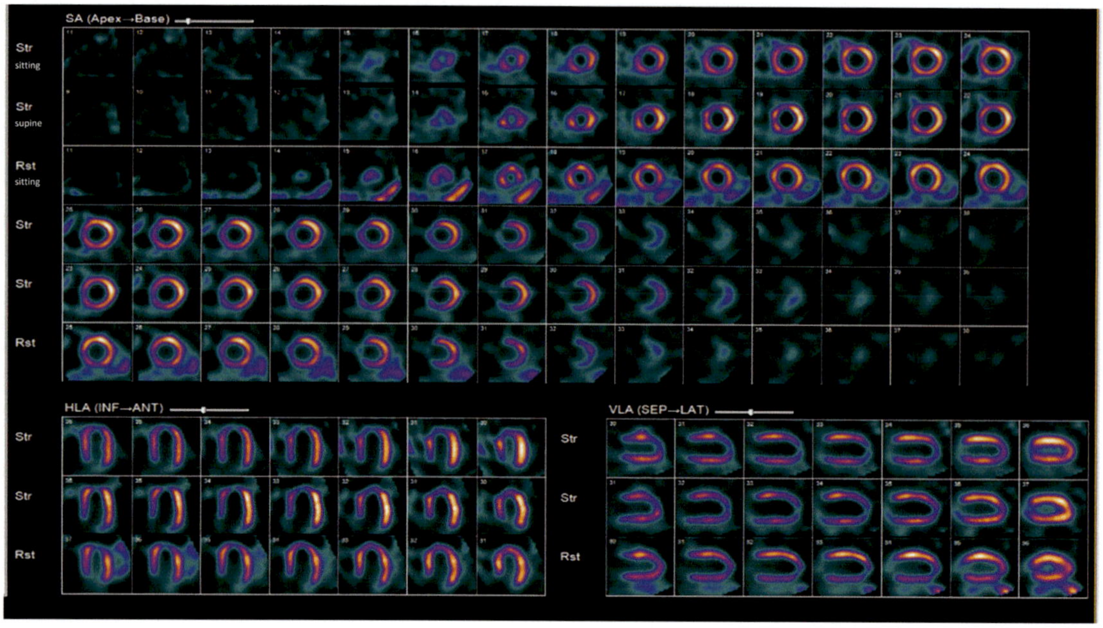

Figure 15.6. SPECT MPI (stress sitting and supine and rest sitting).

CASE 3

A 78-year-old man was evaluated by his cardiologist prior to knee surgery. He had a past medical history of previous smoking (1 pack per day, having quit 15 years prior), hypertension, and hyperlipidemia. He denied chest pain but he was not very active given his knee arthritis. He had a surgical history of gallbladder resection. His medications included atorvastatin 20 mg daily, levothyroxine 150 mcg daily, atenolol 50 mg daily, amlodipine 10 mg daily, and valsartan/HCTZ 160/25 mg daily. His baseline EKG showed normal sinus rhythm without baseline ST-segment deviation (Figure 15.4).

The patient exercised for 5 minutes using the Bruce protocol. He reached 85% of his maximum predicted heart rate but had to stop due to limiting chest pain. His post-exercise EKG showed 2-mm downsloping ST depressions in the inferior and anterolateral leads (Figure 15.5).

The nuclear images were abnormal, showing medium-sized, predominately reversible moderate to severe defects in the anterior wall, septum, and apex (Figure 15.6). The rest and post-exercise LVEF was 55%.

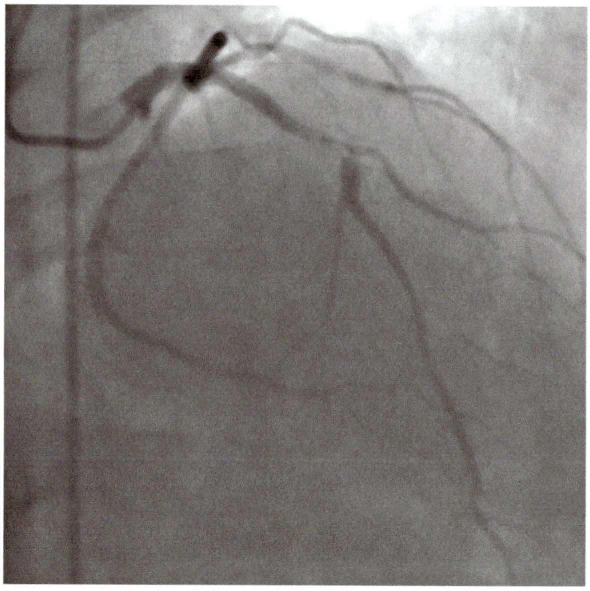

Figure 15.7. Coronary angiography showing 95% stenosis of the left anterior descending artery.

Based on these results, he underwent coronary angiography. The angiogram showed a 95% stenosis in the left anterior descending artery. This lesion was successfully stented and surgery was delayed per guidelines (Figure 15.7).

16.

EVALUATION OF PATIENTS WITH CHEST PAIN IN THE EMERGENCY DEPARTMENT

Elona Rrapo Kaso and Jamieson M. Bourque

CASE 1

A 72-year-old man with a history of hypertension, hyperlipidemia, and esophageal spasms and no known prior CAD presented to the ED with 2 weeks of episodic chest pain. The pain was described as aching with occasional tightness and burning in the upper chest without radiation. He was free from chest pain at the time of evaluation in the ED. His physical exam and ECG were unremarkable. The patient presented to the ED in the evening and underwent two serial negative troponins. He was seen by the cardiology consult service in the ED. Per the current ACC/AHA/ASNC Guidelines[1] and the multisociety recommendations on Appropriate Utilization of Cardiovascular Imaging in Emergency Department Patients with Chest Pain,[2] a stress radionuclide MPI study was recommended for further risk stratification of this intermediate-risk patient with negative ECG and troponin who presented in the ED after resolution of chest pain. In the morning, he underwent an exercise gated ^{99m}Tc sestamibi SPECT MPI study using a 1-day rest–stress imaging protocol. Prone imaging was performed for AC. The patient exercised on the treadmill for 9 minutes, achieving 10.1 METS and >85% of his maximum age-predicted heart rate on a Bruce protocol. The test was stopped due to development of chest discomfort and dyspnea during peak exercise. In addition, the patient developed ECG abnormalities, including 1-mm ST-segment elevation in lead III, <1-mm elevation in lead aVR, and 1-mm horizontal ST depression in V2 and V3. His MPI images revealed a moderate reduction in tracer uptake in the apical to basal inferoseptal, inferior, and inferolateral segments at stress that resolved at rest (Figure 16.1). The perfusion defect persisted despite AC on prone imaging. The percentage LV ischemia was quantified at 18% and abnormal wall motion was confirmed in the defect area (Figure 16.2). Global LV function post stress was normal at 72%. ICA showed 80% stenosis of the distal right coronary artery (RCA) and no other significant obstructive disease (Figure 16.3A,B). Successful percutaneous coronary intervention of the RCA was performed with a drug-eluting stent (Figure 16.3C). The patient completed a cardiac rehabilitation program and was started on appropriate guideline-directed medical therapy for CAD. On his follow-up visit in the cardiology clinic, the patient reported feeling well without any symptom recurrence.

QUESTION

1. Prone imaging was used for AC. How does prone imaging improve SPECT MPI accuracy?
   a. Distinguishes residual liver activity
   b. Improves recognition of diaphragmatic attenuation
   c. Corrects for breast attenuation
   d. Decreases patient motion

ANSWER

1b. Prone imaging is used to distinguish a true perfusion defect in the inferior wall from artifacts, particularly diaphragmatic attenuation. On prone imaging, the patient lies on their abdomen, creating greater separation between the heart and diaphragm as the heart shifts anteriorly and upward, whereas the diaphragm is pushed down. This technique allows for less inferior wall attenuation as compared to supine imaging. As shown in the first case, radionuclide imaging is performed in both supine and prone positions. A comparison is made between the two images. A true inferior perfusion defect will persist on prone imaging as opposed to a diaphragmatic attenuation artifact, which can resolve with attenuation imaging. Thus, prone imaging decreases the false-positive rate of inferior wall perfusion defects. Current guidelines

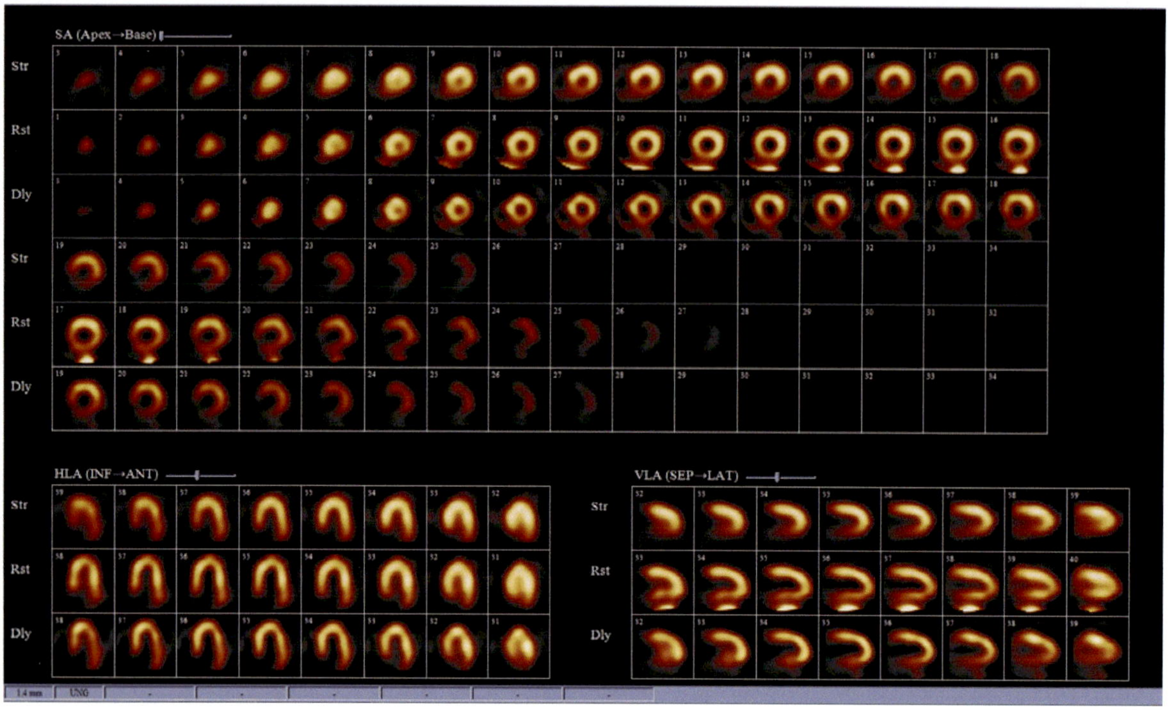

Figure 16.1. Case 1. Gated SPECT MPI with AC showing a reversible perfusion abnormality in the RCA territory. Images in the third row are obtained in prone position.

recommend prone imaging to supplement supine SPECT imaging.[3] However, prone imaging is not reliable in distinguishing liver activity, breast attenuation, or patient motion, and these artifacts can be seen on both supine and prone imaging. Prone imaging can result in artifactual anterior defects and only the inferior wall should be evaluated.

Improving SPECT imaging technique with AC to accurately identify low- and high-risk patients is particularly helpful in rest-only imaging during acute chest pain or when stress-only imaging is performed in the ED setting. AC improves diagnostic and prognostic accuracy.[4,5] Routine use of this practice would lead to improved clinical outcomes and better efficiency of SPECT MPI in the ED by discharging appropriately low-risk patients and hospitalizing those at high risk.

CASE 2

A 77-year-old female with a history of hypertension, stage 3 chronic kidney disease (CKD), chronic obstructive pulmonary disease, former tobacco use, and no known prior CAD

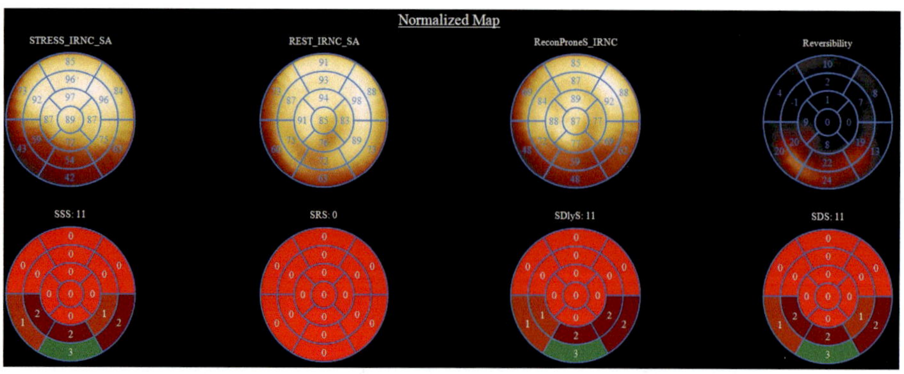

Figure 16.2. Case 1. The polar map showing the extent of the perfusion abnormality compared with a database of normal subjects (the percentage LV ischemia was 18%).

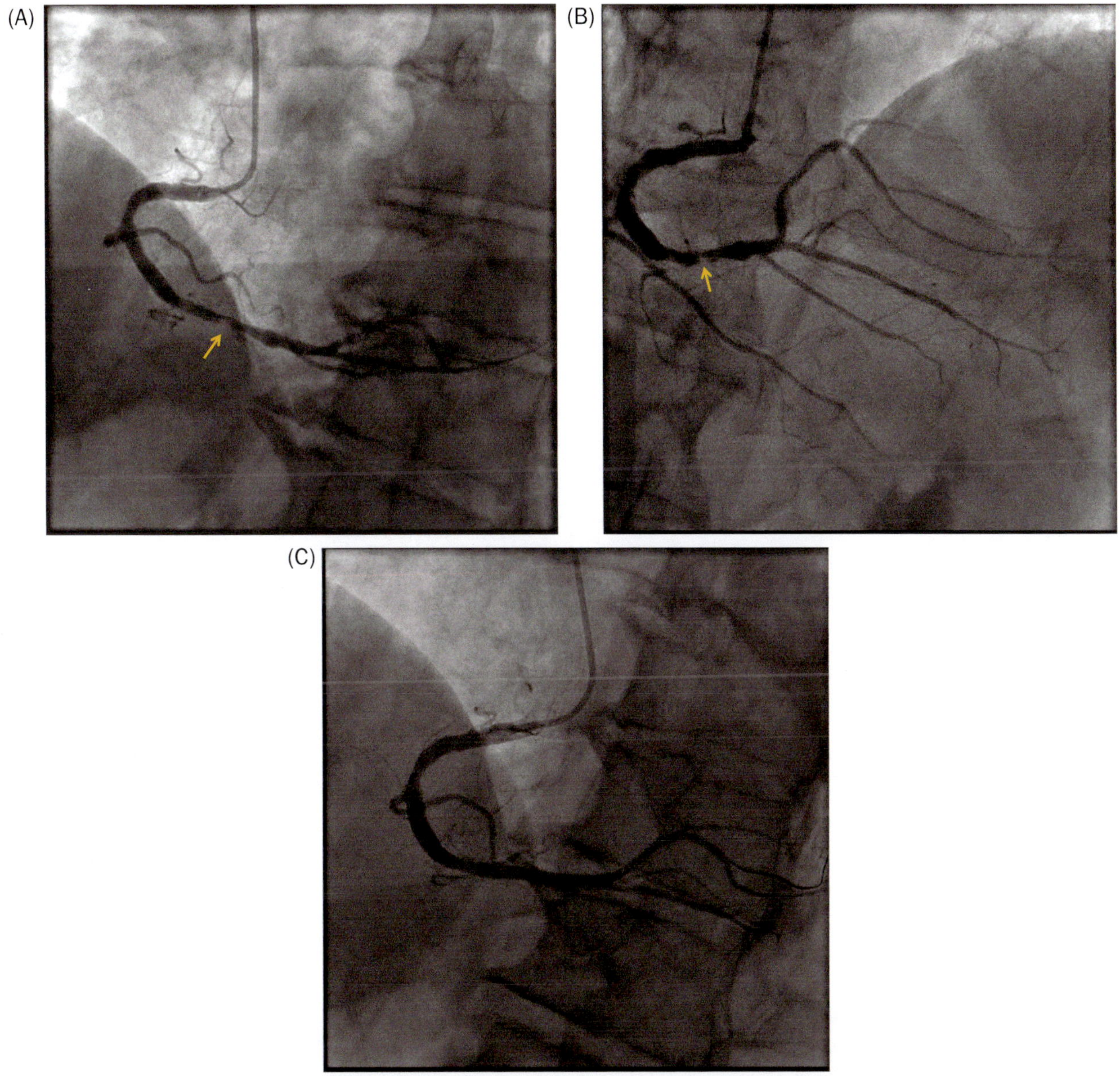

Figure 16.3. Case 1. (A, B) RCA LAO (Left Anterior Oblique)/cranial views showing an 80% distal RCA stenosis (arrows). (C) The RCA after percutaneous coronary intervention.

presented to an outside ED with an episode of chest pain. The pain was described as retrosternal pressure without radiation. The chest pain was intermittent and resolved within 30 minutes. Her ECG showed left anterior fascicular block and left ventricular hypertrophy with diffuse T-wave inversions in leads II, III, avF, I, and V4–V6. There was no prior ECG available for comparison. An initial troponin was negative. Her chest x-ray revealed emphysema. Given that this patient was at intermediate risk for ACS, she was transferred to our tertiary-care ED with coronary angiography capabilities for further risk stratification. Her physical exam upon transfer to our ED was significant for a blood pressure of 158/78 mmHg. A second troponin was negative. The patient remained free of chest pain. She underwent a pharmacologic stress test with regadenoson. A gated ^{99m}Tc sestamibi SPECT MPI study with a 1-day, rest–stress imaging protocol was performed. This imaging revealed a small-sized region with moderate reduction in uptake in the apical to mid anteroseptal segments that was reversible (Figure 16.4). There was normal wall motion in the defect area. The perfusion defect was visualized on perfusion images; however, it did not flag as abnormal compared with a database of normal subjects on quantitative analysis. Global and regional LV function post stress was normal with an EF of 66%. The small reversible perfusion defect was favored to represent a change in the position

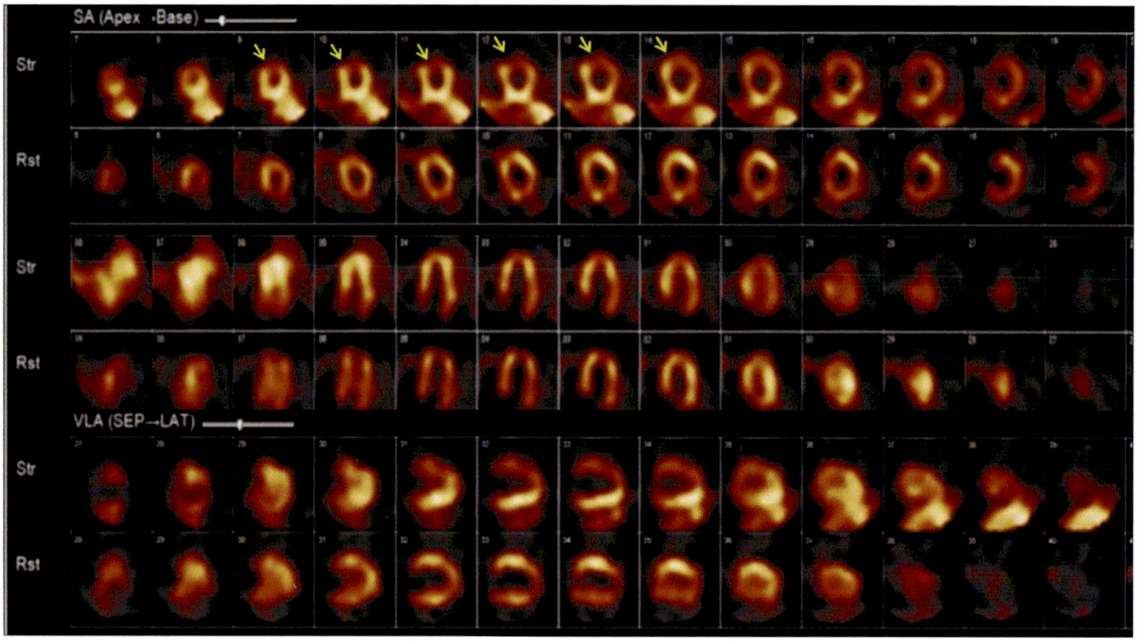

Figure 16.4. Case 2. Anteroseptal artifact (arrows) on perfusion imaging.

of the breast on stress versus rest images rather than inducible ischemia (Figure 16.5). Myocardial wall thickness appeared to be increased, consistent with LV hypertrophy as also suggested by her ECG. She followed up with her primary care physician for management of her hypertension and reported no chest pain recurrence.

QUESTION

1. The patient had significant risk factors for CAD. Since she presented in the ED after resolution of symptoms, a stress–rest SPECT MPI protocol was performed. Which of the following statements is correct if the SPECT MPI results were abnormal in this patient with CKD?
   a. Both ischemia and scar on SPECT MPI are predictors of events.
   b. Annual death rate with a normal SPECT MPI is <1% per year.
   c. Only ischemia on SPECT MPI is a predictor of events.
   d. Only infarct on SPECT MPI is a predictor of events.

ANSWER

1a. SPECT MPI is an ideal diagnostic and prognostic test, particularly for patients with CKD who present to the ED with chest pain. Patients with impairments in renal function and chest pain have limited options for CAD assessment and have relative contraindications for CCTA, CMR, and diagnostic ICA. Accordingly, patients with renal impairment have been excluded from studies pertaining to these modalities. SPECT MPI can be performed safely in patients with CKD and chest pain in the ED setting.

As demonstrated in Case 2, it is important to risk stratify intermediate- to high-risk patients with significant risk factors with testing such as a stress–rest SPECT MPI protocol. A study of 1,652 patients who underwent stress SPECT MPI showed that the presence of either myocardial ischemia or scar is a strong predictor of cardiac events (cardiac death, all-cause mortality, and nonfatal MI) in patients with CKD.[6] In addition, patients with CKD have a higher annual cardiac death rate even with a normal SPECT MPI (2.7%) as compared to patients without CKD and normal SPECT MPI (<1%).

Furthermore, regarding the SPECT MPI protocol, a stress–rest protocol is necessary to increase the sensitivity of the test in patients who present in the ED after the chest pain has resolved. If the radionuclide tracer is injected during active chest pain, the sensitivity of SPECT MPI is very high, almost 100%, with a negative predictive value for ruling out MI over 99%, and for future adverse cardiac events over 97%. However, the sensitivity of rest SPECT MPI to detect perfusion abnormalities decreases as more time passes since symptom resolution. In Case 2, a small perfusion defect was seen with stress but not rest imaging; this was due to shifting breast artifact, which occurs due to

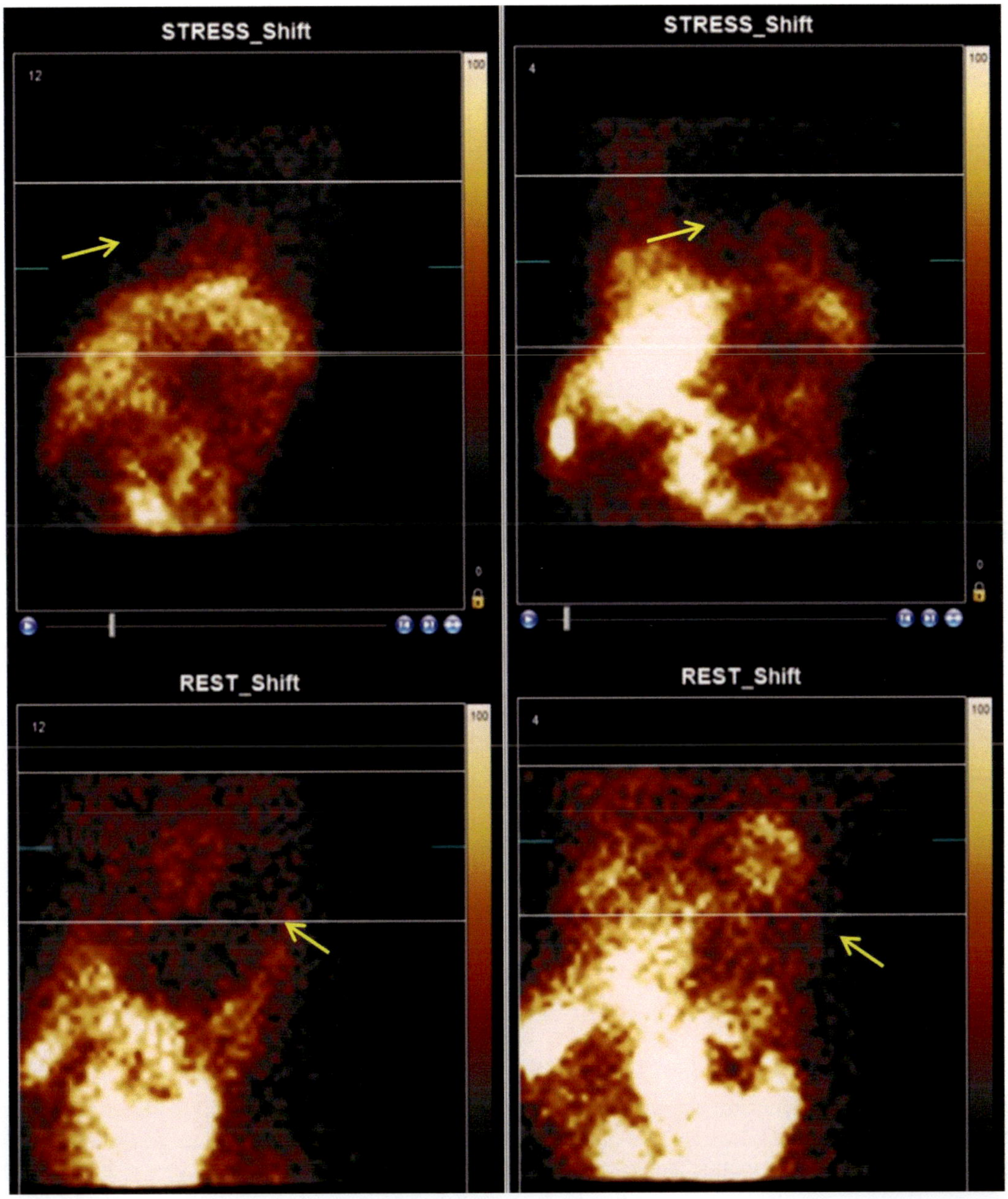

Figure 16.5. Case 2. Shifting breast artifact showing different positions of breast (arrows) with stress and rest images. In the stress images, the bottom edge of the breast is at the level of the inferior wall. At rest, the bottom edge of the breast is substantially below the heart. This leads to different attenuation patterns.

the breast moving from stress to rest images. One way to address shifting breast artifact is by taping the breast to minimize breast position changes.

CASE 3

A 64-year-old female with a history of hypertension, prediabetes, morbid obesity, hypothyroidism, and rheumatoid arthritis presented to the ED with chest tightness and palpitations. Her chest tightness resolved after a few minutes. The patient's family history was significant for early-onset CAD, with her father dying at age 51 and mother at age 62, both from MIs. Physical exam revealed morbid obesity with a body mass index (BMI) of 54. Her ECG was normal and serial troponins were negative. A chest x-ray showed no pulmonary edema or pleural effusions. The patient reported physical limitation due to rheumatoid arthritis and was unable to exercise on a treadmill. Given her intermediate risk for ACS and her significant BMI, she underwent ammonia PET MPI. Perfusion images showed a significant reversibility in the inferior and lateral walls in addition to

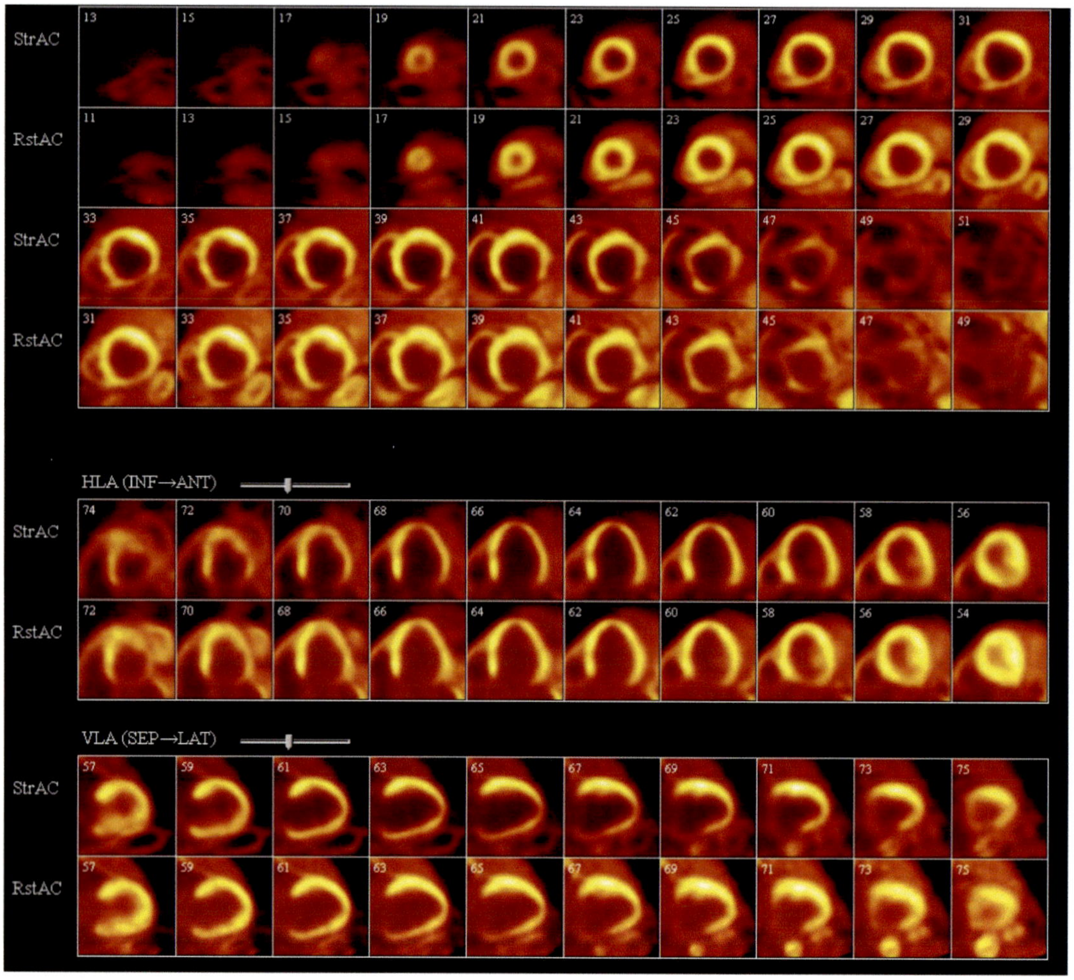

Figure 16.6. Case 3. Ammonia PET MPI showed significant reversibility in mid to base inferior and lateral walls in addition to a fixed inferior defect that is also accompanied by TID.

a fixed inferior defect, which is also accompanied by TID, and gated imaging showed wall-motion abnormality in the same region concerning for infarct (Figures 16.6 and 16.7). Also, systolic function was severely reduced with stress and rest. Absolute flows were reduced globally in all three coronary territories (Figure 16.8). The patient underwent ICA, which showed a total occlusion of the RCA with collaterals and significant stenosis of LAD and LCX. The patient underwent coronary artery bypass grafting with improvement of symptoms.

QUESTION

1. After reviewing the ammonia PET MPI images, which of the following statements is true?
   a. TID and reduced LV function predict worse prognosis and outcomes.
   b. Relative perfusion images can underestimate the extent and severity of CAD.
   c. Absolute flow evaluation by PET provides incremental information.
   d. All of the above are correct.

ANSWER

1d. In the ED setting, immediate accessibility to a PET camera for evaluation of chest pain may be challenging in some centers. However, certain patient populations, such as patients who have large body mass index or patients who may have coronary microvascular disease, would get a better evaluation with PET imaging. PET image quality is better than SPECT given the greater spatial and temporal resolution as well as more reliable AC. In the presence of collateral blood flow, relative perfusion images can

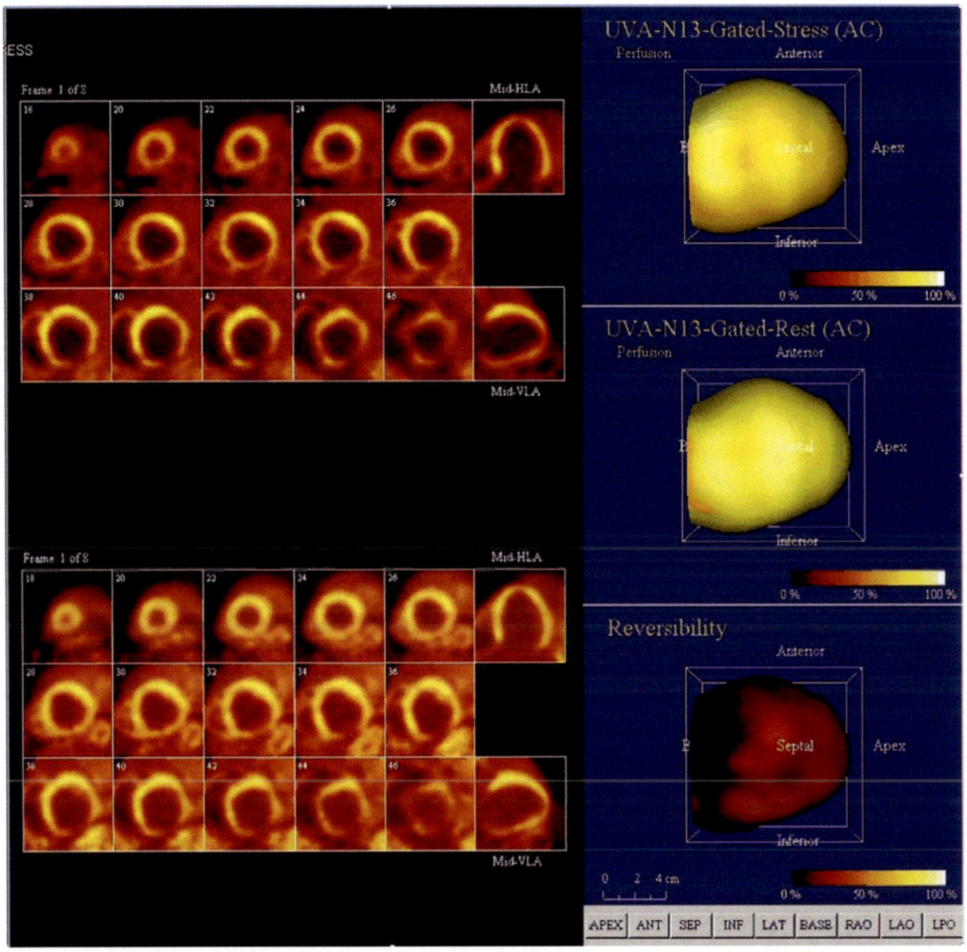

Figure 16.7. Case 3. Gated imaging showed wall-motion abnormality in inferior region and reduced systolic function with stress and rest.

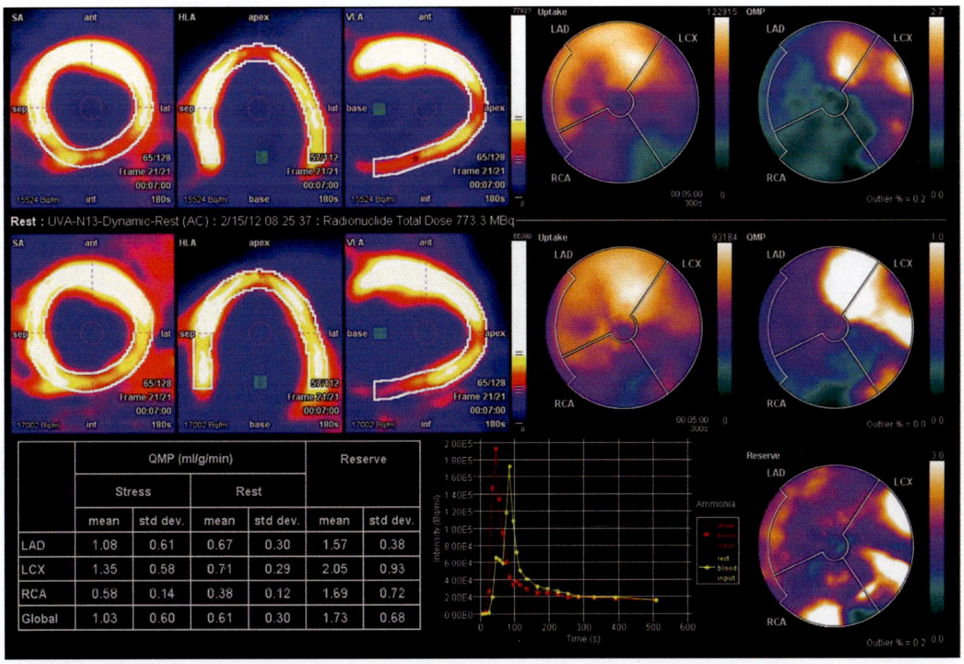

	QMP (ml/g/min)				Reserve	
	Stress		Rest			
	mean	std dev.	mean	std dev.	mean	std dev.
LAD	1.08	0.61	0.67	0.30	1.57	0.38
LCX	1.35	0.58	0.71	0.29	2.05	0.93
RCA	0.58	0.14	0.38	0.12	1.69	0.72
Global	1.03	0.60	0.61	0.30	1.73	0.68

Figure 16.8. Case 3. Absolute flows are reduced globally.

underestimate the extent and severity of CAD. Assessment of absolute myocardial blood flow and a true stress LVEF by PET MPI have incremental value in identification of left main multivessel obstructive CAD.[7]

CASE 4

A 62-year-old male with a history of hypertension and no known cardiac history presented to the ED for evaluation of a burning sensation in his chest associated with diaphoresis, lightheadedness, and loss of appetite. His ECG was unchanged from prior (Figure 16.9). Two serial troponin I levels performed 6 hours apart were both 0.05 (reference range < 0.02 ng/mL). His TIMI risk score was 2. He underwent a stress SPECT MPI study (Figure 16.10).

QUESTION

1. What is the best next step?
   a. Discharge from the ED without further workup
   b. ICA
   c. Resting transthoracic echocardiogram
   d. CCTA
   e. Empiric medical treatment for CAD

ANSWER

1c. The stress SPECT MPI shows normal perfusion; however, the borderline ECG changes (TWI in the anterolateral leads) and his inconclusive troponin are concerning despite a low TIMI score. Patients with a positive troponin of unclear significance have an increased risk of mortality. The TACTICS-TIMI-18 trial showed that patients with a positive troponin and no obstruction on coronary angiogram had a 6-month mortality or re-infarction rate.[8] A similar adverse prognosis is present in those with an elevated cardiac troponin of unclear etiology, a population whose prevalence has increased in the era of hs-TnT. Lee et al. found that one in eight patients without suspected ACS seen in the ED who received troponin testing had an elevated level. They added to the research showing an association of troponin rise with mortality independent of age, sex, and renal function.[9] Therefore, this patient with a positive troponin needs further workup. A closer look at the SPECT MPI reveals increased myocardial wall thickness consistent with LV hypertrophy. Global and segmental LV function was normal. The differential diagnosis for LV hypertrophy includes hypertensive heart disease, hypertrophic cardiomyopathy, cardiac amyloid or other infiltrative heart disease. Therefore, an echocardiogram would be the next step.

This patient underwent echocardiography (Figure 16.11), which was significant for moderate apical asymmetric hypertrophy without a gradient, suggestive of apical hypertrophic cardiomyopathy. CMR was performed that confirmed this diagnosis. It showed severe apical hypertrophy with cavity obliteration (Figure 16.12A, B), consistent with the apical variant of hypertrophic cardiomyopathy as well as severe basal and mid-inferoseptal hypertrophy. In addition, there was patchy late gadolinium enhancement in the mid-ventricular segment (Figure 16.12C) and diffuse enhancement at the apex.

As demonstrated in this case, abnormal troponin levels with a nondiagnostic ECG do not automatically equate to acute myocardial ischemia (MI), and therefore

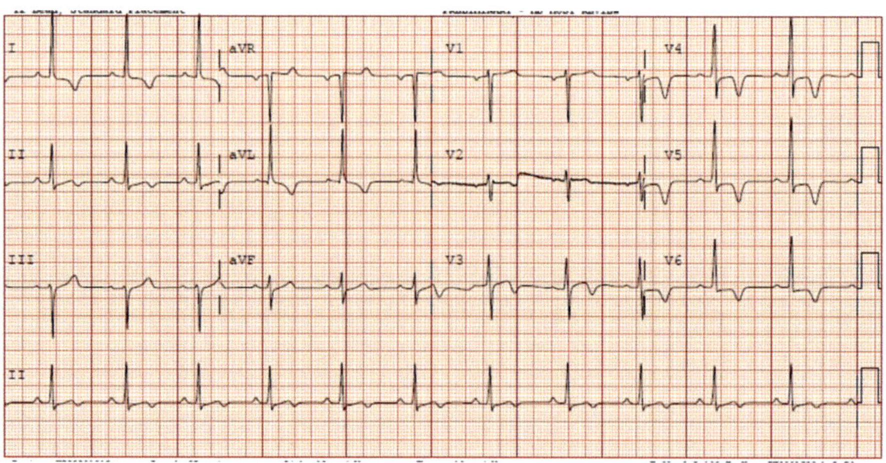

Figure 16.9. Case 4. ECG on initial presentation to the ED. This ECG is unchanged from a prior one obtained 1 year ago.

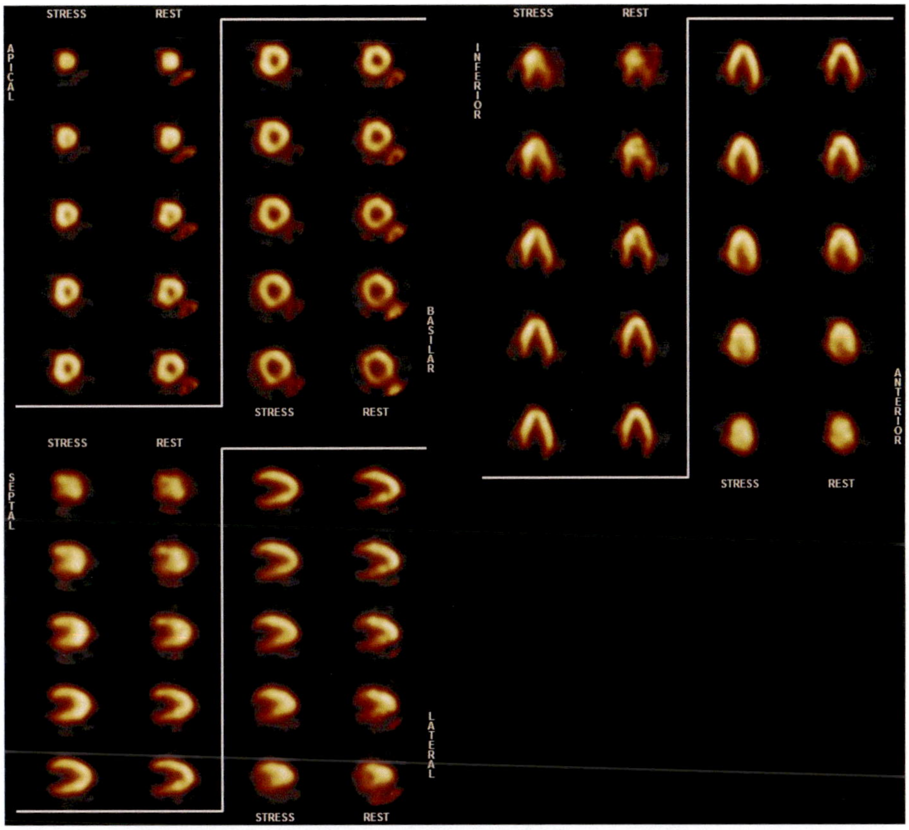

Figure 16.10. Case 4. Stress and rest SPECT MPI.

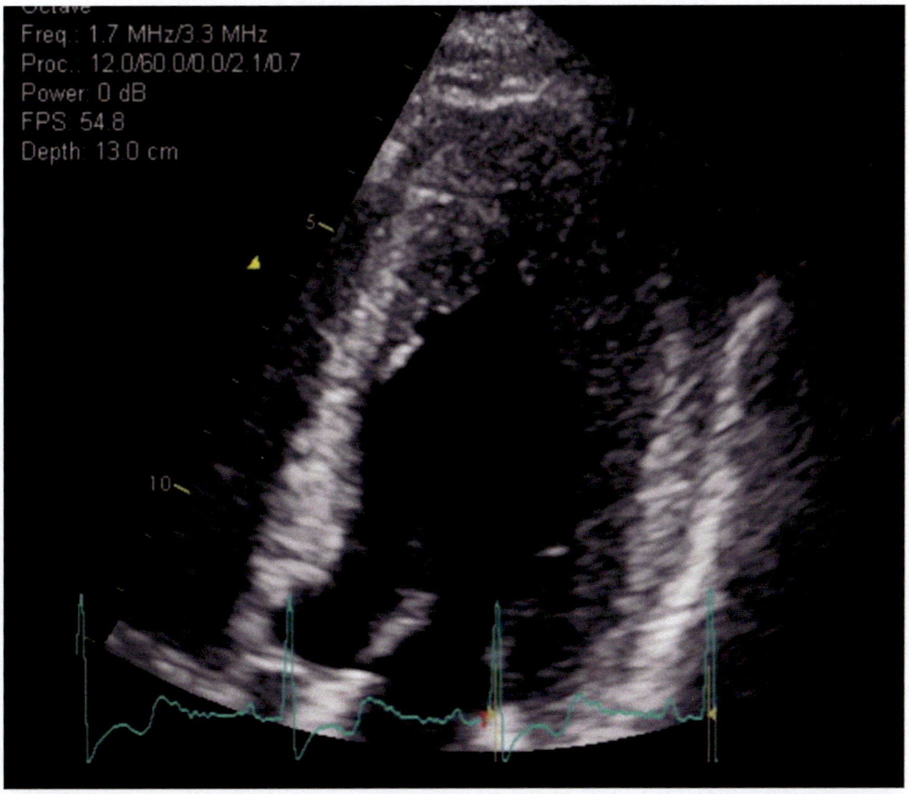

Figure 16.11. Case 4. Four-chamber apical view of a resting transthoracic echocardiogram revealing apical focal hypertrophy concerning for the apical variant of hypertrophic cardiomyopathy.

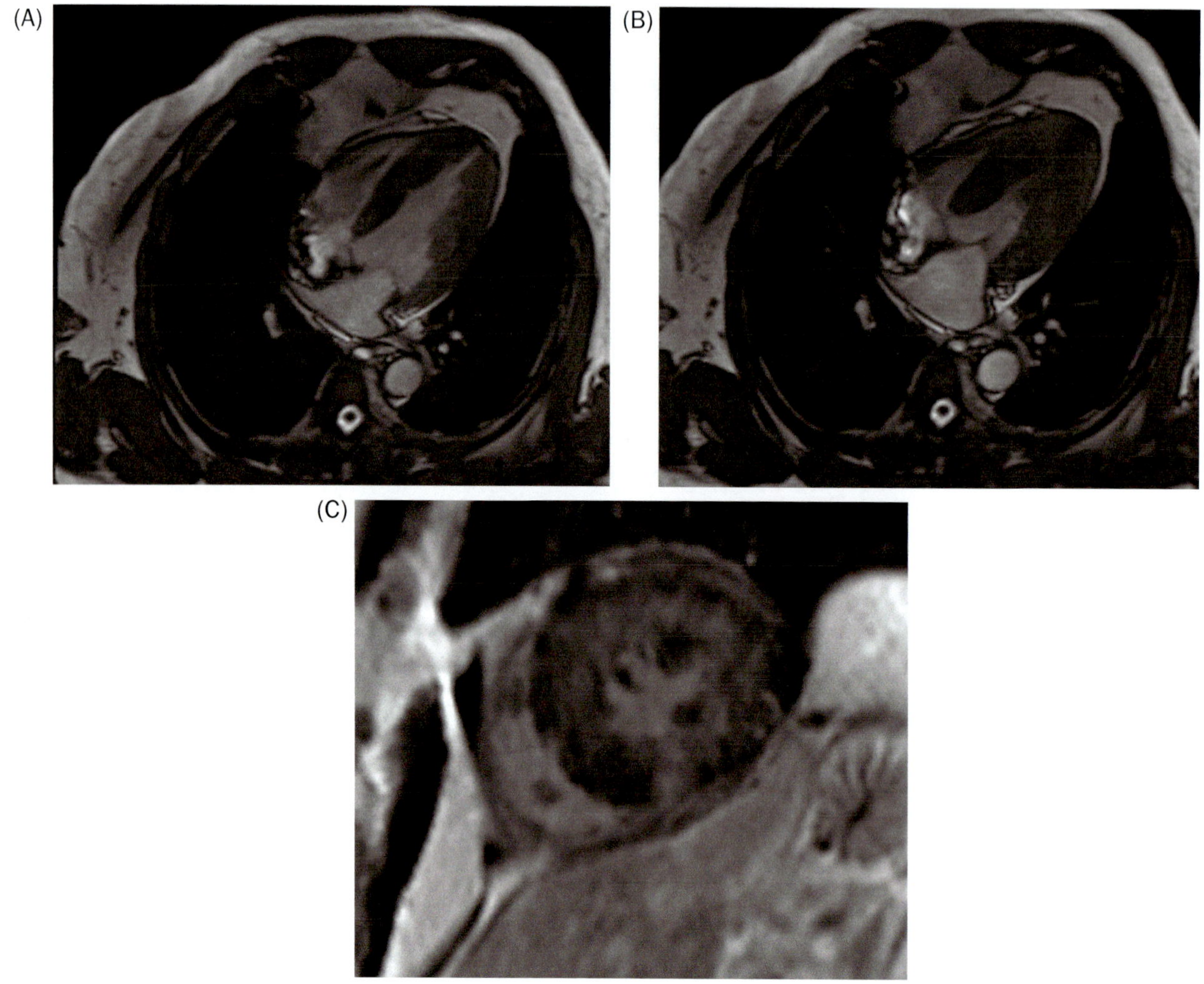

Figure 16.12. Case 4. (A) CMR still image at diastole of a four-chamber SSFP cine acquisition. Marked apical hypertrophy is appreciated. (B) CMR still image at systole of a four-chamber SSFP (Steady-State Free Precession) cine series showing cavity obliteration. (C) CMR late gadolinium enhancement imaging in the mid short axis showing patchy uptake.

more sophisticated ways that utilize imaging are appropriate for accurate diagnosis and prognosis of patients with chest pain in the ED. It is important to point out that the specificity of a positive troponin is low and ED physicians are challenged to accurately diagnose chest pain, which may or may not be due to acute MI or may stem from other conditions such as myocarditis, cardiomyopathy, severe hypertension, renal failure, PE, or other chronic conditions.[10,11] SPECT MPI measures various scintigraphic variables, including extent and severity of perfusion defects and their reversibility, multivessel disease patterns, TID, LVEF, and end-diastolic and end-systolic volumes. It is a robust tool for evaluation of chest pain in the ED as it can identify risk of cardiac events and mortality. In Case 4, the SPECT MPI did not show a perfusion defect or any high-risk features for CAD, and therefore ICA and CCTA are not the next best steps. Similarly, SPECT MPI was not suggestive of ischemia or infarction, and therefore empiric treatment for CAD would not be an appropriate step.

REFERENCES

1. Klocke FJ, Baird MG, Lorell BH, et al. ACC/AHA/ASNC guidelines for the clinical use of cardiac radionuclide imaging—executive summary. *J Am Coll Cardiol.* 2003;42(7):1318–1333. doi:10.1016/j.jacc.2003.08.011
2. Rybicki FJ, Udelson JE, Peacock WF, et al. 2015 ACR/ACC/AHA/AATS/ACEP/ASNC/NASCI/SAEM/SCCT/SCMR/SCPC/SNMMI/STR/STS Appropriate Utilization of Cardiovascular Imaging in Emergency Department Patients with Chest Pain. *J Am Coll Cardiol.* 2016;67(7):853–879. doi:10.1016/j.jacc.2015.09.011
3. Holly TA, Abbott BG, Al-Mallah MH, et al. ASNC imaging guidelines for nuclear cardiology procedures: Single photon-emission computed tomography. *J Nucl Cardiol.* 2010;17:941–973.

4. Garcia EV. SPECT attenuation correction: An essential tool to realize nuclear cardiology's manifest destiny. *J Nucl Cardiol.* 2007;14(1):16–24.
5. Mathur S, Heller GV, Bateman TM, et al. Clinical value of stress-only Tc-99m SPECT imaging: Importance of attenuation correction. *J Nucl Cardiol.* 2013;20(1):27–37.
6. Hakeem A, Bhatti S, Dillie KS, et al. Predictive value of myocardial perfusion single-photon emission computed tomography and the impact of renal function on cardiac death. *Circulation.* 2008;118(24):2540–2549. doi:10.1161/CIRCULATIONAHA.108.788109
7. Dorbala S, Di Carli MF, Beanlands RS, et al. Prognostic value of stress myocardial perfusion positron emission tomography: Results from a multicenter observational registry. *J Am Coll Cardiol.* 2013;61(2):176–184. doi:10.1016/j.jacc.2012.09.043
8. Dokainish H, Pillai M, Murphy SA, et al. Prognostic implications of elevated troponin in patients with suspected acute coronary syndrome but no critical epicardial coronary disease: A TACTICS-TIMI-18 substudy. *J Am Coll Cardiol.* 2005;45:19–24.
9. Lee KK, Noaman A, Vaswani A, et al. Prevalence, determinants, and clinical associations of high-sensitivity cardiac troponin in patients attending emergency departments. *Am J Med.* 2019;132:110.e8–110.e21.
10. de Lemos JA, Drazner MH, Omland T, et al. Association of troponin T detected with a highly sensitive assay and cardiac structure and mortality risk in the general population. *JAMA.* 2010;304(22):2503–2512.
11. Mueller C. Biomarkers and acute coronary syndromes: An update. *Eur Heart J.* 2014;35(9):552–556.

17.

ROLE OF PET IN DIAGNOSIS AND RISK ASSESSMENT IN PATIENTS WITH KNOWN OR SUSPECTED CAD

Christiane Wiefels, Brian A. Mc Ardle, Jennifer M. Renaud, Robert A. deKemp, Rob S. B. Beanlands, and Steven Promislow

CASE 1

Mrs. C is a 71-year-old female referred for MPI after undergoing an exercise treadmill test that was felt to be likely electrocardiographically positive for ischemia but confounded by significant artifact at peak exercise. Her relevant past medical history is notable only for being an active smoker of approximately a half-pack of cigarettes a day. On history, she describes feeling well up until 4 months prior to her test, able to walk for up to 45 minutes at a time with no exertional chest discomfort or shortness of breath. However, over the few months leading up to her test, she notes gradually progressive exertional chest discomfort such that she would develop symptoms with 5 minutes of walking or going up and down one flight of stairs; the symptoms would resolve after 5 to 10 minutes, and she had never experienced any symptoms of more prolonged duration nor any symptoms at rest. Her cardiovascular exam was unremarkable.

She underwent dipyridamole ^{82}Rb-PET MPI, which demonstrated moderate reduction in tracer uptake in the mid to apical anterior wall and apex that normalized on rest imaging (Figure 17.1), consistent with ischemia in the LAD territory (11.8% LV ischemia).

Gated images demonstrate normal LV size, EF, and wall motion at rest. With stress, mild anteroapical hypokinesis is noted, consistent with the perfusion findings suggestive of ischemia in the LAD territory (▶ Video 17.1).

LV function is as follows:

Stress LVEF: 74%, EDV: 43 mL, ESV: 11 mL

Rest LVEF: 71%, EDV: 42 mL, ESV: 12 mL

On review of the CT images acquired for AC, coronary calcification is noted in the LAD (Figure 17.2).

Polar maps demonstrating rest and stress MBF along with MFR are provided in Figure 17.3.

QUESTION

1. Regarding the flow quantification results, what can we describe?
   a. There is normal global MFR, but there is relative reduction in MFR and stress MBF in the LAD territory.
   b. There is global reduction of MFR in the three coronary territories, compatible with triple-vessel disease.
   c. There is normal global MFR and normal regional stress MBF.
   d. There is global reduction of MFR due to severely reduced MFR in the LAD territory.

ANSWER

1a. MFR is determined by the ratio of absolute hyperemic (stress) MBF and rest MBF in mL/min/g tissue and can be quantified globally, by coronary territory, or on a segmental level. The measurements are derived from dynamic acquisition resulting in measurable time–activity curves of the myocardium uptake and blood pool.[1] At a regional level, reductions in both stress MBF and MFR provide information on the physiologic functional significance of an epicardial stenosis, especially when of intermediate severity.[2,3] Many studies have defined <2.0 as the cut point for reduced MFR in PET imaging.[4–6] Regarding stress MBF, Gupta et al. defined <1.8 as the cut point for prognostic significance.[5] In this case (Figure 17.3), there is globally normal MFR (2.34). However, there is reduced MFR and stress MBF in the LAD territory (MFR 1.73, stress MBF 1.17 mL/min/g). This regionality is in accordance with the perfusion findings, emphasizing the presence of ischemia in this region. Simply reporting the global MFR as being normal would be misleadingly reassuring.

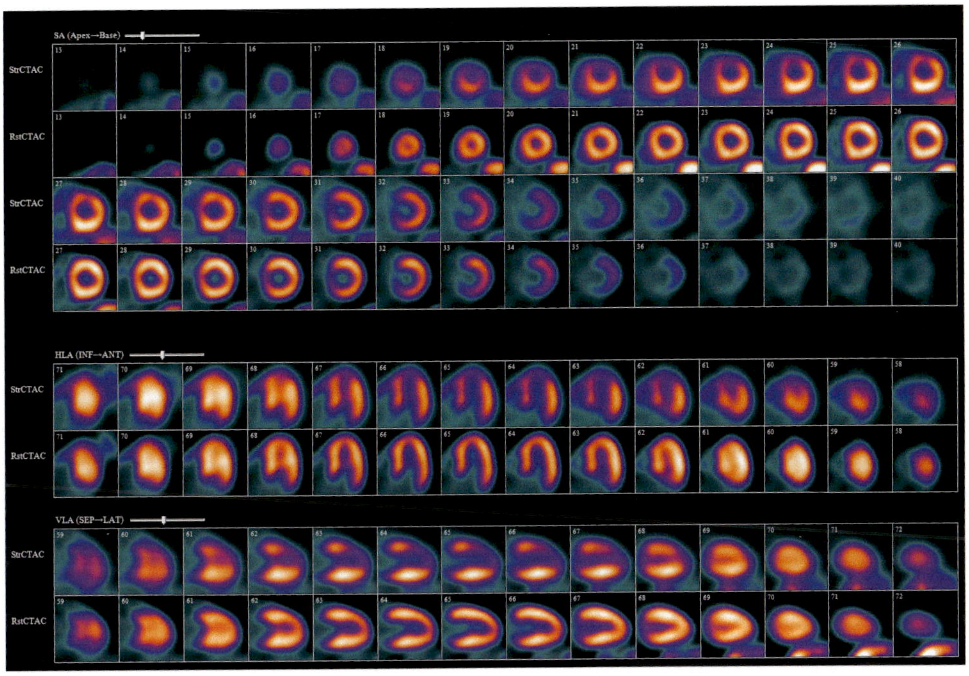

Figure 17.1. Case 1. Stress (Str, top row) and rest (Rst, bottom row) ^{82}Rb PET MPI in corresponding short-axis (SA), horizontal long-axis (HLA), and vertical long-axis (VLA) slices.

Given her progressive symptoms and significant ischemia noted in the LAD territory on her PET imaging, Mrs. C was referred for coronary angiography, which demonstrated obstructive CAD involving the proximal and mid LAD as well as the first diagonal (see Figure 17.4 and ▶ Video 17.2). These lesions were all treated with a total of three drug-eluting stents, with resolution of her symptoms.

CASE 2

Mrs. L is a 64-year-old female with equivocal previous stress testing. Given the presence of multiple cardiac risk factors, she underwent dipyridamole ^{82}Rb-PET MPI to evaluate for ischemia. Her ECG during dipyridamole infusion was unremarkable. Perfusion images are provided in Figure 17.5,

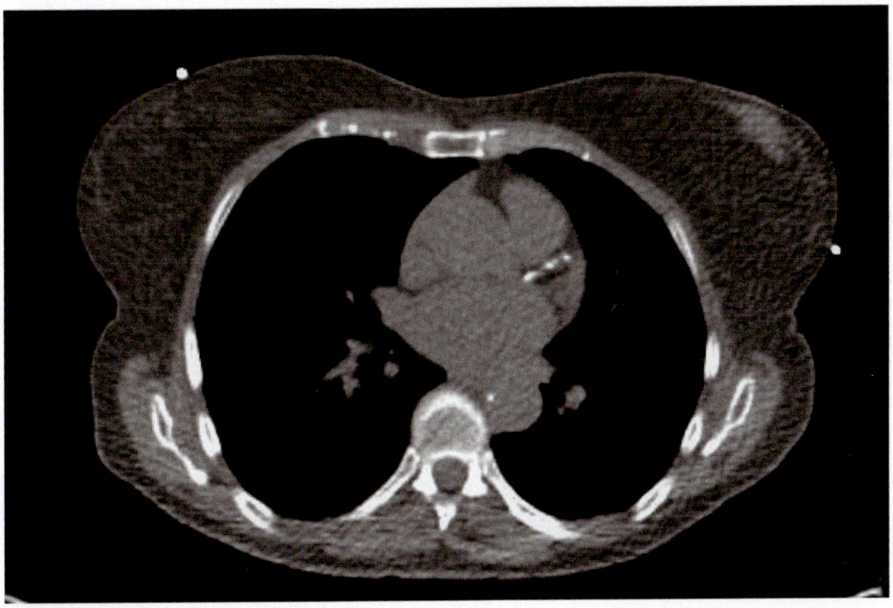

Figure 17.2. Case 1. CT chest used for AC.

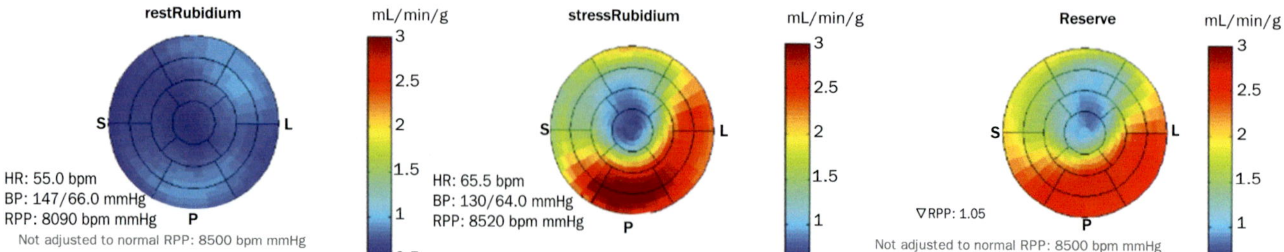

	LV	LAD	LCx	RCA
MBF	0.73	0.68	0.81	0.76

	LV	LAD	LCx	RCA
MBF	1.75	1.17	2.18	2.34

	LV	LAD	LCx	RCA
MFR	2.34	1.73	2.73	3.03

Figure 17.3. Case 1. Corresponding polar maps of rest flow (restRubidium), stress flow (stressRubidium) and myocardial flow reserve (Reserve).

demonstrating ischemia in the LAD territory (32.4% LV ischemia).

Her LVEF was normal at rest. With stress, there was development of hypokinesis in the mid to apical anterior and anteroseptal walls, consistent with ischemia. However, no significant reduction in LVEF was noted (▶ Video 17.3).

The CT images acquired for AC demonstrated coronary calcification in the LAD (Figure 17.6).

Polar maps demonstrating rest and stress MBF along with MFR are provided in Figure 17.7.

QUESTION

1. Which of the following high-risk features of PET imaging is NOT present in this case?
   a. Large perfusion defect (with >20% LV ischemia)
   b. Presence of transient ischemic dilatation

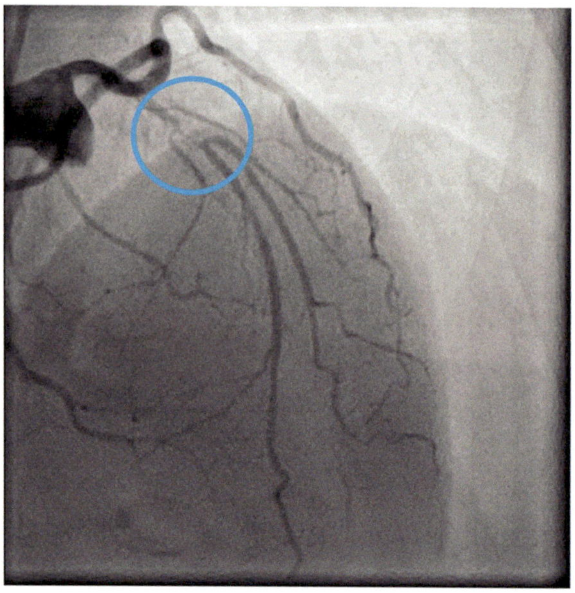

Figure 17.4. Case 1. Coronary angiogram demonstrating severe LAD stenosis (circled).

   c. Reduced stress LVEF
   d. Reduced MFR (<2.0) AND reduced stress MBF (<1.8)

ANSWER

1c. This case demonstrates a number of high-risk features present in someone with disease in the LAD territory. The patient had a large perfusion defect of moderate to severe degree in the LAD territory, consistent with >20% of the LV being ischemic, as well as evidence of transient ischemic dilatation (TID = 1.31). Global MFR was reduced (1.57), driven by a relative severe reduction in MFR in the LAD territory (MFR = 0.92), as was global stress MBF (stress MBF = 1.33). While no significant decrease in LVEF at stress was noted in this particular study, Dorbala et al.[7] demonstrated the incremental value of the LVEF reserve in predicting the risk of future adverse events, with a decrease in stress LVEF compared to rest LVEF being significantly associated with adverse cardiac events and mortality. Table 17.3 in the accompanying textbook shows several features of PET MPI that portend high risk for subsequent adverse events.

This patient was subsequently referred for coronary angiography, which demonstrated a 60% distal left main stenosis and severe stenoses of the mid LAD and a large septal branch off the LAD (Figure 17.8, ▶ Video 17.4).

CASE 3

Mrs. A is a 79-year-old female with a past medical history of dyslipidemia and chronic obstructive pulmonary disease. She described gradually progressive shortness of breath on exertion, and a chest CT performed to evaluate for other causes of her dyspnea demonstrated severe coronary calcification. Given her progressive symptoms and the CT

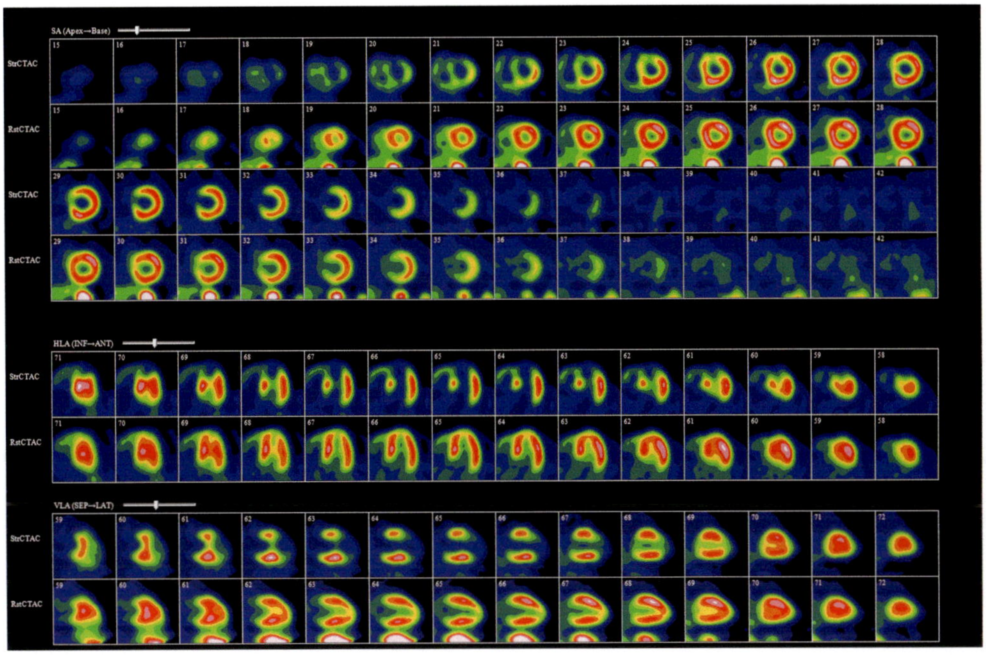

Figure 17.5. Case 2. Stress (Str, top row) and rest (Rst, bottom row) ^{82}Rb-PET MPI in corresponding short-axis (SA), horizontal long-axis (HLA), and vertical long-axis (VLA) slices. Transient ischemic dilatation ratio: 1.31 (normal < 1.20).

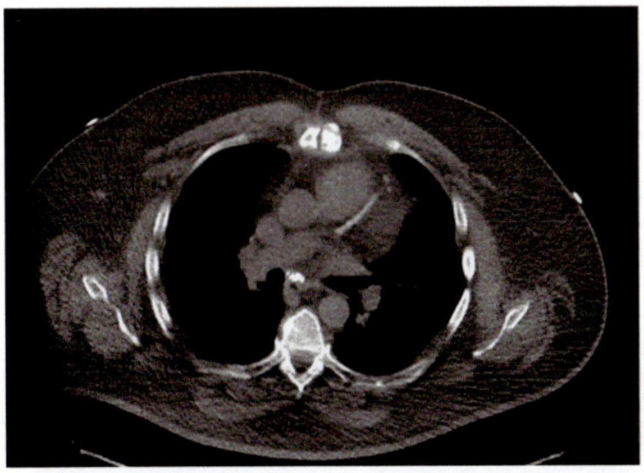

Figure 17.6. Case 2. CT chest used for AC.

findings, she underwent dipyridamole ^{82}Rb-PET MPI to evaluate for ischemia.

Perfusion images are provided in Figure 17.9. Of note, transient ischemic dilatation is present, with a ratio of 1.22.

Additionally, review of her ECG during dipyridamole infusion demonstrates 1 mm of downsloping ST-segment depression relative to baseline in multiple leads (Figure 17.10).

Her LVEF was normal at both rest and stress, with no obvious stress-induced wall-motion abnormalities (▶ Video 17.5).

The CT images acquired for AC confirmed the presence of coronary calcification in the LAD, LCx, and RCA as had been previously demonstrated on her initial chest CT.

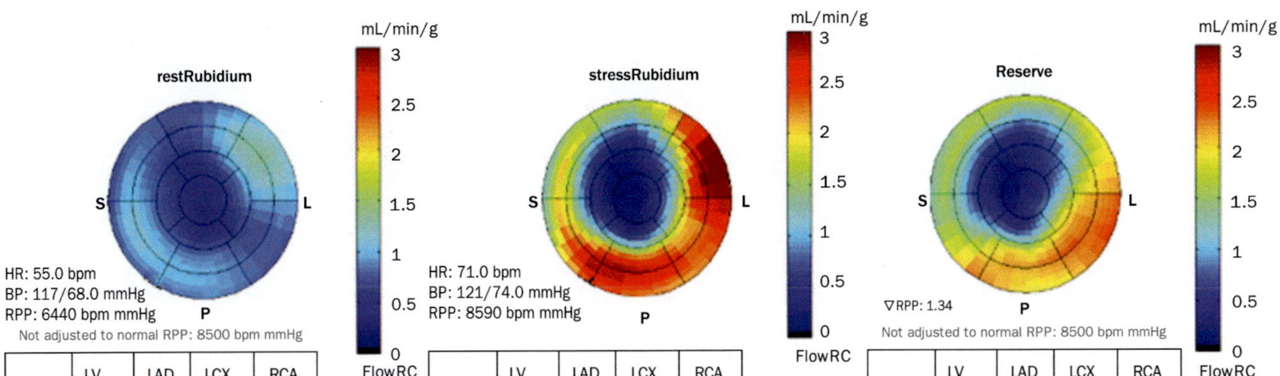

	LV	LAD	LCX	RCA
MBF	0.77	0.66	0.90	0.83

	LV	LAD	LCX	RCA
MBF	1.33	0.68	2.04	1.74

	LV	LAD	LCX	RCA
MFR	1.57	0.92	2.28	2.00

Figure 17.7. Case 2. Corresponding polar maps of rest flow (restRubidium), stress flow (stressRubidium) and myocardial flow reserve (Reserve).

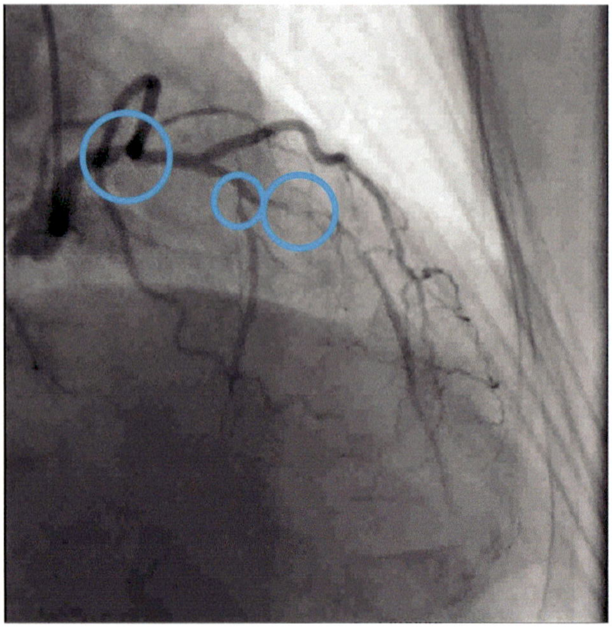

Figure 17.8. Case 2. Coronary angiogram demonstrating (circles from left to right) 60% stenosis of the left main artery, severe stenosis of a septal branch off the LAD, and severe stenosis of the mid LAD.

Polar maps demonstrating rest and stress MBF along with MFR are provided in Figure 17.11.

QUESTION

1. Which of the following conclusions is most appropriate?
   a. The study is equivocal; consider repeat PET with dobutamine.
   b. The study is normal, other than the presence of coronary calcification.
   c. There is ischemia in the RCA territory.
   d. Obstructive multivessel disease should be considered.

ANSWER

1d. This case is a good example of the value of flow quantification. In Figure 17.9 we can see that there is only mild

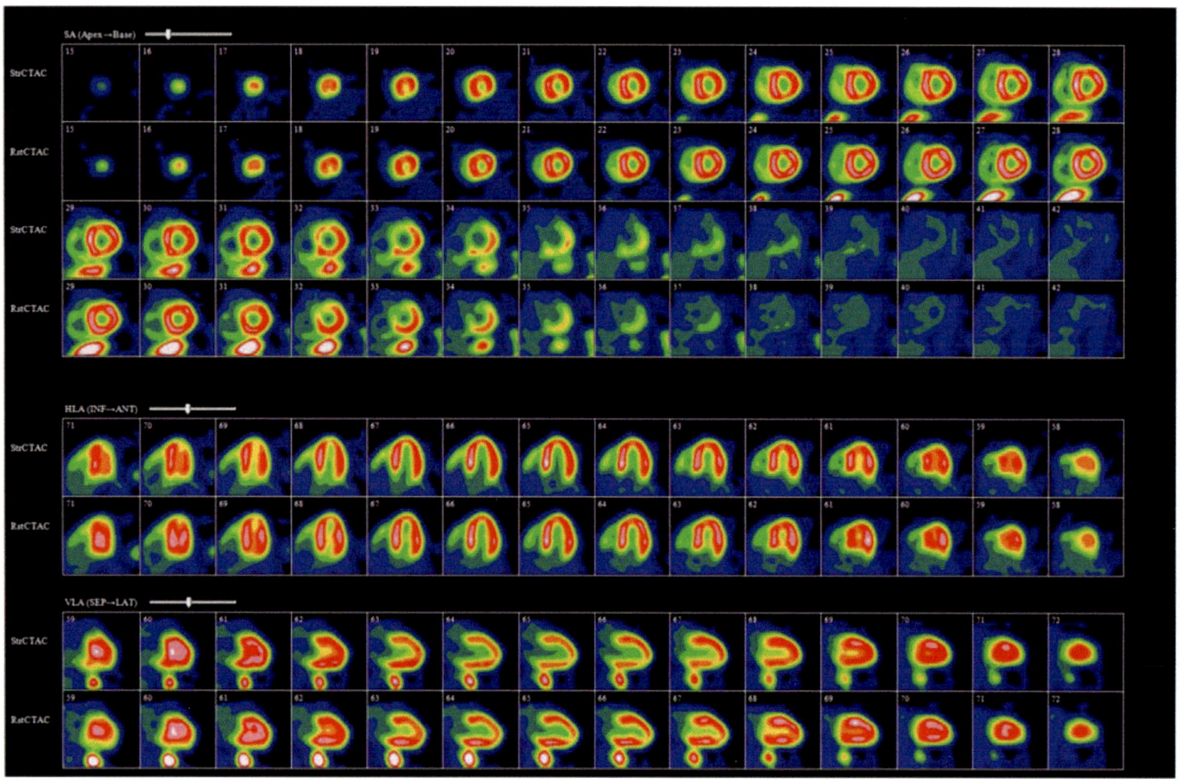

Figure 17.9. Case 3. Stress (Str, top row) and rest (Rst, bottom row) ^{82}Rb-PET MPI in corresponding short-axis (SA), horizontal long-axis (HLA), and vertical long-axis (VLA) slices. Transient ischemic dilatation ratio: 1.22 (normal <1.20).

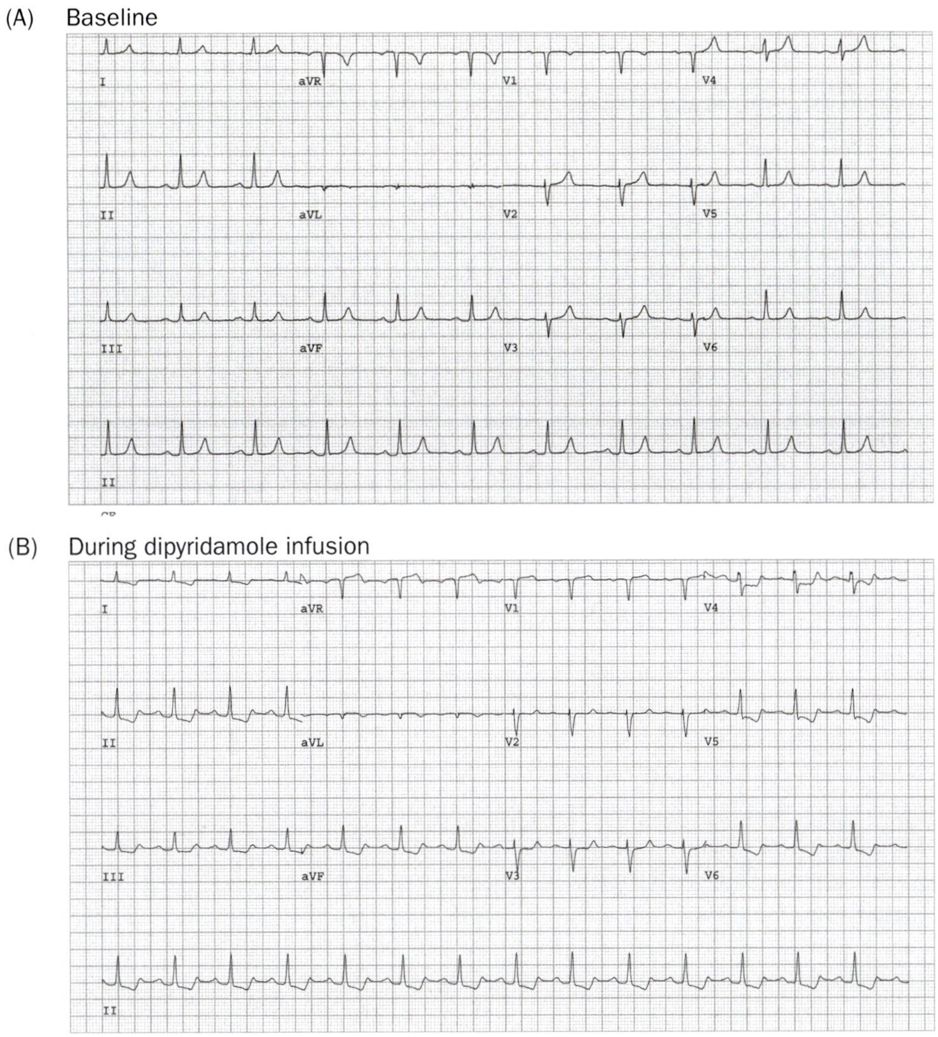

Figure 17.10. Case 3. ECG (A, at baseline; B, during dipyridamole infusion).

reduction in uptake in the apical inferior wall, with improvement at rest, consistent with a small area of mild ischemia in the distal RCA territory (1.5% LV ischemia). However, some high-risk features are present in this study that raise the suspicion for more extensive CAD: There are ECG changes suggestive of ischemia during dipyridamole infusion (see Figure 17.10) and transient ischemic dilatation is present on perfusion imaging (see Figure 17.9), all in the setting of the known diffuse coronary calcification on CT. The flow quantification polar maps (see Figure 17.11)

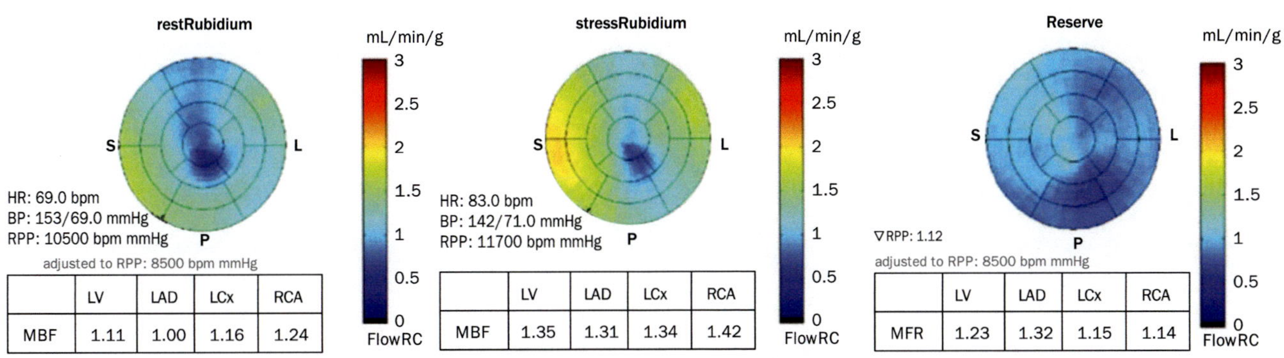

Figure 17.11. Case 3. Corresponding polar maps of rest flow (restRubidium), stress flow (stressRubidium) and myocardial flow reserve (Reserve).

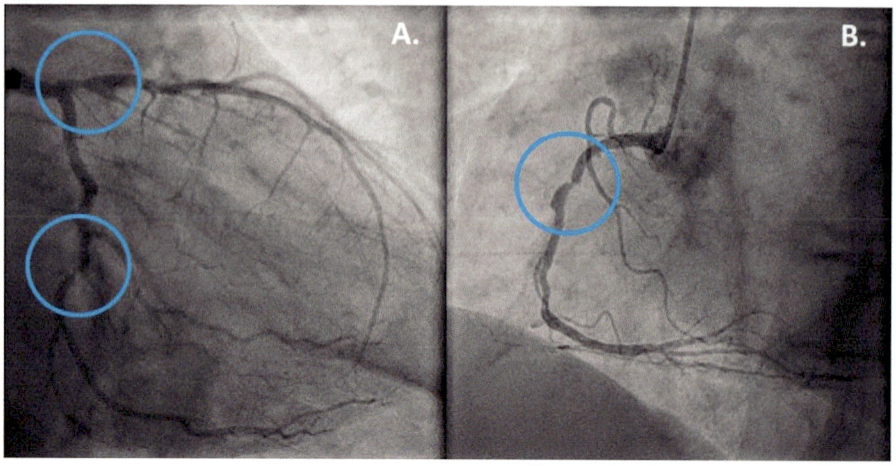

Figure 17.12. Case 3. Coronary angiogram demonstrating (A) significant stenosis of the ostial LAD and mid LCx and (B) significant stenosis of the RCA.

show globally reduced MFR (1.23) and stress MBF (1.35). In the appropriate context, diffusely reduced MFR can represent balanced ischemia or microvascular dysfunction. Given the presence of multivessel coronary calcification and other higher-risk features identified above, obstructive multivessel disease should be a strong consideration. As such, the patient was referred for coronary angiography, which showed obstructive disease in the ostial LAD, mid LCx, and proximal and mid RCA (Figure 17.12 and ▶ Videos 17.6 and ▶ 17.7).

REFERENCES

1. Dilsizian V, Bacharach SL, Beanlands RS, et al. ASNC imaging guidelines/SNMMI procedure standard for positron emission tomography (PET) nuclear cardiology procedures. *J Nucl Cardiol.* 2016;23:1187–1226.
2. Gould KL, Johnson NP, Bateman TM, et al. Anatomic versus physiologic assessment of coronary artery disease: Role of coronary flow reserve, fractional flow reserve, and positron emission tomography imaging in revascularization decision-making. *J Am Coll Cardiol.* 2013;62(18):1639–1653.
3. Danad I, Uusitalo V, Kero T, et al. Quantitative assessment of myocardial perfusion in the detection of significant coronary artery disease: cutoff values and diagnostic accuracy of quantitative [(15)O] H2O PET imaging. *J Am Coll Cardiol.* 2014;64(14):1464–1475.
4. Ziadi MC. Myocardial flow reserve (MFR) with positron emission tomography (PET)/computed tomography (CT): Clinical impact in diagnosis and prognosis. *Cardiovasc Diagn Ther.* 2017;7(2):206–218.
5. Gupta A, Taqueti VR, van de Hoef TP, et al. Integrated noninvasive physiological assessment of coronary circulatory function and impact on cardiovascular mortality in patients with stable coronary artery disease. *Circulation.* 2017;136(24):2325–2336. CIRCULATIONAHA.117.029992
6. Murthy VL, Bateman TM, Beanlands RS, et al. Clinical quantification of myocardial blood flow using PET: Joint position paper of the SNMMI Cardiovascular Council and the ASNC. *J Nucl Med.* 2018;59(2):273–293.
7. Dorbala S, Vangala D, Sampson U, et al. Value of vasodilator left ventricular ejection fraction reserve in evaluating the magnitude of myocardium at risk and the extent of angiographic coronary artery disease: A 82Rb PET/CT study. *J Nucl Med.* 2007;48(3):349–358.

18.

NUCLEAR CARDIAC IMAGING IN WOMEN

Viviany R. Taqueti and Ana Carolina do A. H. de Souza

CASE 1

A 68-year-old woman (G2P2) with a history of hypertension and dyslipidemia and a family history of premature coronary atherosclerosis was referred for an exercise stress test for evaluation of chest pain. Her symptoms had begun 3 weeks prior following a hospital admission for her younger brother who had sustained a heart attack resulting in urgent percutaneous coronary intervention. Chest pain was characterized by a squeezing substernal tightness that was unrelated to exertion and worse in the evenings. During her treadmill stress test, she exercised for 10 minutes on a Bruce treadmill protocol, achieving 11.7 METs with normal heart rate and blood pressure response, stopping for fatigue. Her ECG response to exercise demonstrated some motion artifact with beat-to-beat variation and 1- to 2-mm horizontal ST-segment depression in leads II, III, aVF, and V4–V5 beginning 6 minutes into the test and resolving within 1 minute into recovery (Figure 18.1). She then underwent CCTA for further evaluation. Her CCTA demonstrated a left dominant coronary circulation with a large amount of diffuse calcified and noncalcified plaque along the LAD resulting in focal areas of minimal (<25%) proximal stenosis followed by sequential tubular mid and mid-distal moderate (50–70%) stenoses prior to and after the diagonal 2 artery takeoff (see Figure 18.1). There was also a small amount of partially calcified plaque in the distal left main coronary artery extending into the ostial LAD. In addition, the CT was notable for a small hiatal hernia with associated mild circumferential thickening of the distal esophageal wall. She was then referred for evaluation with N-13 ammonia cardiac PET-CT. The ECG response to vasodilator stress with regadenoson demonstrated up to a horizontal ST-segment depression of up to 1 mm in lead V4, which was not associated with symptoms. MPI was normal, with no evidence of regional flow-limiting CAD and normal ventricular volumes and function. Furthermore, quantitative assessment of regional and global myocardial blood flow demonstrated a robust global peak stress value of 2.64 mL/min/g and global coronary flow reserve of 3.18 with no regional variation (see Figure 18.1).

In summary, this symptomatic patient with multiple cardiac risk factors, perhaps unsurprisingly, has evidence of coronary atherosclerosis. Reassuringly, she also demonstrated a high capacity for exercise and normal cardiac PET results with no ischemic sequelae of her anatomic disease. Despite the extent and severity of her CAD, she demonstrated normal regional and global stress myocardial blood flow and coronary flow reserve, with no evidence of coronary microvascular dysfunction. As such, her stress ECG findings likely represented falsely positive results. Although she may be at increased risk for future IHD events, there is no indication for invasive angiography or revascularization at this time. She was continued on preventive therapy with low-dose aspirin, high-intensity atorvastatin, and antihypertensive medications, and was referred for further evaluation and management of her hiatal hernia, which was likely contributing to symptoms of gastroesophageal reflux.

CASE 2

A 73-year-old woman with a history of diabetes mellitus, hypertension, dyslipidemia, obesity, and heart failure with preserved ejection fraction was referred for a vasodilator stress myocardial perfusion PET-CT study to evaluate dyspnea, which had begun 2 months prior. A transthoracic echocardiogram confirmed LVEF of 55% to 60% with no regional wall-motion abnormality, moderate bi-atrial enlargement, and diastolic dysfunction. Cardiac PET-CT demonstrated normal regional myocardial perfusion on both stress and rest images, with an LVEF of 58% and no regional-wall motion abnormalities but with severely increased RV tracer uptake post-stress, consistent with stress-induced pulmonary hypertension (Figure 18.2). Her quantitative

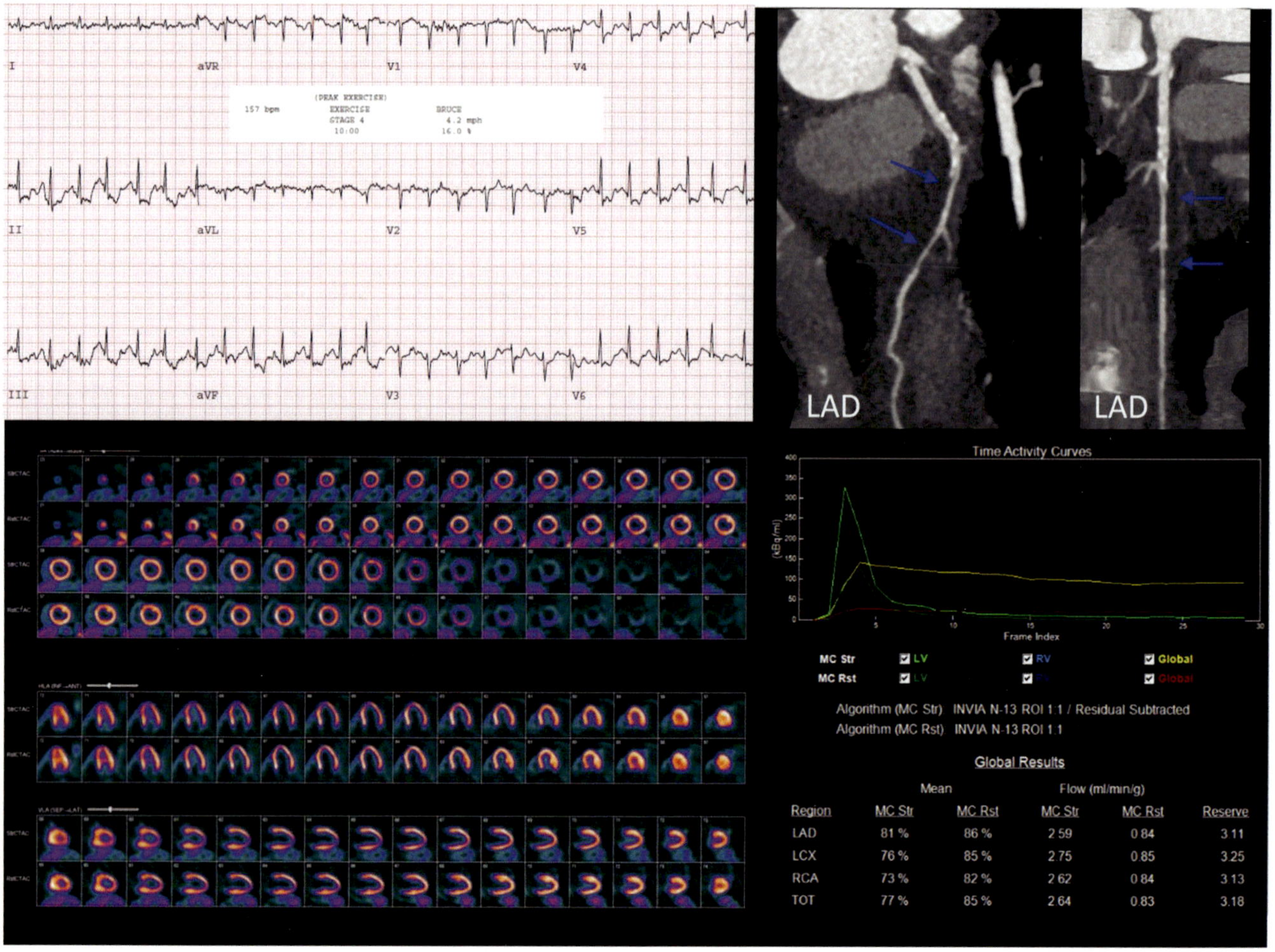

Figure 18.1. Case 1. Exercise ECG at peak stress. CCTA multiplanar reconstructions (curved and straight) of the left anterior descending artery (LAD) with blue arrows demonstrating areas of focal stenosis. Stress and rest ^{13}N-ammonia myocardial perfusion PET images and quantitative myocardial blood flow values.

stress myocardial blood flow was severely reduced at 1.19 mL/min/g with minimal regional variation, with an abnormal global coronary flow reserve of 1.50 (see Figure 18.2). The limited CT transmission scan for AC demonstrated extensive, severe multivessel coronary calcifications. Given concern for diffuse high-grade CAD, the patient underwent invasive coronary angiography, which demonstrated a mid-LAD stenosis of 50% with an instantaneous wave-free ration (iFR) 0.97, confirming absence of flow-limiting disease (see Figure 18.2).

In summary, this patient with multiple cardiac comorbidities and heart failure with preserved ejection fraction has coronary microvascular dysfunction and ischemia with no obstructive coronary artery disease (INOCA). As in her counterpart with obstructive CAD in Case 1, this patient requires aggressive medical therapy and risk factor reduction, including optimal management of blood pressure, lipids, weight, and glycemia. Efforts are ongoing to more precisely phenotype patients like this one who have nonobstructive CAD and CMD, many of whom are women, to determine which additional interventions may be effective. Newer therapies targeting residual cholesterol and inflammatory risk, neurohormonal activation and glucose handling in the kidneys, and even surgical weight loss may demonstrate improved outcomes in these patients. This case illustrates how defining CAD as not only an anatomic problem but also a functional one (for which modern tools may be leveraged in future clinical trials to interrogate the full extent of the coronary circulation) may lead to a more complete understanding of the pathobiology of IHD, with the goal of improving outcomes for all patients.

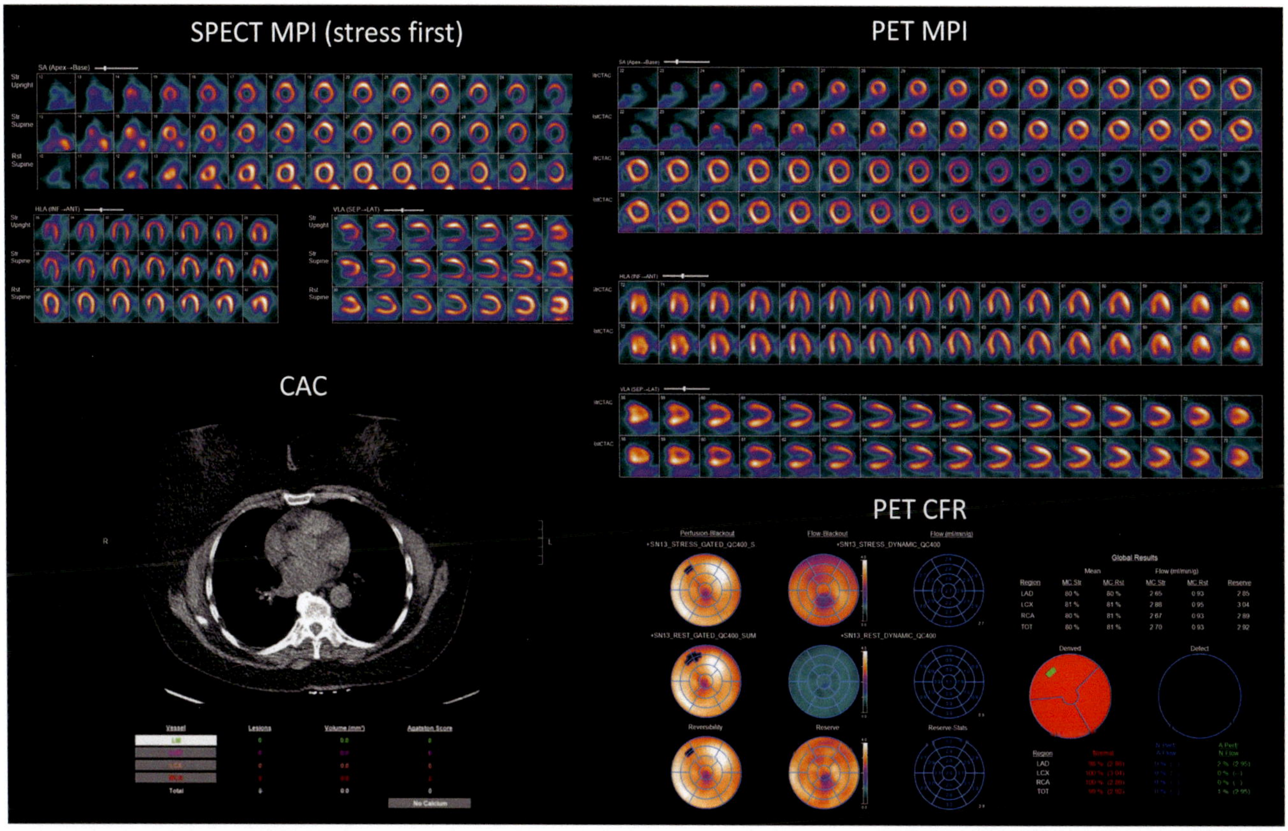

Figure 18.2. Case 2. Stress and rest ^{13}N-ammonia myocardial perfusion PET images and quantitative myocardial blood flow values. Coronary angiographic images and invasive instantaneous wave-free ratio (iFR) measurement of the proximal LAD confirming absence of flow-limiting disease despite a focal stenosis (arrow).

CASE 3

A 62-year-old woman with a history of hypertension and severe obesity and prior abnormal SPECT imaging was referred for a vasodilator stress myocardial perfusion PET-CT study to evaluate for dyspnea and decreased exercise tolerance. Her prior SPECT study had been performed 1 week ago as a stress-first study (Figure 18.3). It had demonstrated a reversible defect involving the inferior wall and was reported as an equivocal study due to possible subdiaphragmatic soft tissue attenuation artifact, which was well appreciated on a rest–stress study from 2 years before. The PET myocardial perfusion images were normal (demonstrating a basal lateral N13 ammonia PET artifact), and no evidence of ischemia or scar, with an LVEF of 74% and no regional wall-motion abnormalities. Quantitative assessment of regional and global myocardial blood flow demonstrated a normal global peak stress value of 2.70 mL/min/g and global coronary flow reserve of 2.92 with no regional variation (including along the segment of visual perfusion artifact) (see Figure 18.3). Furthermore, gated cardiac CT images demonstrated no coronary artery calcification, with an Agatston coronary calcium score of 0 (see Figure 18.3).

In summary, this obese patient with cardiac risk factors was found to have normal myocardial perfusion with no evidence of calcified atherosclerosis. In this case, stress testing with cardiac PET-CT provided a comprehensive diagnostic evaluation, confirming no evidence of flow-limiting CAD or coronary microvascular dysfunction, and normal global LV systolic function, allowing the patient to move forward with supervised exercise training as part of a comprehensive weight loss program.

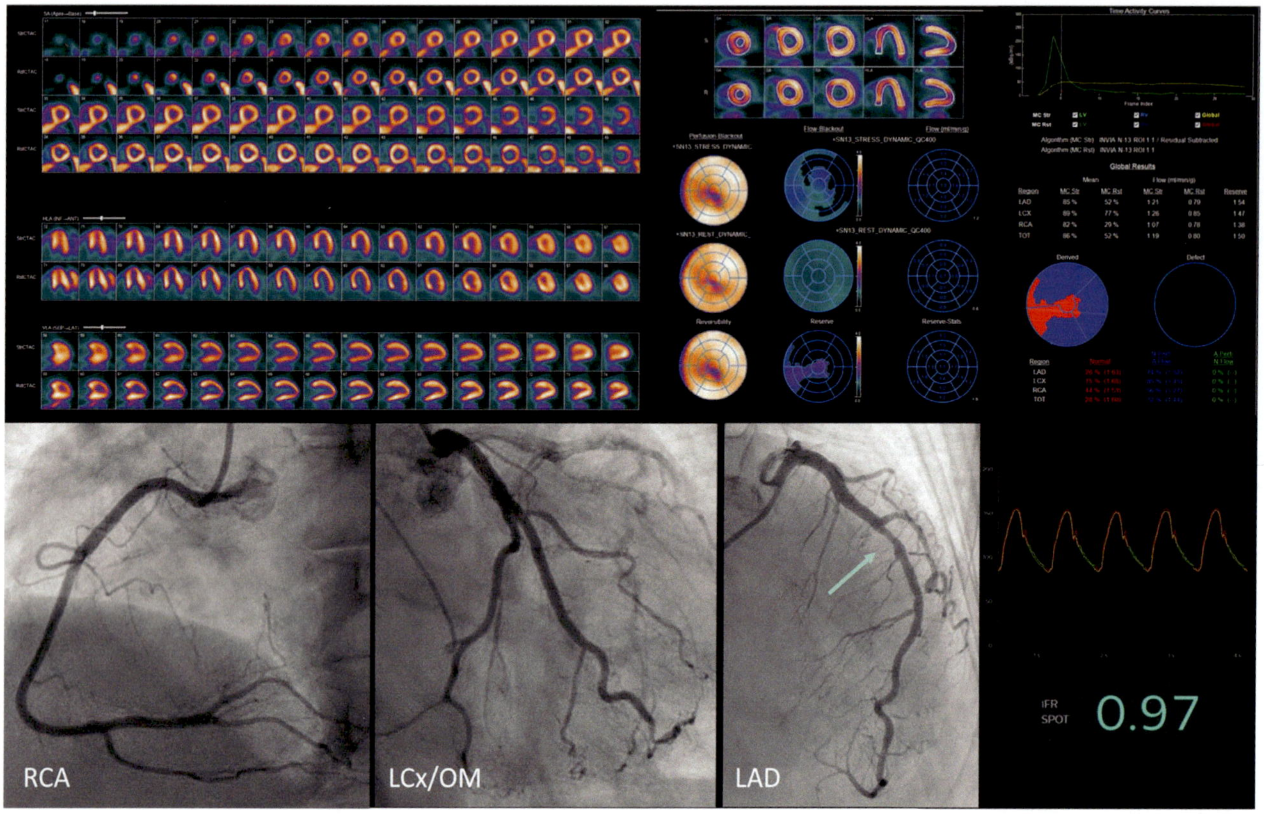

Figure 18.3. Case 3. Stress-first stress and rest Tc-99m sestamibi myocardial perfusion SPECT images. Non-contrast gated CT scan for calcium scoring obtained at time of PET-CT. Stress and rest ^{13}N-ammonia myocardial perfusion PET images and quantitative myocardial blood flow values.

19.

MYOCARDIAL VIABILITY ASSESSMENT BY NUCLEAR TECHNIQUES

Vasken Dilsizian, Ines Valenta, and Thomas H. Schindler

CASE 1

A 78-year-old man presented with increasing shortness of breath during daily activities and more recently also at rest. Cardiovascular risk profile with type 2 diabetes mellitus and arterial hypertension. Physical examination with jugular venous distention, lungs bilateral inspiratory moisture crackles in the basal segments, and pitting edema pre-tibiae. Auscultation with silent heart sounds and mild decrescendo second intercostal space left with punctum maximum apical compatible with mild mitral regurgitation. ECG with sinus rhythm 89 bpm, normal axis deviation and PQ interval, qs in v1–3, sudden R/S transition in v4, and diffuse T flattening. Findings were compatible with old anteroseptal infarction. Subsequent echocardiography showed a marked decrease in LVEF of 28% with akinesis of the mid to apical segments. In addition, mild mitral valve regurgitation was noted. Invasive coronary angiography was performed showing a normal left mainstem but lesions in the proximal LAD of ~90%, RD1-2 of ~40–50%, proximal LCx ~85%, and RCA of ~80%. Given the presence of severe three-vessel CAD, reduced LVEF, and regional wall-motion abnormalities, the patient was referred for viability assessment in view of potential revascularization strategies. ^{99m}Tc-SPECT/CT rest perfusion with short, vertical, and horizontal long axis demonstrates a severe perfusion defect in the antero-septo-apical and apical and also of the infero-lateral wall but of less severity that is accompanied by widely normal FDG uptake (Figure 19.1A). Thus, there is a large area of viable but ischemic compromised myocardium in the LAD and LCx distribution, or so-called mismatch between reduced perfusion and FDG uptake. This corresponds to a severe mismatch score of 28 on polar map analysis and 3D display of rest perfusion and viability images (Figure 19.1B), consistent with hibernating-stunned myocardium. Given the disproportionately high FDG uptake in the mismatch regions (antero-septo-apical, apical and infero-lateral), reflecting 100% reference for signal normalization, some of the remaining myocardium demonstrates mildly lower FDG signal (e.g., basal-mid segments anteriorly and inferiorly) associated with normal rest perfusion to confirm also normal viability in these segments. Given the large size of hibernating-stunned myocardium in the LAD and LCx distribution, and potential stunning in the RCA distribution, the patient underwent successful surgical intervention with multivessel CABG.

QUESTION

1. A "mismatch" finding between reduced resting myocardial perfusion and reduced but maintained viability (FDG uptake > 50%) in an akinetic regions reflects which of the following?
   a. No ischemic component and non-transmural necrosis
   b. Substantial amount of viable myocardium that is ischemic compromised
   c. Transmural necrosis
   d. Concordant decrease in regional perfusion and FDG uptake

ANSWER

1b. Answer b is correct, as a "mismatch" is defined as a segmental hypoperfusion with FDG uptake that substantially exceeds the degree of hypoperfusion. In other words, there is a substantial amount of viability (FDG uptake) that is ischemic compromised (hypoperfusion). Answers a and c are not correct, as there is no ischemic component. Regarding answer a, it describes a concordant reduction in perfusion and viability ("match" finding). Thus, there may be some viable rim but no ischemic component. Answer c is also not correct, as transmural necrosis precludes any

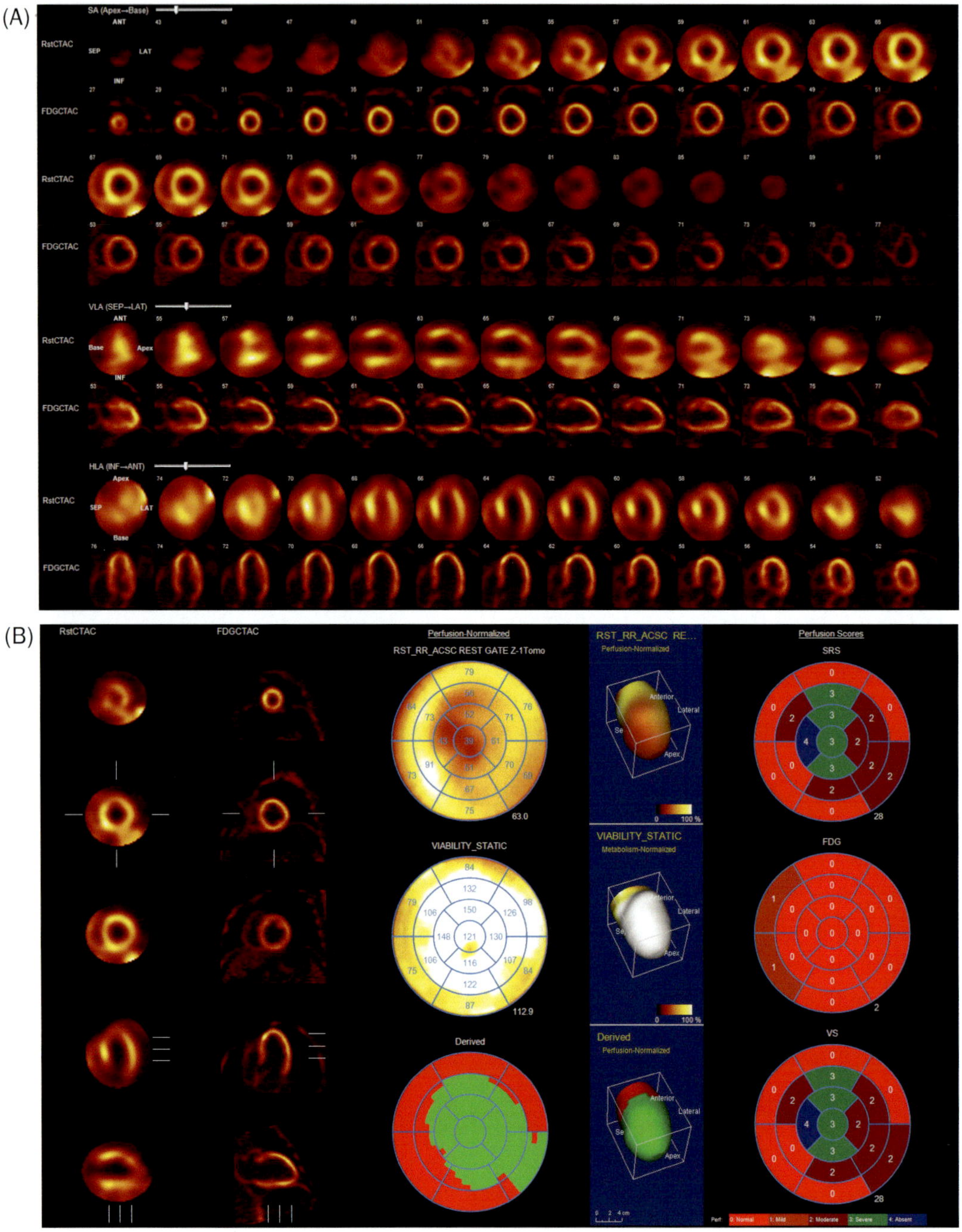

Figure 19.1. Case 1. Images of rest myocardial perfusion with ^{99m}Tc-SPECT/CT and viable myocardium with ^{18}F-FDG-PET/CT in a patient with ischemic cardiomyopathy, demonstrating a "mismatch."

viability. Answer d is not correct, as it describes a "match" finding like in answer a but formulated differently.

CASE 2

A 66-year-old woman presented with shortness of breath during daily activities. She has known CAD with status post serial PCI of lesions in the LAD, LCx, and RCA with stent employment. Cardiovascular risk profile with arterial hypertension, hyperlipidemia, and a positive family history. Physical examination with borderline jugular venous distention, lungs clear to auscultation bilaterally, and discrete pitting edema pre-tibiae. Auscultation with silent heart sounds but no murmurs or rubs. ECG with sinus rhythm 65 bpm, normal axis deviation and PQ interval, qs in v1–5,with mild ST elevation and T inversion, sudden R/S transition in v6, and diffuse T flattening in remaining leads. Findings were compatible with old anterior infarction. Echocardiogram reported severe hypokinesis to akinesis in the antero-septo-apical and dyskinesis in the apical walls. Mild hypokinesis of the remaining myocardium paralleled by an LVEF of ~33%. No significant stenosis or regurgitation of both the aortic and mitral valves. Subsequent invasive coronary angiography demonstrated patent stents in the LCx and RCA, while the LAD stent was occluded. Viability assessment was performed in view of the predominant akinesis in the distal LAD distribution subtended to the described mid-LAD occlusion. ^{99m}Tc-SPECT/CT rest perfusion with short, vertical, and horizontal long axis demonstrated a severe perfusion defect in the antero-septo-apical and apical walls that is associated with predominant absence of FDG uptake (Figure 19.2A). Thus, there is widely a "match" finding with concordant absence of perfusion and viability to signify predominant transmural necrosis in the antero-septo-apical and apical

(A)
(B)
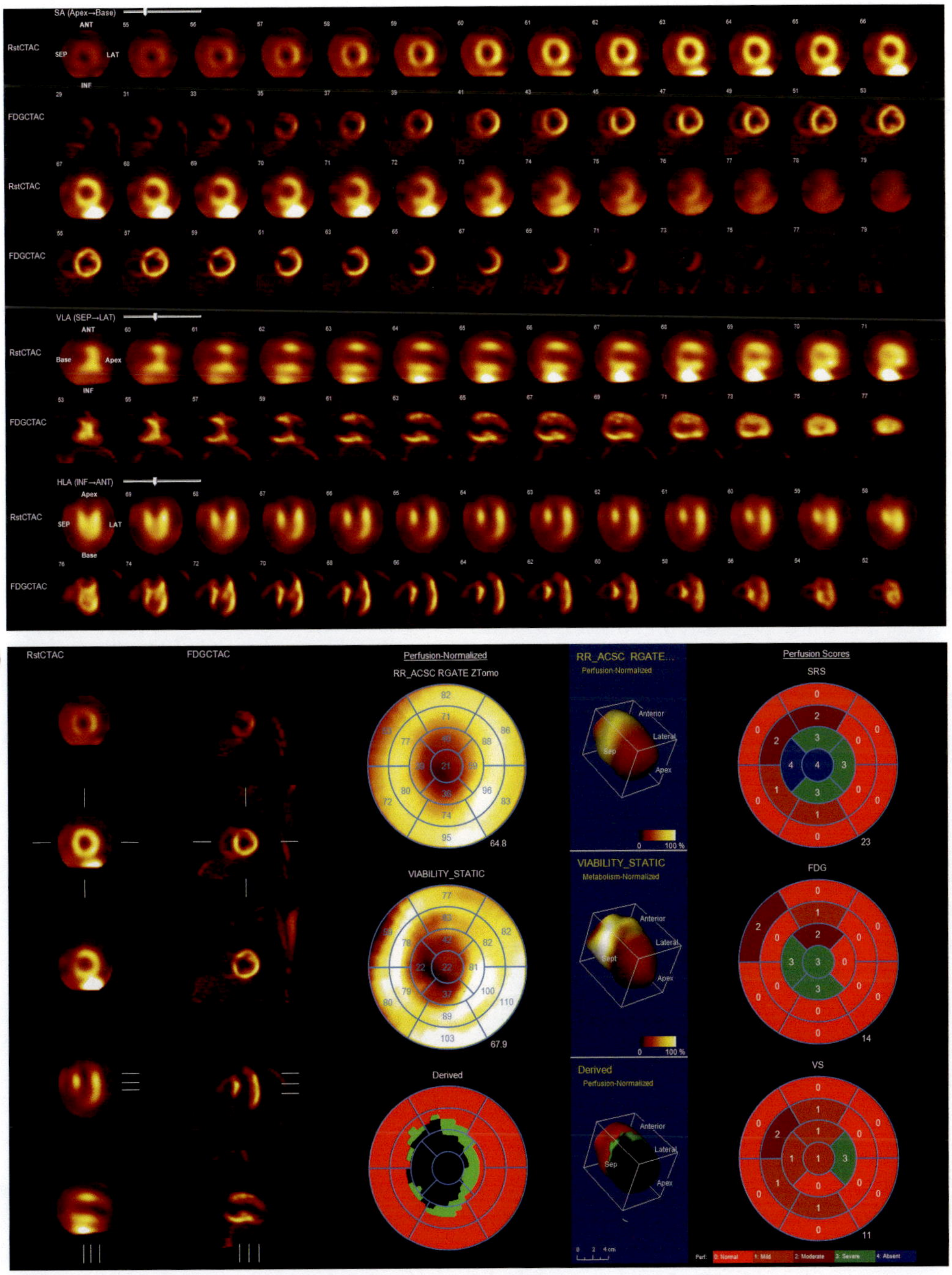

Figure 19.2. Case 2. Images of rest myocardial perfusion with ^{99m}Tc-SPECT/CT and viable myocardium with ^{18}F-FDG-PET/CT in a patient with ischemic cardiomyopathy, showing a "match."

walls as also evident on polar map analysis and 3D display (Figure 19.2B). Given these findings, a reopening of the mid-LAD occlusion was deferred and heart failure treatment intensified.

QUESTION

1. A match finding between reduced resting myocardial perfusion and reduced FDG uptake in an akinetic regions may reflect which two of the following conditions?
   a. Transmural necrosis
   b. Ischemic compromised viable myocardium
   c. Concordant decrease in regional perfusion and FDG uptake
   d. Normal perfusion and viability

ANSWER

1a and c. Answers a and c are correct, as any "match" findings between reductions in perfusion and FDG uptake preclude the presence of resting ischemia. Transmural necrosis implies a severe perfusion defect with widely no FDG uptake, while a concordant decrease in regional perfusion matching some FDG uptake signifies non-transmural necrosis but no ischemic component. Answer b is not correct, as it reflects a classical "mismatch." Answer d is also not correct, as normal perfusion implies normal viability. Thus, when perfusion is normal, no additional viability assessment is needed.

CASE 3

An 80-year-old man with heart failure–related shortness of breath presented to the emergency department with ongoing chest pain. Cardiovascular risk profile with arterial hypertension and hyperlipidemia. Physical examination with jugular venous distension, lungs bilateral with inspiratory moisture crackles in the basal segments, and pitting edema pre-tibiae. Auscultation with silent heart sounds but no murmur or rubs. ECG demonstrated sinus rhythm 85 bpm, left axis deviation and normal PQ interval, no R-progression until v6, ST-segment elevations in the anterior leads and DII-III, AvF, and downsloping ST in aVL. Findings were compatible with ST-elevation myocardial infarction (STEMI), and the patient underwent immediate invasive coronary angiography. Invasive catheterization showed distal occlusion of the LAD and a 90% lesion in the distal LCx. Echocardiography showed mild global hypokinesis with severe hypo-/akinesis in the antero-septo-apical and infero-apical walls associated with an LVEF of 36%. No stenosis or regurgitation of both the aortic and mitral valves was noted. Viability assessment was conducted in view of the predominant akinesis in the distal LAD distribution. ^{99m}Tc-SPECT/CT rest perfusion with short, vertical, and horizontal long axis demonstrates a severe perfusion defect in the antero-septo-apical and infero-apical walls that is paralleled by widely maintained FDG uptake (Figure 19.3A). Thus, there is widely a "mismatch" finding between reduced perfusion and FDG uptake in a predominant akinesis region indicative of hibernating-stunned myocardium in the distal LAD distribution. Interestingly, the FDG images demonstrate predominant FDG uptake in the distal LAD distribution but none in the remaining, normally perfused myocardium and thus viable myocardium (Figure 19.3B). The exact reason why FDG may accumulate only in hibernating-stunned myocardium remains uncertain but necessitates perfusion imaging for an optimal diagnostic yield. Given these findings, however, the patient underwent successful PCI and stent employment of the distal LAD lesion.

QUESTION

1. Concurrent myocardial perfusion imaging to FDG-PET is needed for which two purposes?
   a. Identification of segmental resting perfusion deficit to be compared to FDG uptake to signify a "mismatch" or "match" among both
   b. Accurate assessment of the extent of necrosis
   c. Accurate quantification of viable myocardium
   d. Confirmation of normal viable segments (reflected by normal perfusion) in case of relatively lower FDG signal adjacent to a FDG "hot spot" in a "mismatch" region

ANSWER

1a and d. Answer a is correct, as perfusion assessment is needed to compare the degree of reduced perfusion to the extent of viable myocardium in order to identify "mismatch" (ischemic compromised viable myocardium) or "match" (wide absence of viability or some viability but no

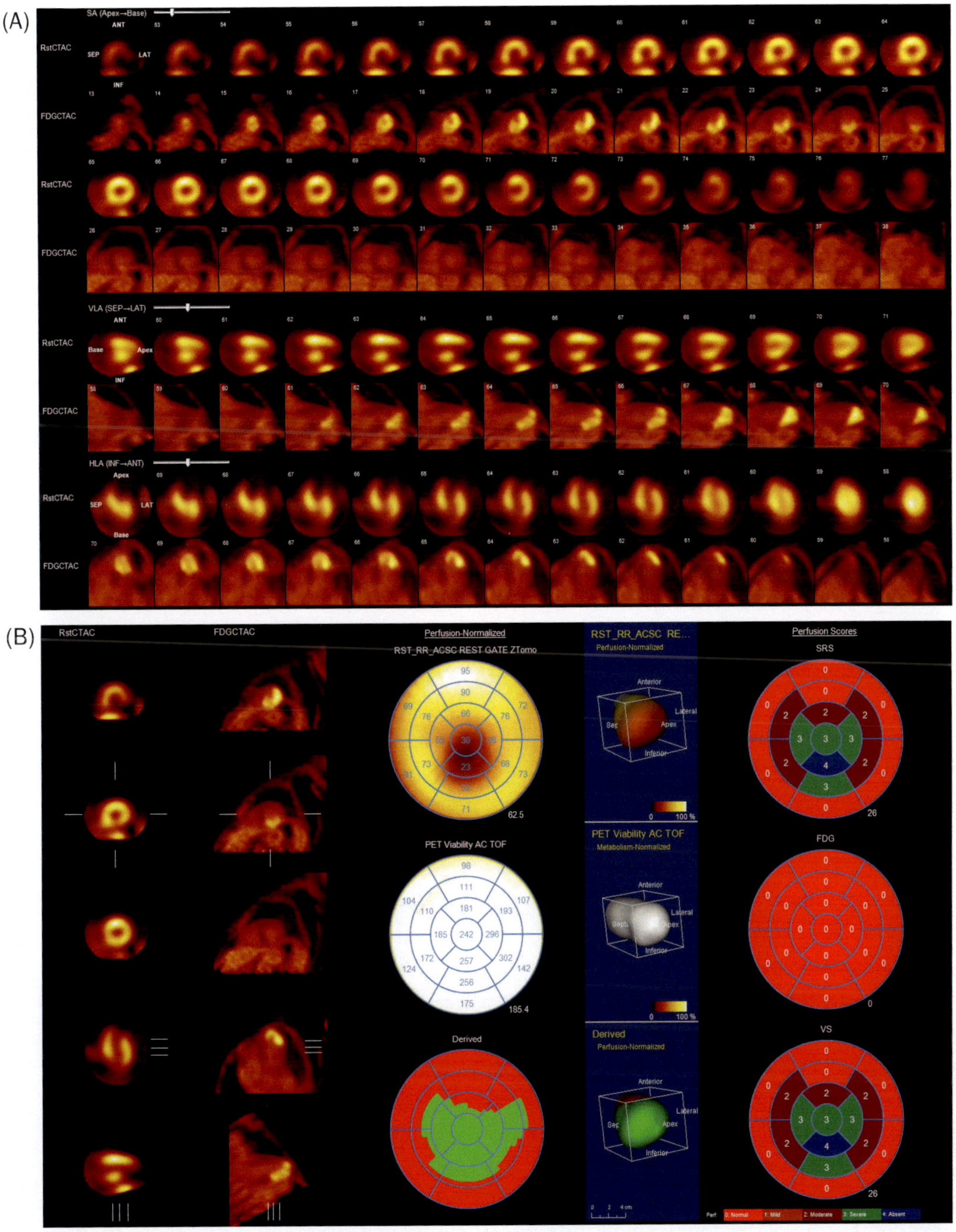

Figure 19.3. Case 3. Images of rest myocardial perfusion with ^{99m}Tc-SPECT/CT and viable myocardium with ^{18}F-FDG-PET/CT in a patient with ischemic cardiomyopathy, showing a "mismatch."

ischemia). Answer d is also correct, as FDG uptake may predominantly accumulate in regions with pronounced "mismatch" (hibernating-stunned myocardium) findings. This can then serve as a reference (100% of signal intensity) and the FDG uptake in the remaining myocardium may be downscaled or even absent, as in this case. Here, normally perfused segments then signify normal viability in these regions with downscaled or absent FDG signal. Answers b and c are not correct, as resting perfusion defects may signify the presence of infarction but not the accurate extent of viable myocardium. For example, in about 30–40% of patients with regional perfusion defect, maintained viability (FDG uptake > 50%) can be found in an akinetic region.

20.

IMAGING DYSSYNCHRONY

Alessia Gimelli and Riccardo Liga

CASE 1

A 56-year-old man had a history of hypertension and dyslipidemia and prior acute anterior myocardial infarction 5 years ago, treated with percutaneous coronary intervention (PCI) of the left anterior descending (LAD) coronary artery. 2D echocardiography (2DE) showed mild LV systolic dysfunction with an EF of 47% and apical akinesia. He was treated with an angiotensin-converting enzyme (ACE) inhibitor, a beta-blocker, low-dose aspirin, and a statin.

He presented with worsening dyspnea on effort and peripheral edema. The ECG showed a new-onset LBBB (Figure 20.1). A repeat 2DE showed more severe LV dysfunction (LVEF = 34%) with more extensive apical akinesia and diffuse hypokinesia of the remaining LV walls and moderate-to-severe mitral regurgitation.

A stress–rest pharmacological gated SPECT MPI was performed to assess the presence of inducible myocardial ischemia. The patient was asymptomatic after a 72-hour washout from his beta-blocker. Dipyridamole was injected at standard dosage (0.56 mg/kg in 4 minutes) without any relevant side effects except for flushing and mild dyspnea, both rapidly reversed with aminophylline. Tc-99m tetrofosmin (187 MBq) was injected intravenously 2 minutes after completion of the dipyridamole infusion.

Stress images were acquired 15 minutes after radiotracer administration with a Discovery NM/CT 530c CZT gamma camera (GE Healthcare, Haifa, Israel). Rest injection (365 MBq) was administered 1 hour after the stress injection and the images were obtained 15 minutes later; the rest of the tetrofosmin injection was performed after administration of sublingual nitrates (Figure 20.2). Both stress and rest studies were acquired using the list mode using a gated 16-frames-per-cycle acquisition with a 20% acceptance window. Acquisition time was 8 minutes for the stress study and 7 minutes for the rest study.

Stress and rest images were reconstructed on a dedicated workstation (Xeleris 4,0 GE Healthcare) using Lister Software from the Alcyone Miscellaneous Tools (GE Healthcare). LV regional perfusion, wall motion, and wall thickening were analyzed with commercially available software (Corridor 4DM, Invia, Ann Arbor, MI) using a 17-segment model. Moreover, the presence of LV dyssynchrony was assessed with phase analysis of gated SPECT images using the same software package and the region of most delayed mechanical contraction was identified.

The analysis of perfusion images demonstrated the presence of an extensive apical scar in the territory of distribution of the LAD coronary artery in the absence of significant reversible myocardial perfusion abnormalities elsewhere. Gated images confirmed the presence of a significantly reduced LV EF, both after stress and during rest, with LV dilation.

Phase analysis showed the presence of significant LV mechanical dyssynchrony with the region of latest mechanical activation located at the level of the viable lateral wall, a pattern consistent with the known LBBB (Figures 20.3 and 20.4).

Cardiac MRI showed the presence of moderate-to-severe LV systolic dysfunction (EF 36%) with a large transmural apical scar. Myocardial inflammation and infiltrative disease were also excluded (Figure 20.5).

^{123}I-metaiodobenzylguanidine (MIBG) imaging (using 3 mCi) after 15 minutes and 4 hours from the tracer injection showed poor visualization of the heart with reduced early and delayed heart-to-ediastinum ratios (1.32 and 1.25, respectively), indicating a significantly increased risk for major adverse cardiac events (Figure 20.6).

The patient underwent implanted cardioverter defibrillator (ICD)/CRT device implantation (Figure 20.7). The LV pacing lead was placed at the lateral wall based on the results of the phase analysis.

After 2 years of follow-up, the patient remained stable and asymptomatic. No major events and/or arrhythmias

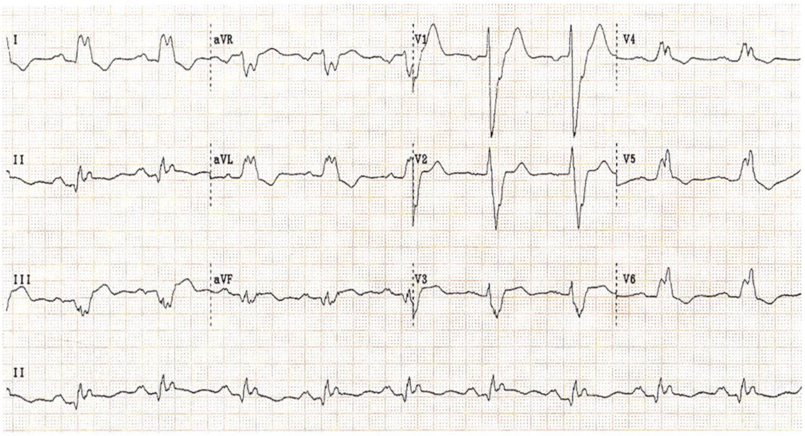

Figure 20.1. Case 1. 12-lead ECG tracing showing a left-bundle branch block.

were recorded. Importantly, a significant LV reverse remodeling was observed, with a consistent reduction of LV volumes coupled with a significant improvement of LV systolic function (EF 41%) as well as a regression of functional mitral regurgitation.

This case demonstrates the usefulness of gated SPECT MPI for the assessment of myocardial perfusion, global LV function, as well as regional wall motion and dyssynchrony, providing relevant prognostic data and potentially guiding clinical management.

CASE 2

A 67-year-old man had a history of premature CAD, hypertension, hypercholesterolemia, and prior inferior acute myocardial infarction 9 years ago treated with PCI of the right coronary artery (RCA). 2DE then showed inferior akinesis and an LVEF of 50%. He was treated with a beta-blocker, an ACE inhibitor, a statin, and low-dose aspirin and was followed regularly in an outpatient setting.

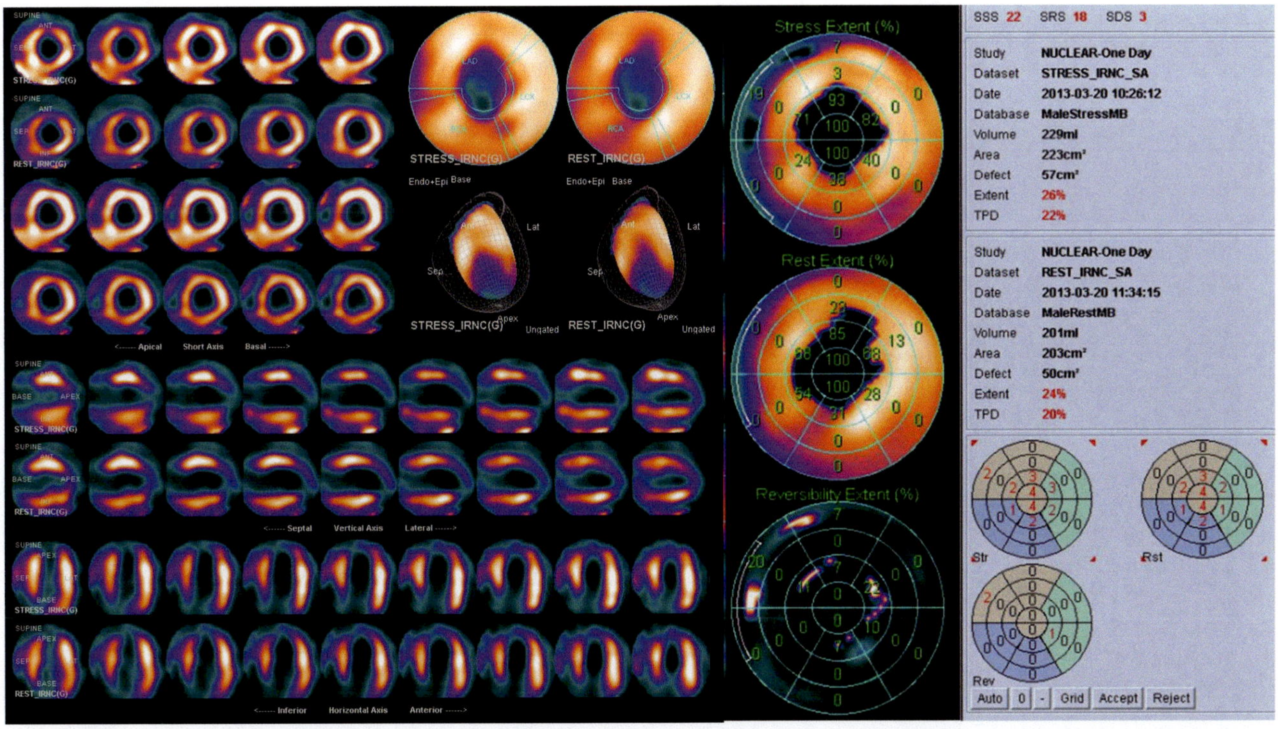

Figure 20.2. Case 1. Stress and rest MPI, acquired with a dedicated CZT cardiac camera (Discovery NM/CT 530c CZT gamma camera; GE Healthcare, Haifa, Israel) showing a large apical non reversible LV perfusion defect.

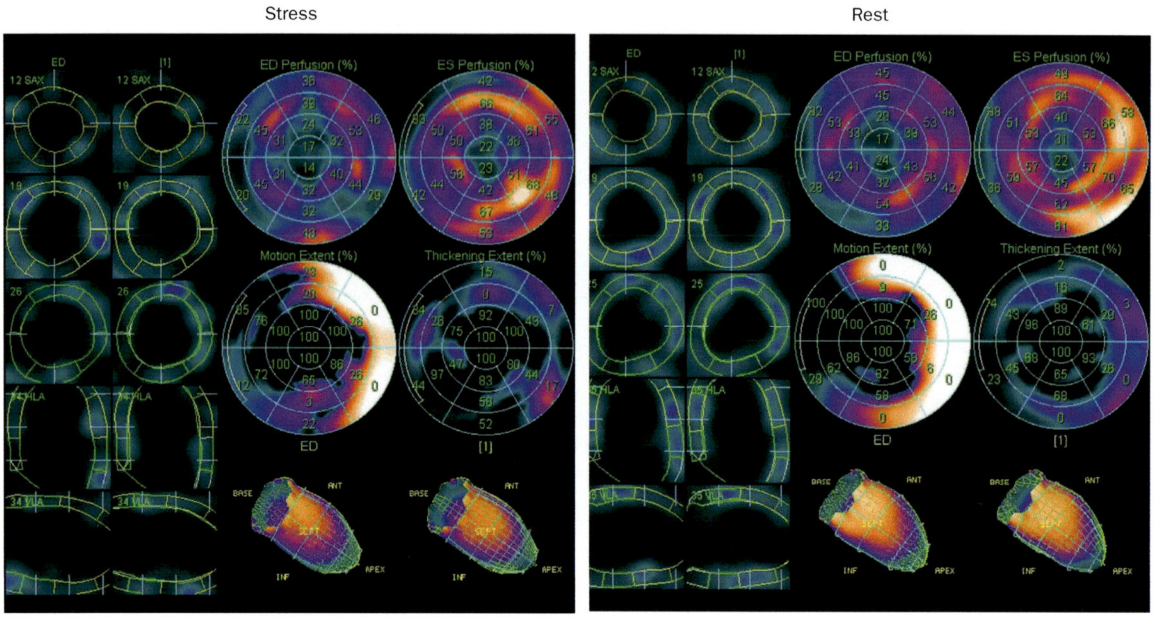

	Stress	Rest
LV-EF (%)	33	35
LV-EDV (ml)	285	270
LV-ESV (ml)	183	167

Figure 20.3. Case 1. Gated CZT images.

He started complaining of progressive dyspnea on effort [New York Heart Association (NYHA) class 2] as well as moderate effort angina [Canadian Cardiovascular Society (CCS) class 2]. Unfortunately, due to the COVID-19 pandemic, cardiology consultation was delayed for many months, at which time his symptoms had progressed (NYHA and CCS class both 3).

A repeat 2DE showed a severely depressed LV systolic function (EF 30%), inferior wall akinesia, and apical and lateral wall hypokinesia. The ECG showed old inferior myocardial infarction but normal QRS duration.

He underwent stress/rest gated SPECT MPI using a similar protocol as outlined in Case 1.

The images demonstrated the presence of a fixed myocardial perfusion defect in the territory of the RCA and reversible perfusion abnormalities in the anteroseptal regions (Figure 20.8). The gated images showed severely reduced LVEF and LV dilatation.

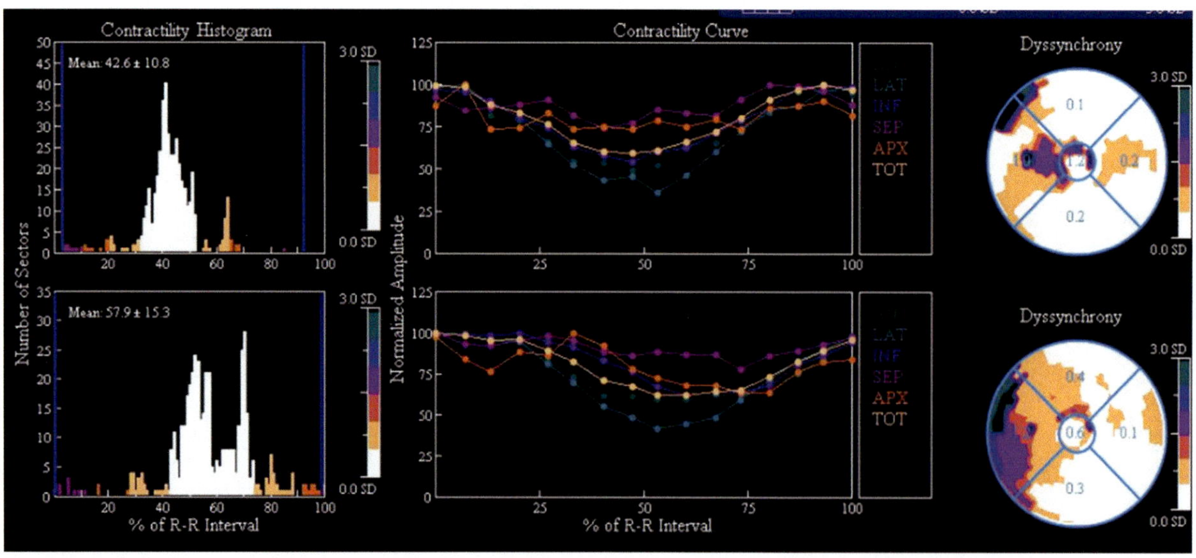

Figure 20.4. Case 1. Results of phase analysis.

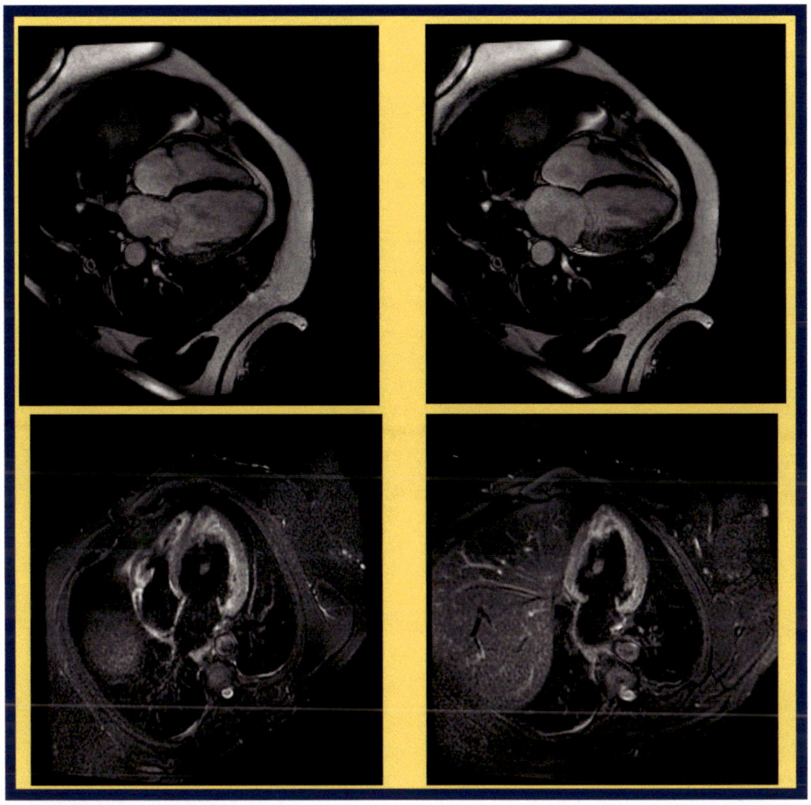

Figure 20.5. Case 1. Cardiac magnetic resonance imaging. End-diastolic (left) and end-systolic (left) LV frames.

Despite the presence of a narrow QRS on a 12-lead ECG, phase analysis showed the presence of significant LV mechanical dyssynchrony, with the region of latest mechanical activation located at the level of the viable anteroseptal wall (Figure 20.9).

Invasive coronary angiography demonstrated the presence of a significant stenosis at the level of the proximal LAD, treated effectively with stenting (Figure 20.10).

After follow-up, a significant improvement in regional and global function was observed with the LVEF of 40%, with a complete resolution of the symptoms.

This case is an example of significant LV mechanical dyssynchrony in a patient with a narrow QRS.

Figure 20.6. Case 1. Planar MIBG images. The heart-to-mediastinum (H/M) ratios and washout rate (WO) are reported.

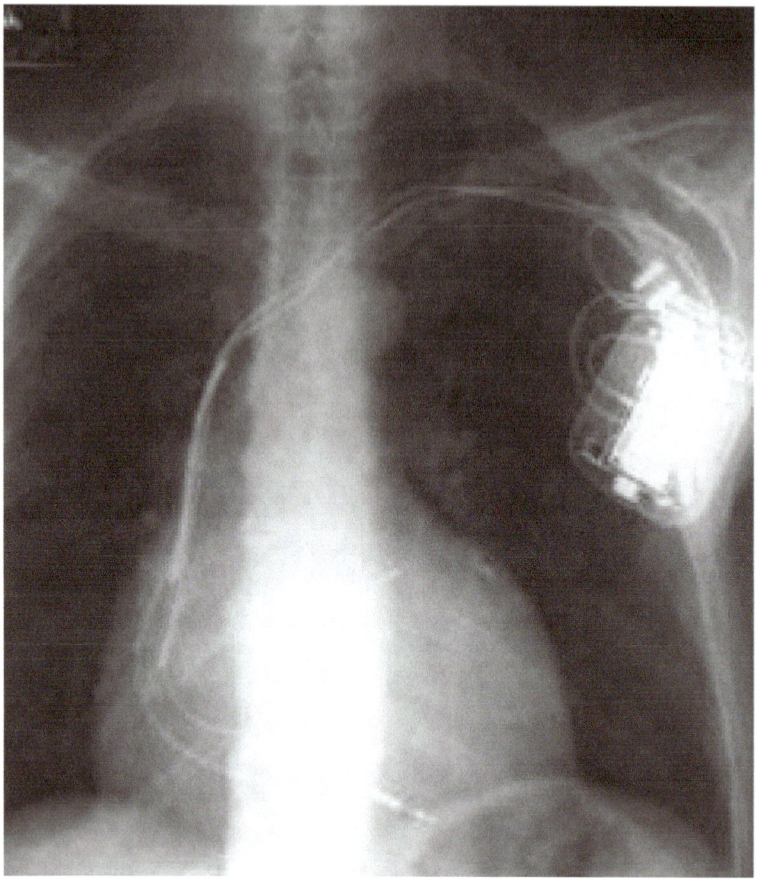

Figure 20.7. Case 1. Postero-anterior chest x-ray showing a ICD/CRT device.

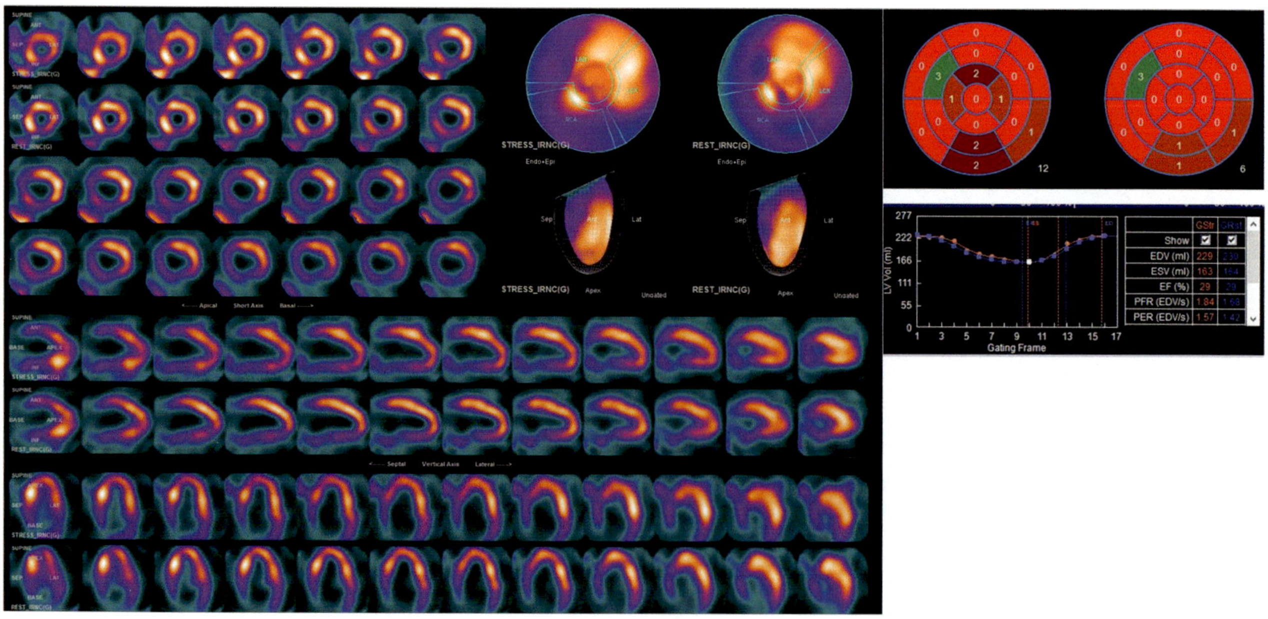

Figure 20.8. Case 2. Gated stress and rest MPI, acquired with a dedicated CZT cardiac camera (Discovery NM/CT 530c CZT gamma camera; GE Healthcare, Haifa, Israel). The results of LV functional analysis is reported on the right.

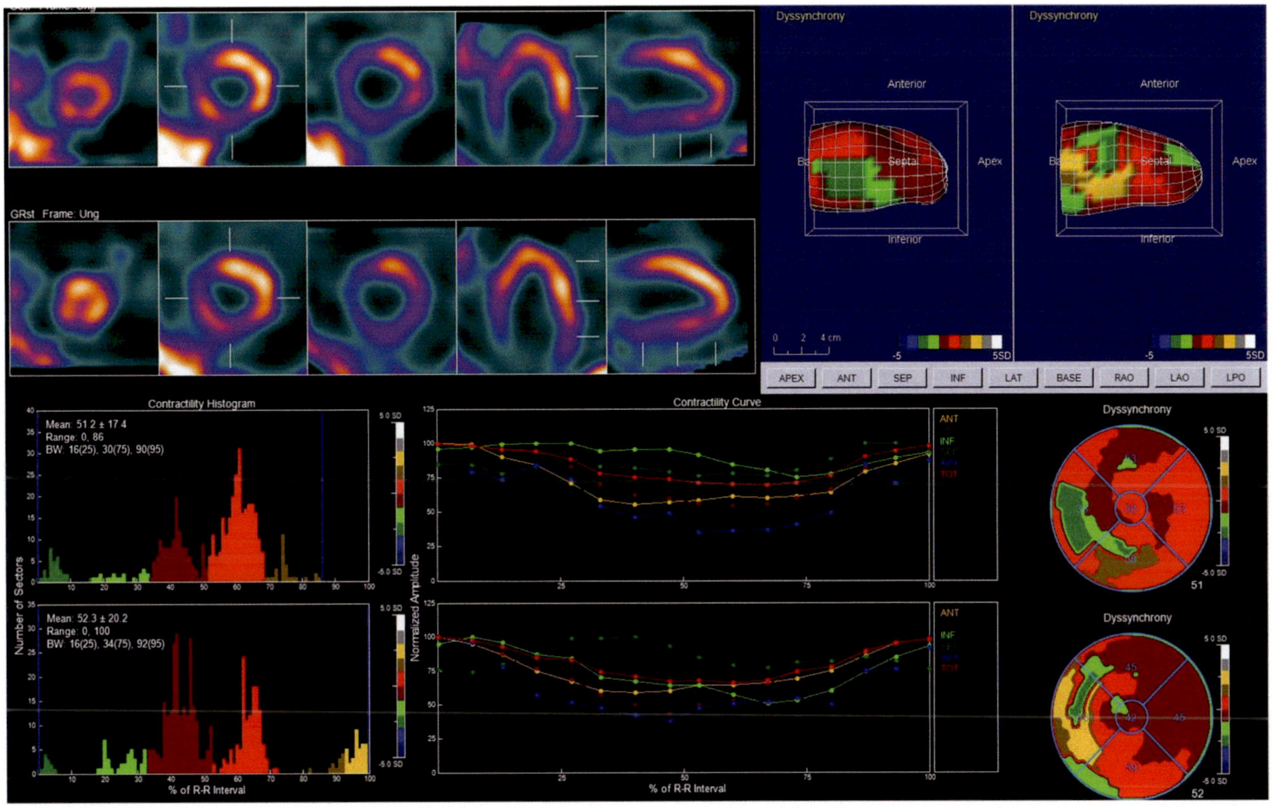

Figure 20.9. Case 2. Results of phase analysis.

CASE 3

A 55-year-old asymptomatic man was seen because he needed clearance to engage in noncompetitive sports. He was mildly obese (BMI 32 kg/m^2) and reported a history of cigarette smoking (20 pack-years), arterial hypertension, and hypercholesterolemia and has been on treatment with ramipril 10 mg, atorvastatin 20 mg, and fenofibrate 145 mg. The physical examination was otherwise normal.

The ECG revealed for the first time the presence of intermittent LBBB by 24-hour Holter monitoring. A transthoracic echocardiogram showed the presence of a slightly enlarged LV (90 ml/m^2) with a mild systolic dysfunction (EF 48%) due to apical hypokinesia.

A stress–rest gated SPECT MPI was performed to rule out the presence of inducible ischemia. At the time of stress testing the ECG showed a normal QRS. Accordingly, a bicycle exercise stress test was performed. Baseline HR was

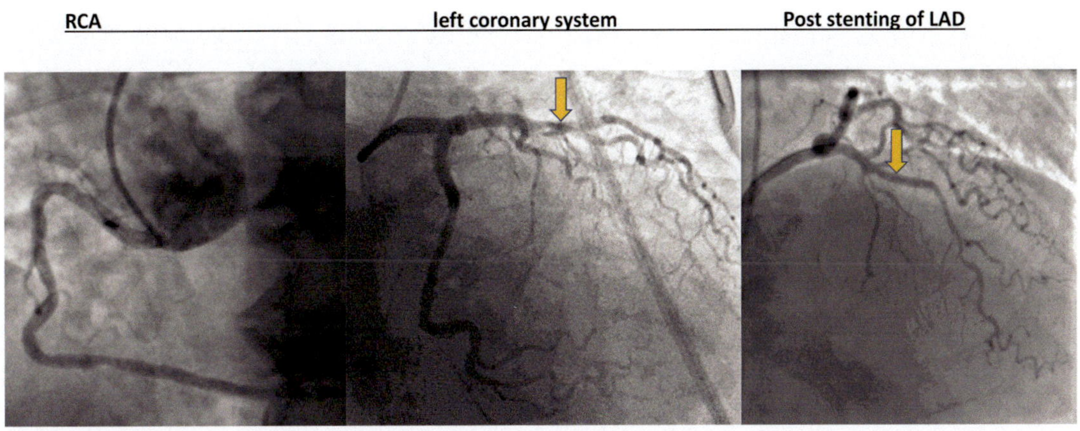

Figure 20.10. Case 2. Invasive coronary angiography showing an obstructive LAD stenosis.

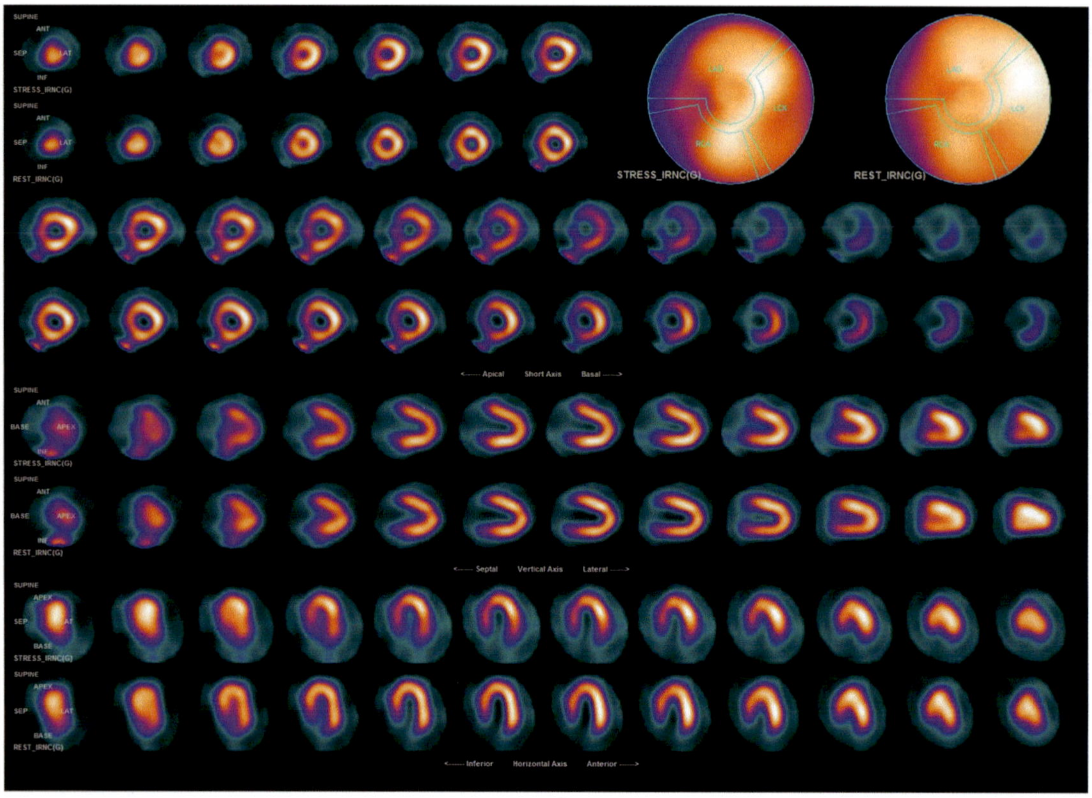

Figure 20.11. Case 3. Stress and rest MPI, acquired with a dedicated CZT cardiac camera (Discovery NM/CT 530c CZT gamma camera; GE Healthcare, Haifa, Israel).

75 bpm and BP was 135/80 mmHg. Tc-99m tetrofosmin (187 MBq) was injected intravenously at peak exercise at 8 minutes of exercise; HR and BP were 165 bpm and 190/100 mmHg, respectively. Transient LBBB appeared shortly before peak exercise and persisted until the third minute of recovery. Image acquisition and processing were similar to those in Case 1.

The stress and rest images demonstrated the presence of a small inducible perfusion defect in the proximal portion of the septal wall (Figure 20.11). Gated images revealed normal LVEF both at rest and after stress with normal volumes. Phase analysis showed that minimal global LV dyssynchrony was detected (SD 51.3 ± 4.1) with septal delayed mechanical activation (Figure 20.12).

Computed tomography coronary angiography revealed the presence of nonobstructive atherosclerosis of the LAD coronary artery (Figure 20.13).

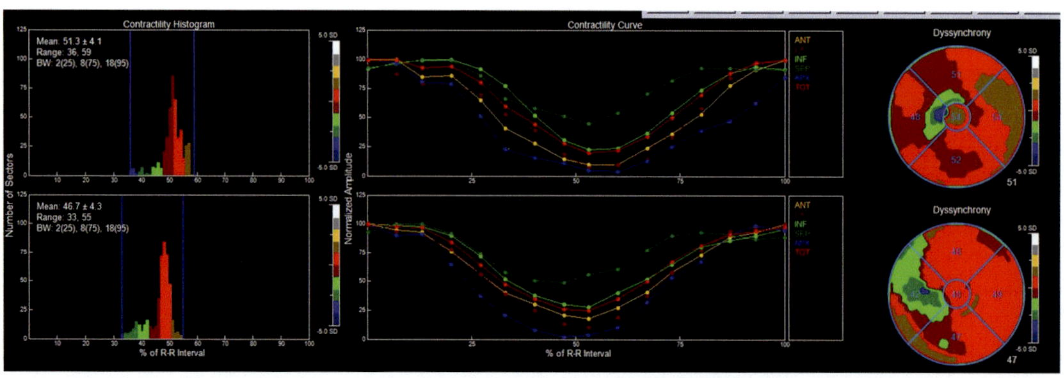

Figure 20.12. Case 3. Results of phase analysis.

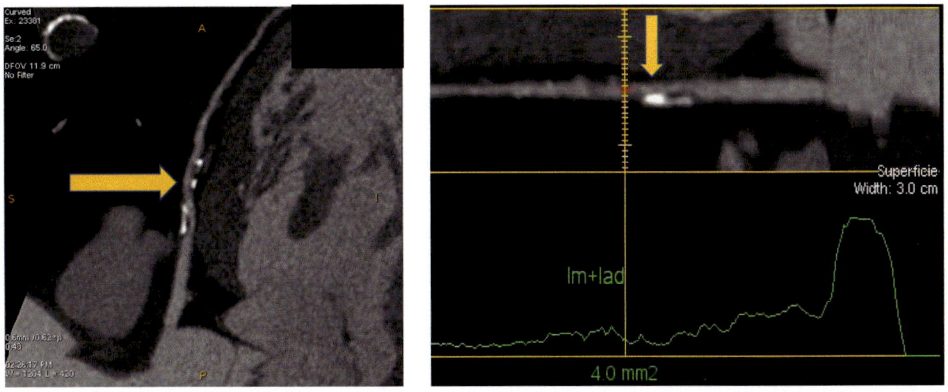

Figure 20.13. Case 3. Computed tomography coronary angiography images showing non-obstructive LAD atherosclerosis.

The septal perfusion abnormality in this patient is most likely due to LBBB, which was not present at the beginning of exercise but appeared at the time of trace injection when the heart rate was high. It is for this reason that current guidelines recommend pharmacologic stress testing in patients with LBBB. Repeat testing in this patient using vasodilator stress (without exercise) would have been another option. The lack of significant mechanical dyssynergy is likely because the LBBB was no longer present at the time of image acquisition.

21.

IMAGING MYOCARDIAL INNERVATION BY SPECT AND PET

Mark I. Travin

CASE 1

CLINICAL PRESENTATION

A 61-year-old diabetic male active smoker with hypertension and chronic kidney disease stage III, with a nonischemic cardiomyopathy (minor coronary changes seen at catheterization 6 years prior), NYHA Class III HF, and LVEF = 25%, was referred for evaluation. His ECG showed normal sinus rhythm, a left anterior hemiblock, and T-wave abnormalities. An ICD had been implanted 9 months prior. He consented to undergo a cardiac ^{123}I-*m*IBG imaging study as part of a clinical research study. Imaging findings are shown in Figure 21.1.

CLINICAL OUTCOME

At 2 years of follow-up, the patient had no adverse cardiac events. Eight years after imaging, he was hospitalized for decompensated HF, and again 4 years later. Approximately 13 years after the imaging study, the patient suffered a cardiac arrest at home, was found have pulseless electrical activity, and expired shortly thereafter.

DISCUSSION

Results of the 961 patient ADMIRE-HF study indicated that this patient's HMR of 1.66 is associated with low risk of an adverse cardiac event (HF progression, a potentially lethal arrhythmia, and cardiac death) for the first 2 years of follow-up,[1] as was the case in this instance. However, it is noteworthy that in several studies[2,3] this patient's SPECT summed dysinnervation score of 27 and the presence of an adrenergic-perfusion mismatch predicted increased arrhythmic risk. Nevertheless, those studies had relatively small sample sizes, and in the larger ADMIRE-HF study the short-term prognostic power of planar image results was superior to that of SPECT. At the same time, with longer follow-up for a patient with heart failure that is likely to progress, the predictive power SPECT findings could potentially increase. A more recent study showed that although the risk-stratification power HMR persisted to at least 5 years,[4] absolute cardiac risk became higher, with an expected increase over time. Repeat imaging at periodic intervals to follow disease progression will likely be necessary for cardiac ^{123}I-*m*IBG imaging to be an effective clinical tool.

CASE 2

CLINICAL PRESENTATION

A 64-year-old diabetic woman with hypertension who presented with a nonischemic cardiomyopathy (no CAD at prior catheterization), NYHA Class III HF, and LVEF = 25% to 30% was referred for evaluation. Her ECG showed normal sinus rhythm with nonspecific ST–T-wave changes. An ICD had been implanted 6 years prior without discharge since. She consented to undergo a cardiac ^{123}I-*m*IBG imaging study as part of a clinical research study. Imaging findings are shown in Figure 21.2.

CLINICAL OUTCOME

Approximately 5 months after the imaging study there were recurrent ICD discharges, and 4 years later the patient underwent a VT ablation procedure. The LVEF deteriorated to 15%, with subsequent HF admissions and frequent ICD discharges. The patient declined advanced care, and expired from pump failure 5 years after the ^{123}I-*m*IBG study.

DISCUSSION

Results of the 961-patient ADMIRE-HF study indicate that the patient's HMR of 1.51 is associated with a significant 2-year risk of adverse cardiac events that include HF progression, a potentially lethal ventricular arrhythmia, or cardiac death.[1] The high dysinnervation SPECT score of

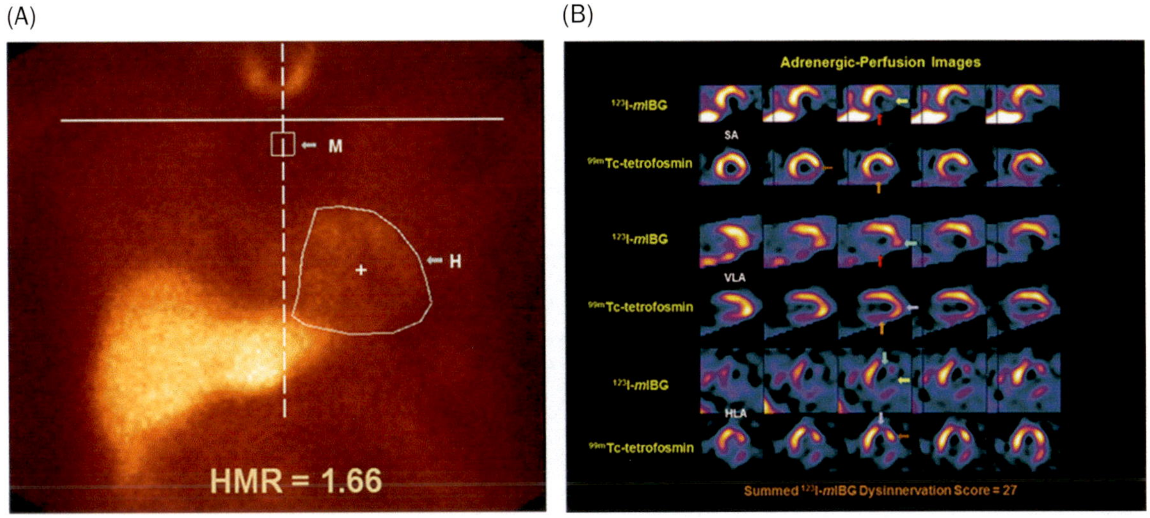

Figure 21.1 In Figure A, anterior planar ^{123}I-*m*IBG images showed a heart (H) to mediastinum (M) ratio of 1.66 that is above the 1.60 normal limit threshold designated by the ADMIRE-HF study.[1] In Figure B, SPECT ^{123}I-*m*IBG adrenergic images showed a large region of abnormal sympathetic innervation involving the inferior (red arrows), lateral (yellow arrows), and apical (green arrows) walls with the summed dysinnervation score determined to be 27. ^{99m}Tc-tetrofosmin perfusion images showed some degree of adrenergic-perfusion mismatch involving the inferior (orange arrows), lateral (gold/brown arrow), and apical (blue arrows) walls.

36 is greater than a reported 26 score threshold for ICD discharges.[2]

CASE 3

CLINICAL PRESENTATION

A 28-year-old morbidly obese (BMI 48) diabetic man with hypertension, obstructive sleep apnea, and chronic kidney disease III with a nonischemic cardiomyopathy (no CAD at catheterization), NYHA Class II HF, and LVEF = 20% was referred for evaluation. The ECG showed an intraventricular conduction delay (IVCD). He consented to undergo a cardiac ^{123}I-*m*IBG imaging study as part of a clinical research study. The patient did not have an ICD at the time of imaging. Imaging findings are shown in Figure 21.3.

CLINICAL OUTCOME

The patient received an ICD 3 months after imaging. Approximately 9½ months after imaging, the patient's

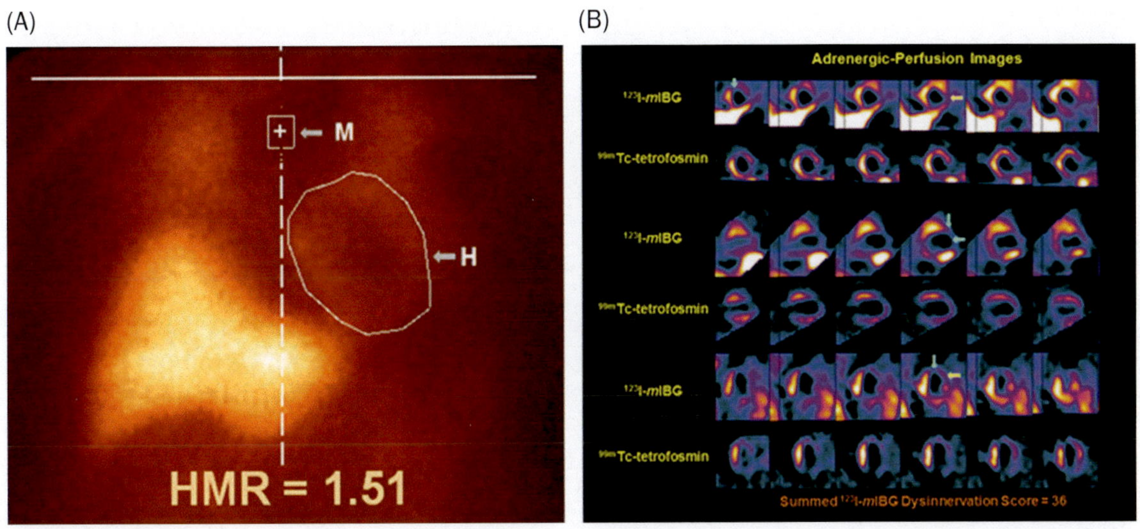

Figure 21.2 In Figure A, anterior planar ^{123}I-*m*IBG images showed an HMR of 1.51 that is below the 1.60 normal limit threshold designated by the ADMIRE-HF study.[1] In Figure B, SPECT ^{123}I-*m*IBG adrenergic images showed a large region of abnormal sympathetic innervation involving the lateral (yellow) and apical/distal anterior walls (green arrows) with the summed dysinnervation score determined to be 36. ^{99m}Tc-tetrofosmin perfusion images showed a pattern similar to that of the ^{123}I-*m*IBG images, thus no significant adrenergic-perfusion mismatch appreciated.

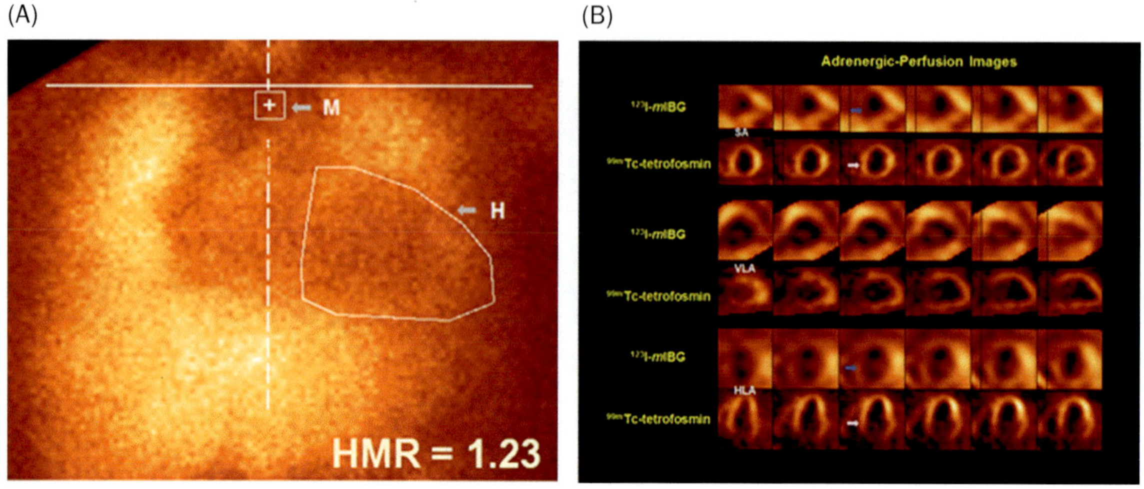

Figure 21.3 In Figure A, anterior planar ^{123}I-*m*IBG images showed an HMR of 1.23 that is well below the 1.60 normal limit threshold designated by the ADMIRE-HF study,[1] and the washout rate was 32.1 (not shown in images) that is abnormal being above a high risk threshold of 27%.[2] In Figure B, SPECT ^{123}I-*m*IBG adrenergic images were of suboptimal quality both because of markedly reduced tracer uptake, patient obesity, and lung uptake overlapping the anterolateral wall. However, a large adrenergic defect is appreciated in the septum (blue arrows), with preserved septal ^{99m}Tc-tetrofosmin uptake (light purple arrows), thus a region of adrenergic-perfusion mismatch, although the IVCD may have contributed to the finding.

HF worsened to NYHA Class III, and biventricular CRT pacing was initiated. He underwent bariatric surgery about 5 years after imaging. Nevertheless, the patient developed progressive systolic dysfunction failure despite the CRT, with the EF deteriorating to 15%. Approximately 12 years after imaging he underwent heart transplantation.

DISCUSSION

The patient had an ^{123}I-*m*IBG scan showing an extremely low HMR (heart counts close to background) and a very high washout rate, findings associated with a worsened outcome.[1,5] The patient developed severe pump failure despite CRT, in accord with evidence of an HMR less than 1.36 decreasing the likelihood of benefit from CRT,[6] necessitating eventual referral for heart transplant.[7]

REFERENCES

1. Jacobson AF, Senior R, Cerqueira MD, et al. Myocardial iodine-123 meta-iodobenzylguanidine imaging and cardiac events in heart failure: Results of the prospective ADMIRE-HF (AdreView Myocardial Imaging for Risk Evaluation in Heart Failure) study. *J Am Coll Cardiol.* 2010;55:2212–2221.
2. Boogers MJ, Borleffs CJ, Henneman MM, et al. Cardiac sympathetic denervation assessed with 123-Iodine metaiodobenzylguanidine imaging predicts ventricular arrhythmias in implantable cardioverter-defibrillator patients. *J Am Coll Cardiol.* 2010;55:2769–2777.
3. Marshall A1, Cheetham A, George RS, et al. Cardiac iodine-123 metaiodobenzylguanidine imaging predicts ventricular arrhythmia in heart failure patients receiving an implantable cardioverter-defibrillator for primary prevention. *Heart.* 2012;98:1359–1365.
4. Agostini D, Ananthasubramaniam K, Chandna H, et al. Prognostic usefulness of planar 123I-MIBG scintigraphic images of myocardial sympathetic innervation in congestive heart failure: Follow-up data from ADMIRE-HF. *J Nucl Cardiol.* 2021;28(4):1490–1503.
5. Ogita H, Shimonagata T, Fukunami M, et al. Prognostic significance of cardiac ^{123}I metaiodobenzylguanidine imaging for mortality and morbidity in patients with chronic heart failure: A prospective study. *Heart.* 2001;86:656–660.
6. D'Orio Nishioka SA, Filho MM, Soares Brandão SC, et al. Cardiac sympathetic activity pre and post resynchronization therapy evaluated by 123I-MIBG myocardial scintigraphy. *J Nucl Cardiol.* 2007;14:852–859.
7. Gerson MC, McGuire N, Wagoner LE. Sympathetic nervous system function as measured by I-123 metaiodobenzylguanidine predicts transplant-free survival in heart failure patients with idiopathic dilated cardiomyopathy. *J Card Fail.* 2003;9:384–391.

QUESTIONS

1. In a patient with NYHA Class II–III HF with a reduced EF (<35%), a planar cardiac ^{123}I-*m*IBG HMR of more than 1.6 is associated with:
   a. A low (<5%) risk of an arrhythmic event over the following 2 years
   b. Increased myocardial tracer washout
   c. Tracer defects on tomographic imaging
   d. A high risk of a cardiac event over the next 10 years

2. In patients with HF with reduced EF, the prognostic significance of a summed dysinnervation score of 30

on tomographic ^{123}I-*m*IBG images is which of the following?

a. Patient risk will depend more on the specific LVEF.
b. Risk of a cardiac event is increased compared with a summed score lower than 10.
c. The score is not associated with increased risk of an adverse cardiac event if the HMR is low (<1.6).
d. The score is associated with lower likelihood of an ICD discharge.

3. On tomographic ^{123}I-*m*IBG imaging, the presence of preserved uptake of perfusion radiotracer in a region with decreased ^{123}I-*m*IBG uptake signifies which of the following?
   a. The ^{123}I-*m*IBG defect is unlikely to predict increased risk.
   b. The presence of preserved perfusion likely increases the risk of a ventricular arrhythmia.
   c. The patient is at lower risk of having an ischemic event.
   d. If in the anterior wall, the ^{123}I-*m*IBG defect is likely to be an artifact.

ANSWERS

1a. In the ADMIRE-HF multicenter study, for 961 patients with NYHA Class II–III HF and reduced EF, an HMR of 1.6 or more was associated with a relatively low risk (3.5%) of an arrhythmic event over approximately 2 years compared with a risk of 10.4% for patients with an HMR of less than 1.6. Tracer washout is not directly related to HMR, and an increased washout is associated with high risk. Findings on tomographic imaging are not specifically related to global tracer uptake on planar images. The most recent follow-up study of ADMIRE-HF patients analyzed follow-up to about 5 years, and continued to find that an HMR of at least 1.6 persisted in predicting a lower cardiac event rate compared with an HMR of less than 1.6. At the time of this writing, there are no reported data on longer follow-up in a large patient cohort.

2b. While compared with planar ^{123}I-*m*IBG imaging there are not as many prognostic data on tomographic imaging, higher defect scores (in one report >26) are associated with increased adverse cardiac events, including a higher likelihood of ventricular arrhythmias and ICD discharges. Patients with tomographic defects and low HMR are likely to be at even higher risk. The predictive value of cardiac ^{123}I-*m*IBG data has been consistently shown to be independent of LVEF.

3b. Animal work and some clinical studies have shown that preserved perfusion in a cardiac region with decreased ^{123}I-*m*IBG uptake (i.e., an adrenergic–perfusion mismatch) produces an area of denervation supersensitivity that increases arrhythmogenicity. In addition, even in the absence of known CAD with no defect seen with a perfusion radiotracer, as neural injury from an ischemic insult persists longer than injury to myocytes, the ^{123}I-*m*IBG defect may indicate a prior ischemic event, such as from an aborted MI or coronary spasm. Given these known circumstances in which an adrenergic defect can be present in the absence of a perfusion defect, without any obvious image-quality issue such as overlying extra cardiac activity or attenuation, an ^{123}I-*m*IBG defect, unless in the inferior wall (sometimes seen in older people without known cardiac pathology), is unlikely to be an artifact.

22.

IMAGING SARCOID HEART DISEASE

David G. Rosenthal and Paco E. Bravo

CASE 1

A 60-year-old man with a history of hypertension and dyslipidemia (treated with simvastatin), previously asymptomatic, experienced a family-witnessed episode of sudden cardiac arrest due to ventricular fibrillation. He was successfully defibrillated and the post-resuscitation ECG (Figure 22.1) revealed normal sinus rhythm, with a right bundle branch block but without evidence of significant ST-segment deviations. The patient underwent a left heart catheterization the same day of the arrest that revealed no significant coronary artery disease. Echocardiography showed a non-dilated LV, with moderate LV hypertrophy, and mild systolic dysfunction, but without obvious regional wall-motion abnormalities. He had a full neurologic recovery and eventually underwent CMR (Figure 22.2) as part of the workup for his cardiac arrest episode. The study showed extensive LGE primarily involving the sub-epicardium and mid-myocardium of the septum and inferior wall from base to apex, in a pattern highly suggestive of CS. There was also a small amount of sub-endocardial LGE at the lateral wall, which can often coexist with sub-epicardial and mid-myocardial involvement of the LV. However, based on current guidelines, the patient did not meet criteria for CS as there was no evidence of biopsy-proven disease.[1] Therefore, an EMB of the right ventricle was pursued, demonstrating non-necrotizing granulomatous inflammation associated with extensive fibrosis and thus confirming the CS diagnosis. At this point, it was clear that sarcoid infiltration was the most likely substrate that triggered the malignant ventricular event. In addition to getting an ICD placed for secondary prevention of cardiac arrest (Class I recommendation),[1] the patient also underwent an F-18 FDG PET/CT scan (Figure 22.3) to assess for the presence and extent of active inflammation in the heart as recommended by an expert consensus.[2] The study was performed in combination with rubidium-82 myocardial perfusion imaging to spatially co-localize FDG activity with perfusion abnormalities. Images showed extensive FDG activity involving most of the septum and extending toward the inferior and anterior wall segments. In addition, there were perfusion defects at the basal and mid-inferior wall, as well as the basal anterior septum. Overall, findings were in keeping with extensive myocardial inflammation from sarcoid infiltration. Following these results, the patient was started on prednisone 40 mg, and the dose was tapered down to 20 mg over the course of weeks. A repeat PET/CT scan 6 months later (Figure 22.4) showed complete resolution of myocardial inflammation. As expected, myocardial perfusion defects remain unchanged. The patient was continued on low-dose prednisone (10 mg/day) and remained without evidence of myocardial inflammation on subsequent PET/CT scans, and free from further ventricular arrhythmic events over the next 2 years of follow-up. During this time, his New York Heart Association functional class ranged between I and II, and his LV function remained mildly reduced, most likely as the result of myocardial fibrosis.

This case summarizes a classic presentation for the leading cause of death in patients with CS, including the typical workup involved, and subsequent management to prevent future adverse events.

CASE 2

A 57-year-old man with a history of diabetes and suspected sarcoidosis presented to the emergency department with back pain, subjective fevers, chills, cough, palpitations, and unintentional weight loss for several weeks. He was presumptively diagnosed with sarcoidosis after the pathology from an enlarging neck mass revealed noncaseating granulomas 2 years prior to this presentation. Treatment was not considered back then as he denied systemic symptoms. However, this time, he was found to have severe hypercalcemia (14.8 mg/dL; upper reference = 10.3 mg/dL) and acute kidney injury (creatinine 4.09 mg/dL; baseline 1.31 mg/dL).

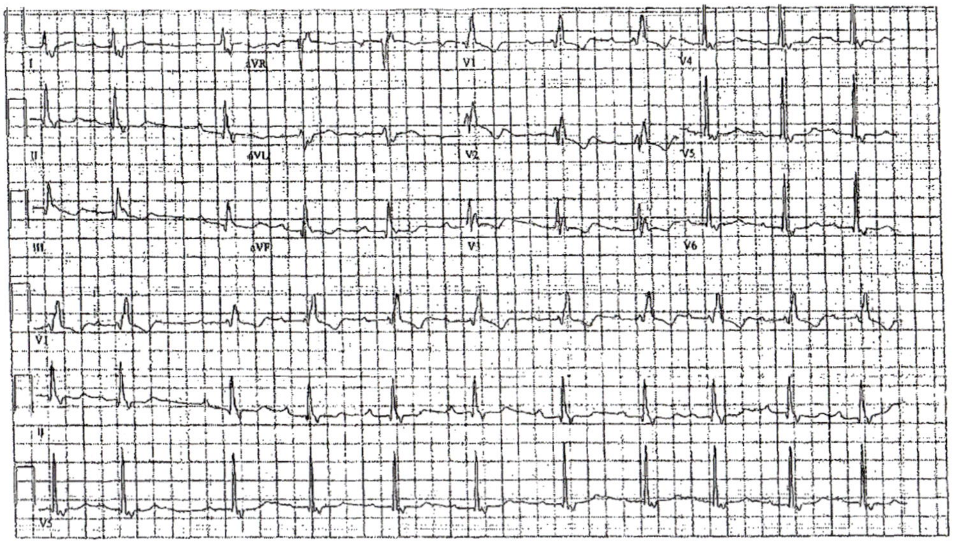

Figure 22.1. Case 1. Post-resuscitation ECG shows normal sinus rhythm and right bundle branch block.

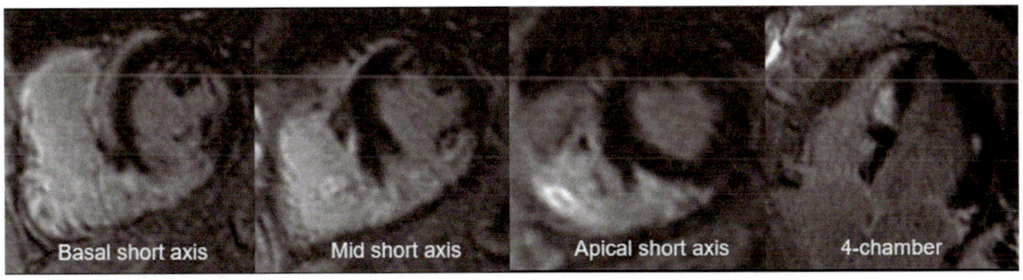

Figure 22.2. Case 1. CMR with extensive LGE.

A chest x-ray showed slight interstitial prominence (Figure 22.5), and a chest CT confirmed numerous pulmonary nodules (Figure 22.6A), and mildly prominent bilateral axillary, cervical, mediastinal, and hilar lymph nodes, possibly related to the patient's presumed sarcoidosis. CT also showed extensive coronary calcification (Figure 22.6B). The patient was started empirically on steroids for presumed sarcoid flare. There was also a concern for cardiac involvement due to the patient's reported history of palpitations, and the capture of short runs of nonsustained VT on telemetry. Echocardiography revealed a non-dilated LV with low-normal systolic function and a possible area of hypo-contractility at the anterior wall. A cardiac MRI would have been the next option to evaluate for CS; however, given his current renal dysfunction, the decision was made to proceed with cardiac PET/CT. The study was performed after the patient followed the ketogenic diet for 24 hours to

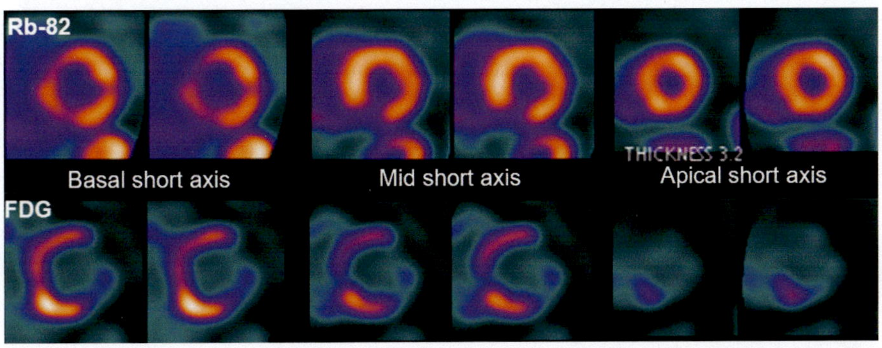

Figure 22.3. Case 1. Baseline cardiac PET/CT with Rb-82 (top row) and F-18 FDG (bottom row) showing typical imaging findings for CS.

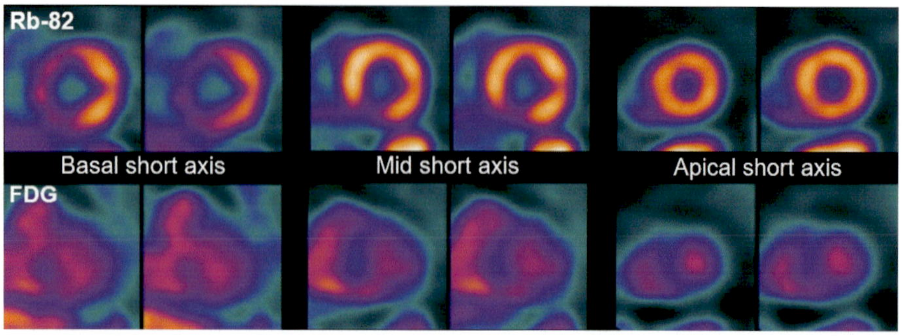

Figure 22.4. Case 1. Follow-up cardiac PET/CT with Rb-82 (top row) and F-18 FDG (bottom row) showing complete treatment response after initiation of prednisone.

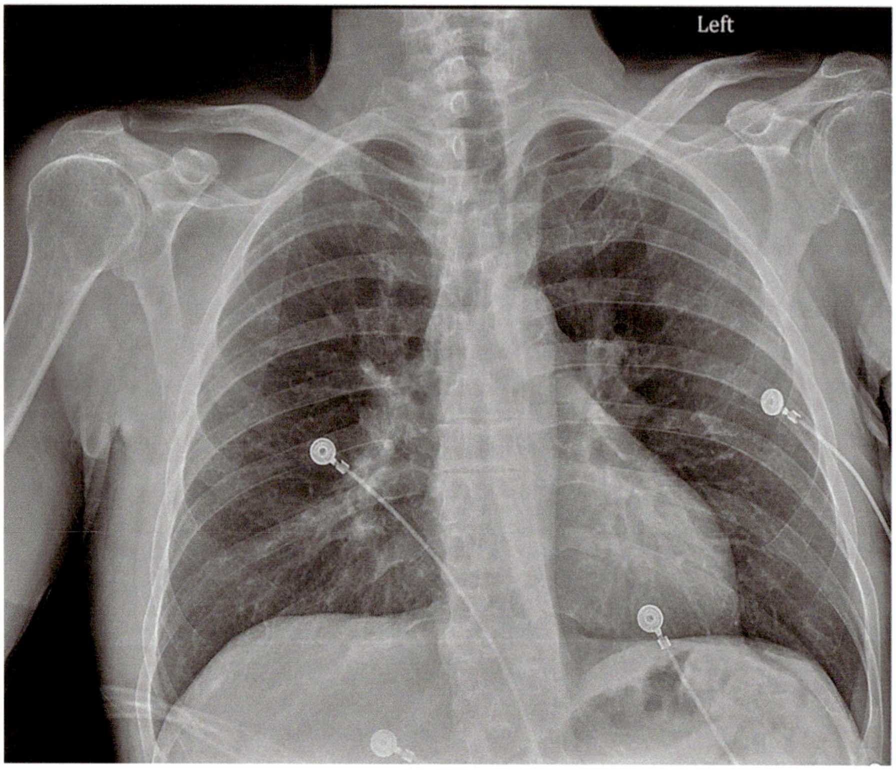

Figure 22.5. Case 2. Chest x-ray suggest the possibility of interstitial prominence bilaterally.

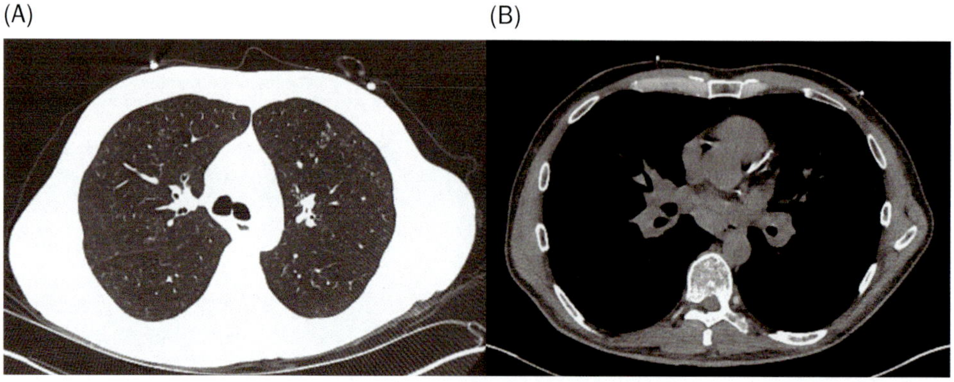

Figure 22.6. Case 2. Chest CT without contrast. (A) Lung window shows numerous pulmonary nodules. (b) Soft tissue window to highlight the extensive coronary calcification present in this patient.

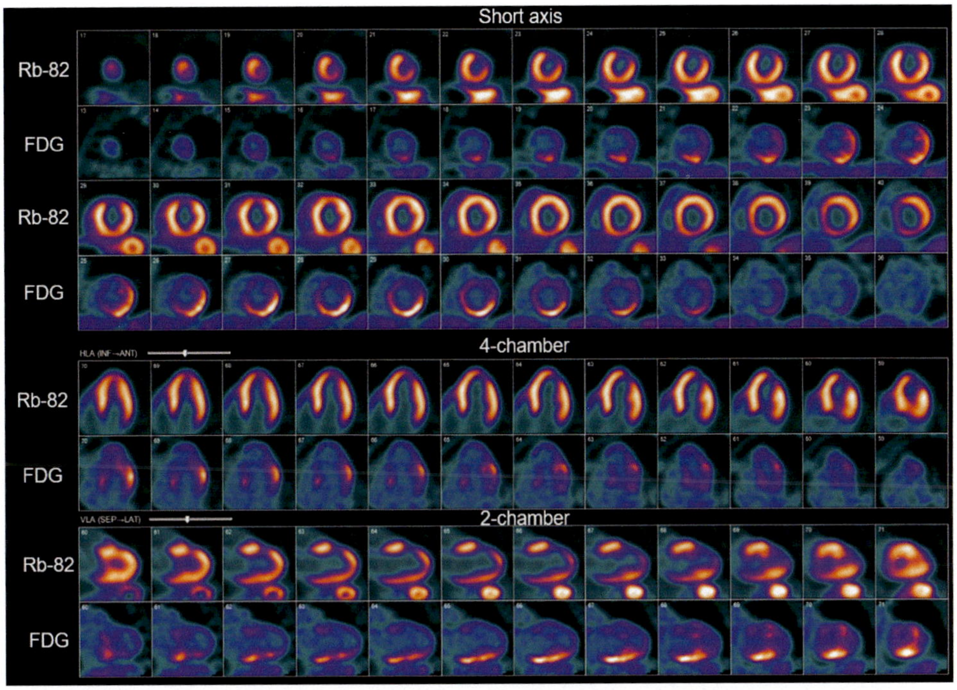

Figure 22.7. Case 2. Initial myocardial perfusion with Rb-82 and metabolic imaging with FDG PET/CT following 24 hours of preparation with the ketogenic diet.

suppress physiologic glucose uptake in the heart (Figure 22.7). Rb-82 perfusion images at rest demonstrated a severe defect at the mid to apical anterior wall, whereas the FDG images showed extensive, heterogeneous uptake along most of the LV in a pattern that was equivocal for inflammation and suspicious for incomplete suppression. Consequently, per our protocol and in light of recent evidence,[3,4] the FDG portion of the study was repeated after the patient followed the ketogenic diet for 72 hours. This repeat study (Figure 22.8) now clearly demonstrated focal FDG activity along the entire inferior wall, extending into the inferior septum, compatible with inflammation in the right clinical context. The patient was discharged home on prednisone (60 mg/day) with the plan to taper down the dose. However, the patient returned to the hospital just 10 days later complaining of shortness of breath and chest heaviness. ECG showed normal sinus rhythm with stable nonspecific ST-T changes, but this time his troponin T level was mildly elevated, eventually peaking at 0.501 ng/mL the following day. He remained with significant renal dysfunction and thus underwent stress testing with Rb-82 PET/CT (Figure 22.9) for further evaluation of this new event. The study showed a medium-sized area of moderate reversibility in the inferior wall suggestive of flow-limiting coronary artery disease in the typical distribution of the right coronary artery. In addition, a fixed defect in the mid-distal anterior wall was again seen, suggestive of a possible prior infarct in a diagonal branch distribution, relatively unchanged compared to the resting perfusion images seen on the baseline exam. Given the clinical picture, the patient underwent invasive coronary angiography despite the resolving renal dysfunction (creatinine down to 2.65 mg/dL), which evidenced the presence of obstructive coronary artery disease in a right dominant system (Figure 22.10). The right coronary artery (see Figure 22.10A) showed a 70% stenosis in the proximal segment (solid arrow) and a chronic subtotal occlusion in its midportion (dashed arrow). The left coronary artery (see Figure 22.10B) was diffusely diseased with up to 50% stenosis in the first diagonal branch and first obtuse marginal. No intervention was performed on the lesion in the right coronary artery, and the decision was made to medically manage the patient. Consequently, and in retrospect, the intense FDG activity seen in the inferior and inferior septum on PET/CT imaging (see Figure 22.8) was most likely the result of ongoing ischemia rather than inflammation.[5,6]

This case vignette highlights the importance of excluding coronary artery disease as a potential driver for myocardial FDG uptake, particularly in patient with cardiovascular risk factors, FDG uptake following a coronary vascular distribution, and presence of extensive coronary calcification on CT.

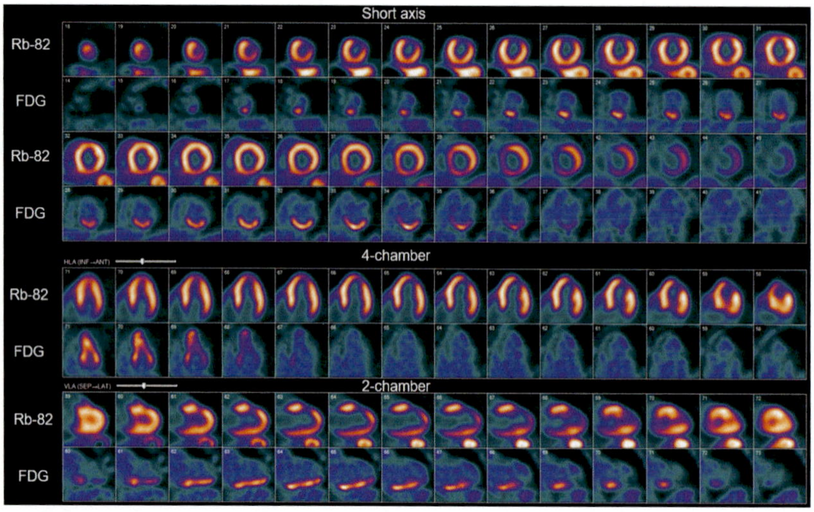

Figure 22.8. Case 2. Repeat FDG PET/CT evaluation 4 days later following 72 hours of preparation with the ketogenic diet. Rb-82 images are the same from the initial evaluation.

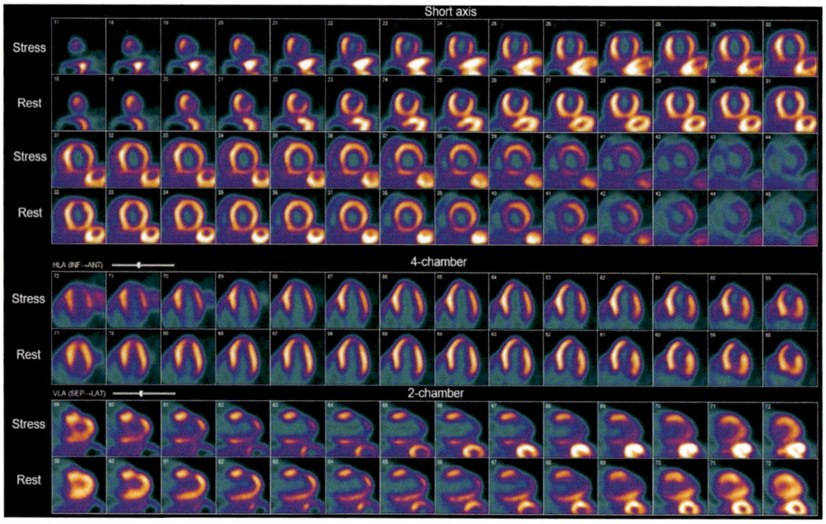

Figure 22.9. Case 2. Rest and stress myocardial perfusion imaging with Rb-82 PET/CT.

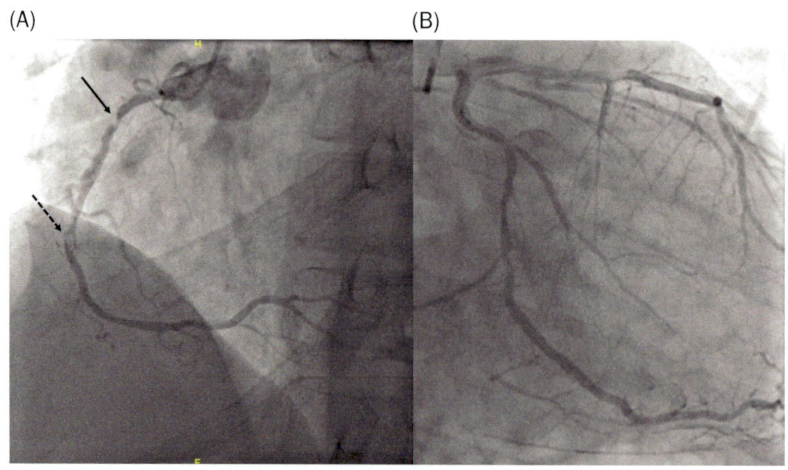

Figure 22.10. Case 2. Invasive coronary angiography. (A) Right coronary with obstructive disease in the proximal (70% stenosis; solid arrow) and mid-segment (subtotal occlusion; dashed arrow). (B) Left coronary system shows diffuse nonobstructive disease.

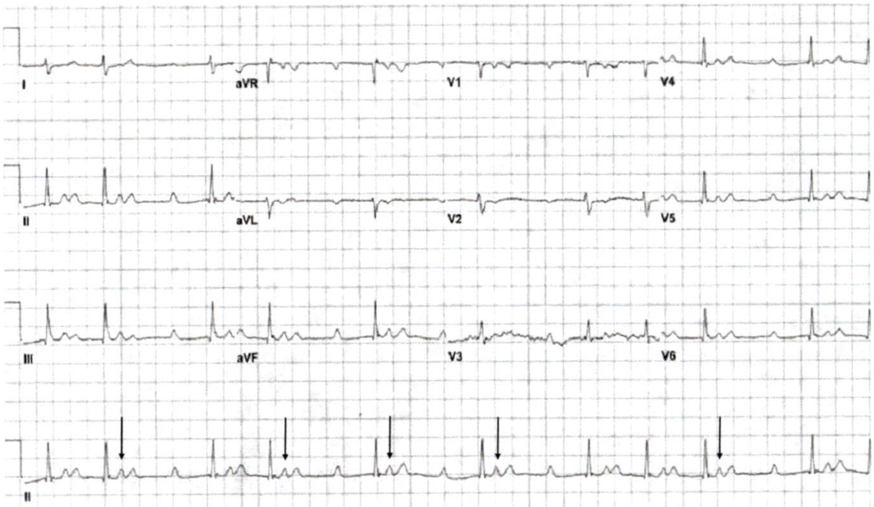

Figure 22.11. Case 3. ECG revealing second-degree Mobitz II AV block. Arrows are pointing at the nonconducting P-waves.

CASE 3

The patient is a 37-year-old woman with new-onset heart block. She had no past medical history and was very active. However, a few weeks prior to her presentation, she started to notice getting easily fatigued and lightheaded. She visited the emergency department and an ECG revealed normal sinus rhythm with Mobitz II second-degree AV block (Figure 22.11). Cardiac markers, complete blood count, and biochemistry findings were unremarkable, and serology was negative for Lyme disease. She underwent cardiac MRI (Figure 22.12) as part of her workup, which revealed an LV that was normal in size and function, without definite evidence of myocardial edema or LGE to suggest

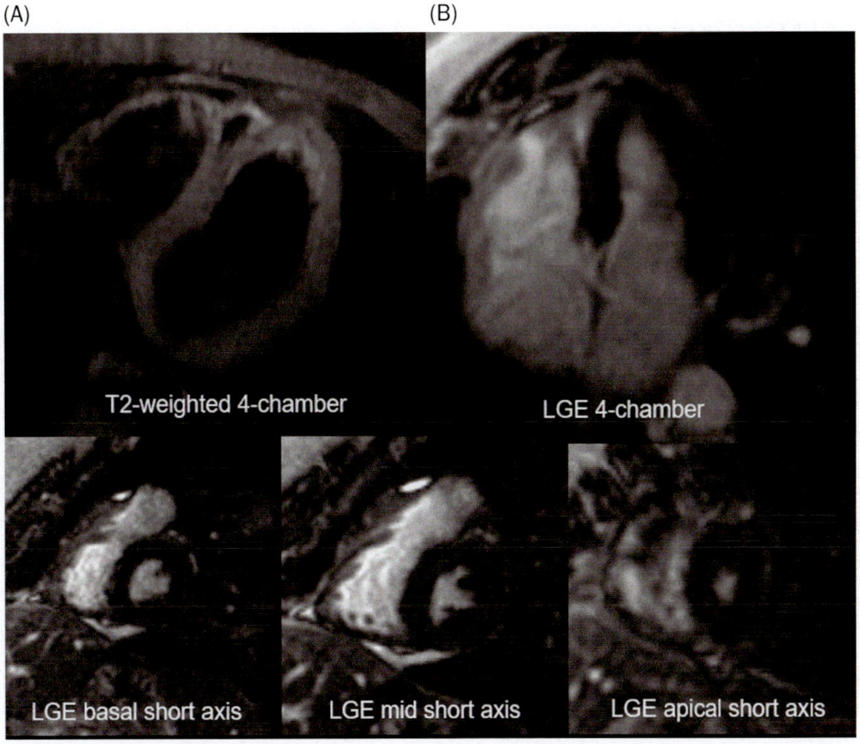

Figure 22.12. Case 3. CMR without evidence of myocardial edema on T2-weighted or scarring on LGE imaging.

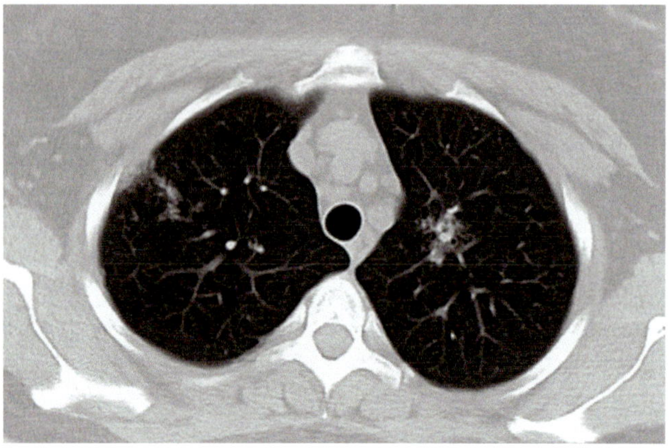

Figure 22.13. Case 3. Chest CT showing ground-glass pulmonary nodules in both upper lobes, suggestive of an inflammatory process.

acute myocarditis or sarcoidosis. A chest CT (Figure 22.13), however, demonstrated predominantly upper lobe pulmonary opacities and mediastinal lymph nodes at the upper limit of normal in size suspicious for sarcoidosis. Her serum angiotensin-1-converting enzyme levels were markedly elevated (354; reference 9–67 U/L). Transbronchial biopsy of some of these nodules showed nonspecific interstitial chronic inflammatory parenchymal changes but failed to reveal granulomas. The patient underwent a dual-chamber pacemaker implantation, without defibrillator capabilities as there was no convincing evidence of CS on MRI. She had a very extensive negative rheumatologic workup as well and was discharged home on a short course of prednisone because of the concern of a nonspecific interstitial pneumonia. However, the patient continued to report some degree of fatigue, and further evaluation with cardiac FDG PET/CT was pursued on an outpatient basis as the clinical suspicion for sarcoidosis remained high. The PET scan (Figure 22.14) showed unequivocal evidence of extensive multi-organ inflammation in the lungs, mediastinum, hilum, bone, liver, spleen, as well as the heart, in a pattern most compatible with metabolically active sarcoidosis. Within the heart, inflammation was most noticeable at the basal-to-mid inferior interventricular septum, the mid-to-apical LV anterolateral wall, and the apical right ventricular free wall. All these areas failed to reveal concomitant LGE on prior CMR and were, consequently, most likely to represent a phenotype of early-stage cardiac sarcoidosis as previously reported (Figure 22.15).[7] The intense inflammation at the interventricular septum corresponded well to the clinical presentation of high-degree AV block. Endobronchial ultrasound-guided lymph node sampling was considered but not pursued. Despite the absence of biopsy-proven disease, there was compelling evidence clinically of the presence of multisystemic sarcoidosis with cardiac involvement. In addition, she has been noted to have runs of nonsustained ventricular arrhythmias on subsequent device interrogations. Therefore, her device was upgraded to an ICD (Class IIa recommendation).[1] Concomitantly, the patient was started on immunotherapy with prednisone (40 mg/day) and methotrexate (15 mg/week) and her treatment response was serially assessed with FDG PET/CT over the next 2 years (Figure 22.16). Throughout this time, she exhibited appropriate response to treatment with evidence of cardiac inflammation relapse at only one point, which resolved after adding leflunomide to her regimen. No episodes of sustained ventricular arrhythmias and/or hospitalizations for HF were recorded during this follow-up time.

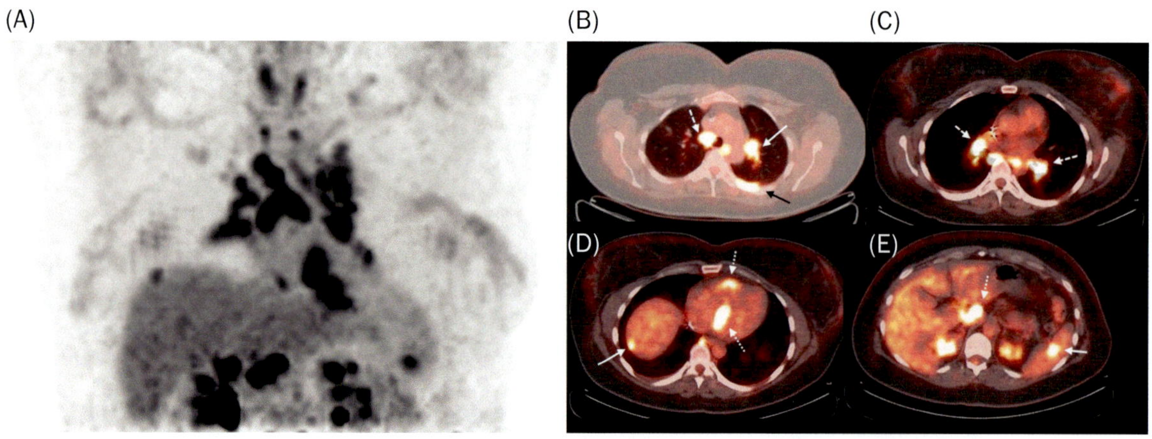

Figure 22.14. Case 3. Maximal intensity projection PET image (A) of the chest and upper abdomen displaying extensive multi-organ inflammation. Fused PET/CT images shows FDG-avid disease in the lung parenchyma (B; solid white arrow), left posterior rib (B; black arrow), mediastinum and hilar nodes (B, C; dashed white arrows), dome of the liver (D; solid arrow), heart (dashed arrows), spleen (E; solid arrow) and abdominal lymph nodes (E; dashed arrow).

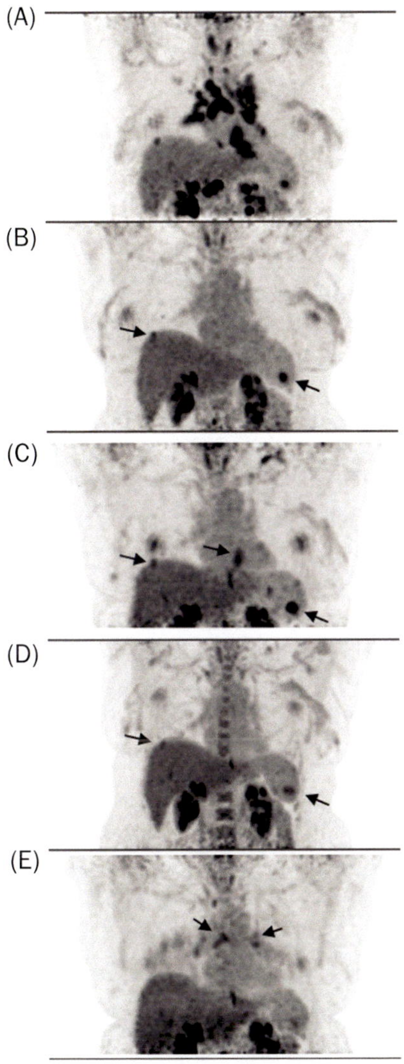

Figure 22.16. Serial FDG PET imaging for the purpose of monitoring therapy response. (A) Baseline scan with extensive extracardiac and cardiac inflammation. (B) 5-month post-therapy scan shows resolution of cardiac inflammation, with only residual inflammation at the dome of the liver and spleen (arrows). (C) 9-month post-therapy scan shows relapse of cardiac inflammation at the interventricular septum, and residual inflammation at the liver and spleen. (D) 15-month post-therapy scan reveals resolution of cardiac inflammation and residual inflammation at the spleen and liver. (E) 24-month post-therapy scan demonstrates resolution of splenic and hepatic inflammation, with some relapse of mediastinal and hilar inflammation. However, the heart remains inactive.

This case illustrates an example that in patients presenting with new-onset high-degree A-V block, and strong clinical suspicion of sarcoidosis, FDG PET may be useful for detecting cardiac involvement in spite of a negative cardiac MRI.

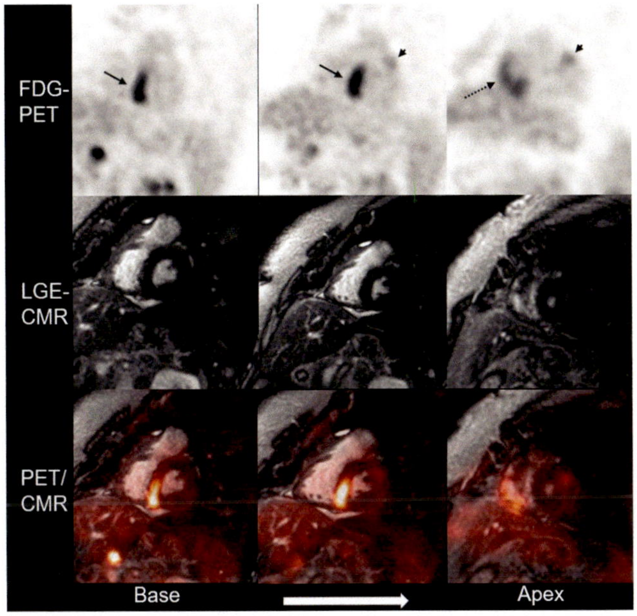

Figure 22.15. Case 3. Co-registration of cardiac FDG PET images with previous cardiac MRI. Notice the FDG uptake in the inferior interventricular septum (solid arrows), LV anterolateral wall (arrowhead), and free right ventricular wall (dashed arrow), without corresponding areas of LGE on CMR.

REFREENCES

1. Birnie DH, Sauer WH, Bogun F, et al. HRS expert consensus statement on the diagnosis and management of arrhythmias associated with cardiac sarcoidosis. *Heart Rhythm*. 2014;11(7):1305–1323.
2. Chareonthaitawee P, Beanlands RS, Chen W, et al. Joint SNMMI-ASNC expert consensus document on the role of (18)F-FDG PET/CT in cardiac sarcoid detection and therapy monitoring. *J Nucl Med*. 2017;58(8):1341–1353.
3. Lu Y, Grant C, Xie K, Sweiss NJ. Suppression of myocardial 18F-FDG uptake through prolonged high-fat, high-protein, and very-low-carbohydrate diet before FDG-PET/CT for evaluation of patients with suspected cardiac sarcoidosis. *Clin Nucl Med*. 2017;42(2):88–94.
4. Ozutemiz C, Koksel Y, Froelich JW, et al. Comparison of the effect of three different dietary modifications on myocardial suppression in (18)F-FDG PET/CT evaluation of patients for suspected cardiac sarcoidosis. *J Nucl Med*. 2021;62(12):1759–1767.
5. Sibille L, Chambert B, Collombier L, et al. False-positive 18F-FDG PET/CT in cardiac sarcoidosis. *J Mol Biol Mol Imaging*. 2015;2(2):1020.
6. Lopaschuk GD, Stanley WC. Glucose metabolism in the ischemic heart. *Circulation*. 1997;95(2):313–315.
7. Ohira H, Birnie DH, Pena E, et al. Comparison of (18)F-fluorodeoxyglucose positron emission tomography (FDG PET) and cardiac magnetic resonance (CMR) in corticosteroid-naive patients with conduction system disease due to cardiac sarcoidosis. *Eur J Nucl Med Mol Imaging*. 2016;43(2):259–269.

23.

IMAGING AMYLOID HEART DISEASE

John P. Bois, Martha Grogan, and Panithaya Chareonthaitawee

CASE 1

A 66-year-old male presents with a 5-year history of unexplained watery diarrhea with accompanying 40-pound weight loss and negative upper and lower endoscopies. He also endorses a history of progressive bilateral upper and lower extremity paresthesia, fatigue, and dysgeusia. He recalls that his father suffered from progressive muscle wasting, lower extremity weakness, and edema before succumbing to HF of unclear etiology at age 73.

Physical examination demonstrates mild muscle wasting with absent biceps and ankle reflexes. Left ankle dorsiflexion weakness was noted on manual muscle testing. Sensory examination showed length-dependent sensory loss to small greater than large fibers. Cardiovascular examination was notable for regular rate and rhythm with no murmurs, gallops, or rubs. No lower extremity edema was appreciated.

Laboratory testing was remarkable for a normocytic anemia (11.7 g/dL), and an elevated creatinine (1.6 g/dL), troponin I (0.05 ng/mL, upper limit of normal [ULN] 0.03 ng/mL), and NT-proBNP (5,540 pg/mL). Renal function, troponin, and NT-proBNP in particular have proven useful in amyloid risk-prediction assessment.[1,2] Monoclonal protein studies were negative: kappa free light chain 1.31 mg/dL (ULN 1.94 mg/dL), lambda free light chain 1.30 md/dL (ULN 2.63 mg/dL), and free light chain ratio 1.0 (normal range 0.26–1.65).

Chest x-ray demonstrated a chronic left rib fracture. Resting 12-lead ECG showed sinus rhythm with first-degree AV block, premature ventricular complexes, and low anterior forces (Figure 23.1). Classic teaching notes discordance between increased LV wall thickness and low-voltage QRS on ECG. However, this finding has limited sensitivity and has been reported in approximately 60% of AL amyloid cases and 20% of ATTR amyloid cases.[3]

Transthoracic echocardiogram revealed severe concentric LV hypertrophy, right ventricular hypertrophy, abnormal longitudinal peak systolic strain (−9%) with apical sparing, severe bilateral enlargement, and increased filling pressures (▶ Videos 23.1 and 23.2 and Figure 23.2). The reduced longitudinal shortening of the basal segments with relative spring of the apical segments is characteristic of both AL and ATTR amyloidosis and can help to differentiate this disease from other cardiac pathologies that also present with LV hypertrophy such as aortic stenosis and hypertrophic cardiomyopathy, which manifest with a strain pattern that is typically reduced in areas of maximal myocardial hypertrophy.[4]

^{99m}Tc-PYP SPECT/CT scan was performed and was positive with a H/CL ratio of 1.84, with confirmed myocardial uptake hybrid SPECT/CT axial fused images (Figures 23.3 and 23.4). ^{99m}Tc-PYP cardiac scintigraphy is recommended if there is a clinical suspicion of cardiac amyloidosis, especially if ATTR subtype is suspected as it can provide critical diagnostic and prognostic information that may guide medical management.[5] Specifically, a positive ^{99m}Tc-PYP scan in the absence of a monoclonal process in the right clinical setting has excellent sensitivity and specificity for cardiovascular involvement of ATTR, and a high burden of disease (as defined by an H/CL ratio of > 1.6), as noted in this case, is associated with decreased survival.[6]

Subsequent fat pad biopsy confirmed familial TTR amyloidosis (T60A mutation) and the patient was initiated on tafamidis therapy.

QUESTION

1. The 1-hour ^{99m}Tc-PYP H/CL ratio is 1.84 in a 66-year-old man with HFpEF. Monoclonal protein studies were negative. What is the next best step among the choices below?
   a. Perform cardiac biopsy
   b. Perform fat aspirate
   c. Perform ^{99m}Tc-PYP SPECT imaging
   d. Re-acquire images at 3 hours after ^{99m}Tc-PYP injection

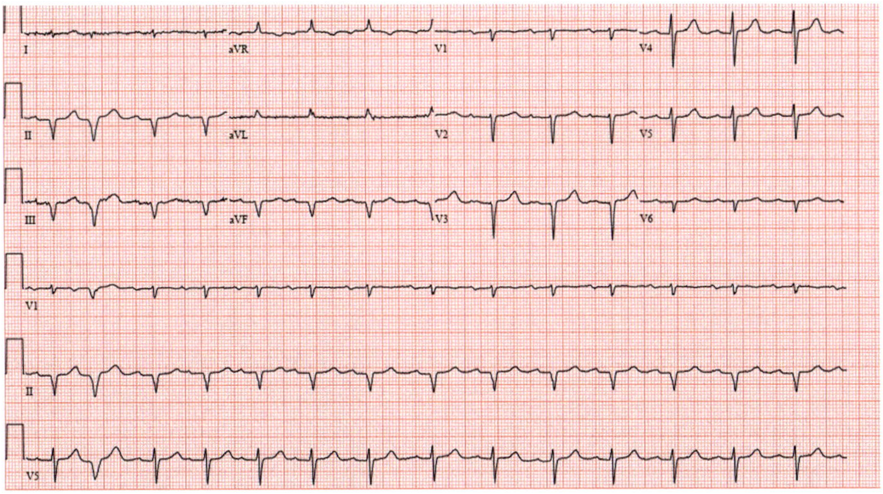

Figure 23.1. Resting twelve-lead ECG demonstrates sinus rhythm, first degree A-V block, a single PVC and low anterior forces.

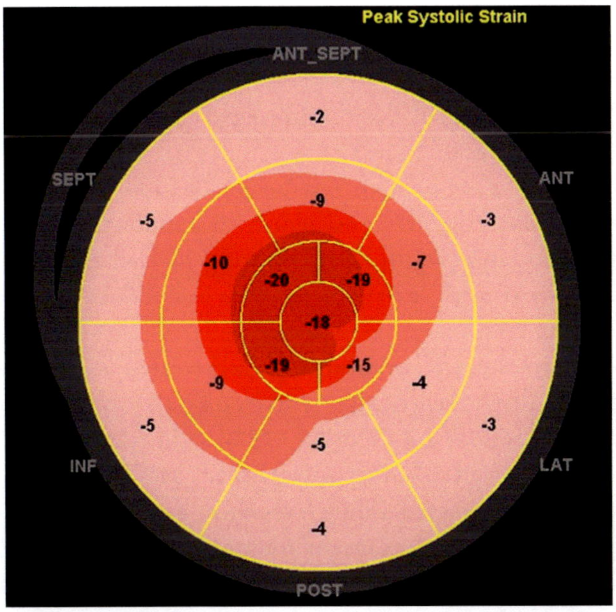

Figure 23.2 Global longitudinal peak systolic strain was reduced with sparing of the apex consistent with cardiac amyloidosis. (abnormal strain with apical sparing).

e. Re-acquire images at 6 hours after ^{99m}Tc-PYP injection

ANSWER

1c. The next best step would be to perform and review ^{99m}Tc-PYP SPECT images to differentiate between blood pool activity and myocardial tracer uptake and look for possible causes of a false-positive H/CL ratio. Cardiac biopsy should be performed in the presence of an abnormal free light chain assay or evidence of a monoclonal protein regardless of the grade of myocardial ^{99m}Tc-PYP uptake, or if high suspicion remains for TTR CA in the presence of a negative ^{99m}Tc-PYP study. The presence of amyloid in noncardiac sites such as the abdominal fat pad along with typical echocardiographic or CMR findings may be sufficient to diagnose CA but is only positive in 15% of ATTRwt cases.[7] A negative fat pad biopsy is therefore insufficient to exclude the diagnosis, and biopsy of an involved organ would offer the highest yield.[8] Re-acquiring the images at 3 hours may reduce blood pool activity, but it would be more efficient to proceed with SPECT images at 1 hour. Even at 3 hours SPECT images should also be used to differentiate between blood pool activity and myocardial tracer uptake and to look for possible causes of a false-positive or a false-negative H/CL ratio. ^{99m}Tc-PYP protocols for CA have mainly used acquisition at 1 hour or 3 hours.

CASE 2

A 70-year-old male with a history of persistent atrial fibrillation/atrial flutter and a remote history of biceps tendon rupture presents with a 6-month history of exertional dyspnea, orthopnea, and presyncope. Atrial fibrillation/flutter is the most common arrythmia in ATTR cardiac amyloidosis, occurring in over two-thirds of patients.[9] The loss of atrial kick that accompanies the onset of atrial fibrillation/flutter exacerbates diastolic dysfunction, thereby worsening symptoms of dyspnea and orthopnea.[10] Furthermore, ATTR deposition in the

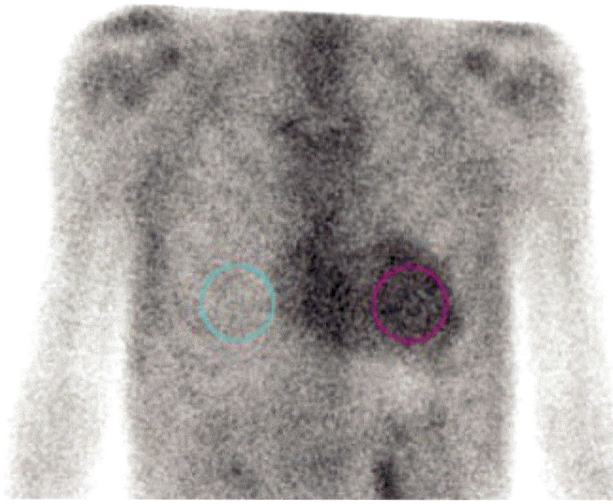

Figure 23.3. 99m Technetium-pyrophosphate SPECT/CT three-hour planar image heart (pink region of interest) to contralateral (turquoise region of interest) ratio is positive (>1.3). Imaging obtained at three hours.

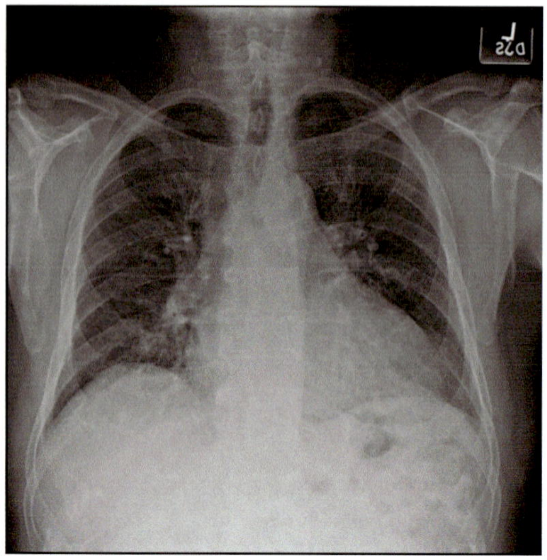

Figure 23.5. Posteroanterior chest x-ray demonstrates cephalization of the pulmonary vasculatures consistent with elevated pulmonary venous pressure.

biceps tendon predisposes amyloid patients to a 15-fold higher risk of tendon rupture compared to the general population, thereby serving as a critical diagnostic clue for the practitioner.[11]

Physical examination showed an irregularly irregular rhythm and mild abdominal distention. Laboratory testing was remarkable for a mild normocytic anemia (13.1 g/dL), an elevated high sensitivity troponin T (32 ng/L, ULN 15 ng/L), and an elevated NT-proBNP (2,118 pg/mL). Serum protein electrophoresis was negative for the presence of a monoclonal protein: kappa free light chain 1.29 mg/dL (ULN 1.94 mg/dL), lambda free light chain 1.10 mg/dL (ULN 2.63 mg/dL), and a free light chain ratio of 1.17 (normal range 0.26–1.65).

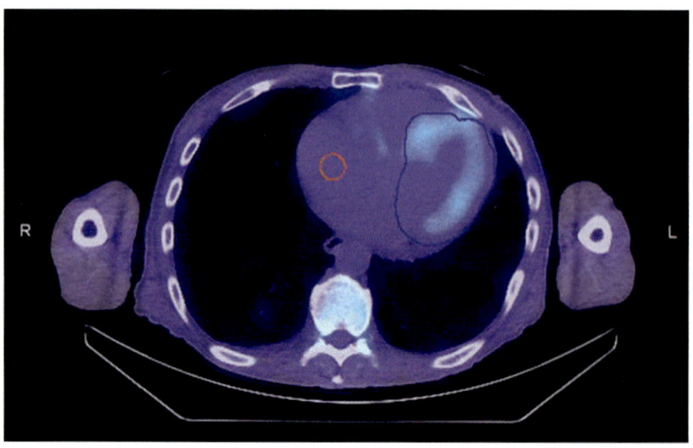

Figure 23.4. Hybrid SPECT/CT axial slice demonstrated myocardial uptake of 99m Technetium-pyrophosphate and confirms the positive planar and 3D scores consistent with ATTR cardiac amyloidosis in the right clinical setting. Imaging obtained at three hours.

Chest x-ray demonstrated cephalization of the pulmonary vasculature consistent with pulmonary venous hypertension (Figure 23.5). Resting 12-lead ECG was consistent with atrial flutter with variable AV block (Figure 23.6).

Transthoracic echocardiogram revealed concentric left and right ventricular hypertrophy, abnormal longitudinal peak systolic strain (−13%) with relative apical sparing, severe bilateral enlargement, small pericardial effusion, increased filling pressures, and a right ventricular systolic pressure of 61 mmHg (▶ Video 23.3 and Figures 23.7 and 23.8). The patient's pulmonary hypertension was likely secondary to increased left-sided filling pressures (type II pulmonary hypertension) rather than as a sequela of possible pulmonary amyloid fibril deposition, which rarely results in pulmonary hypertension.[12]

^{99m}Tc-PYP cardiac scintigraphy H/CL ratio was negative (1.24, positive ≥ 1.3). However, SPECT/CT imaging revealed myocardial PYP uptake consistent with a positive study (Figure 23.9). Reassessment of the planar images suggested that the contralateral ROI was erroneously placed over an area of focal PYP uptake (Figure 23.10), resulting in a false-negative H/CL score. The current case exemplifies the importance of assessing all acquired images and not solely relying on the initial H/CL ratio. The purpose of the contralateral lung ROI is to determine normal background rib uptake. However, if it is erroneously placed

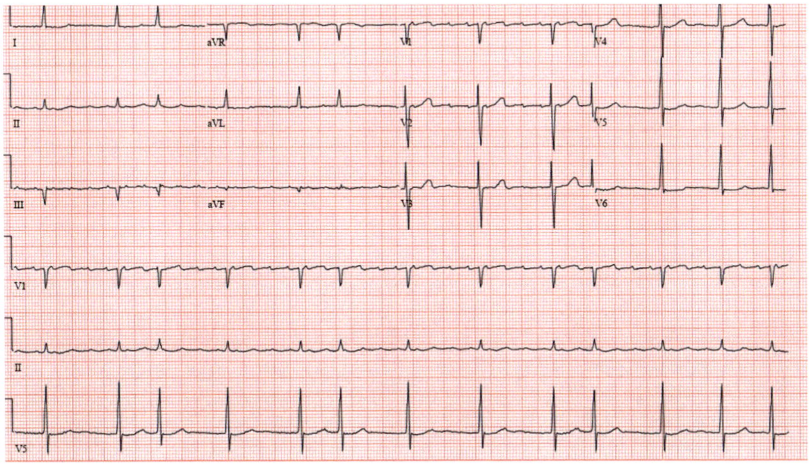

Figure 23.6. Resting 12-lead ECG demonstrates atrial flutter with variable A-V block.

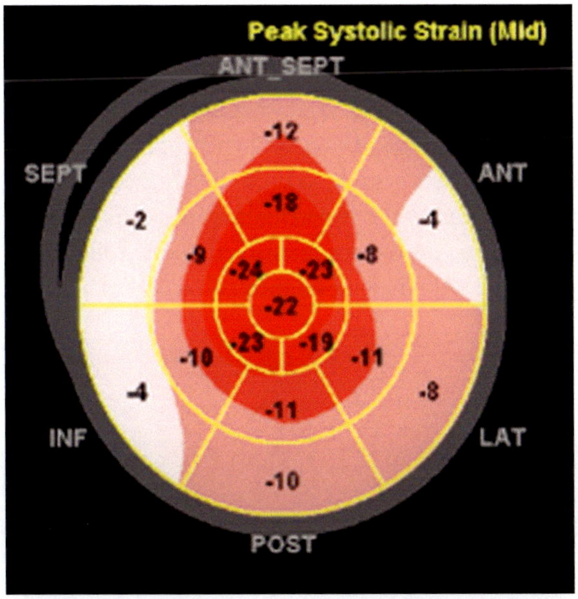

Figure 23.7. Global longitudinal peak systolic strain was reduced with sparing of the apex consistent with cardiac amyloidosis.

over an area with increased blood pool ^{99m}Tc-PYP, such as the right atrium (as most likely was the case in the current scenario), or in other areas of elevated PYP uptake such as a rib fracture, a false-negative result can occur. In the current case, the ROI could have been placed further cephalad to obtain a more accurate planar H/CL. In scenarios where the H/CL and SPECT or fused SPECT/CT images are discordant, the SPECT or SPECT/CT results take priority over the planar findings.[13]

The patient subsequently was enrolled in a therapeutic trial investing an RNA inference agent.

QUESTION

2. Which of the following findings may cause a "false-positive" ^{99m}Tc-PYP H/CL ratio on the 1-hour planar image in the absence of myocardial ^{99m}Tc-PYP uptake on SPECT images?
   a. Persistent blood pool ^{99m}Tc-PYP activity
   b. Rib fracture(s) or calcified costal cartilage overlying the contralateral ROI
   c. Skeletal muscle damage overlying the contralateral ROI
   d. Skin lesions overlying the contralateral ROI

ANSWER

2a. Persistent blood pool ^{99m}Tc-PYP activity is a common pitfall of planar imaging, and myocardial versus blood pool ^{99m}Tc-PYP activity may be challenging to differentiate on planar imaging and generally can be differentiated more easily on SPECT images. In the absence of myocardial ^{99m}Tc-PYP uptake on SPECT images, factors associated with increased activity in the contralateral ROI such as rib fractures, skeletal muscle damage, or skin lesions are more likely to cause a false-negative H/CL ratio, whereas factors associated with increased activity in the heart ROI such as

(A) (B)

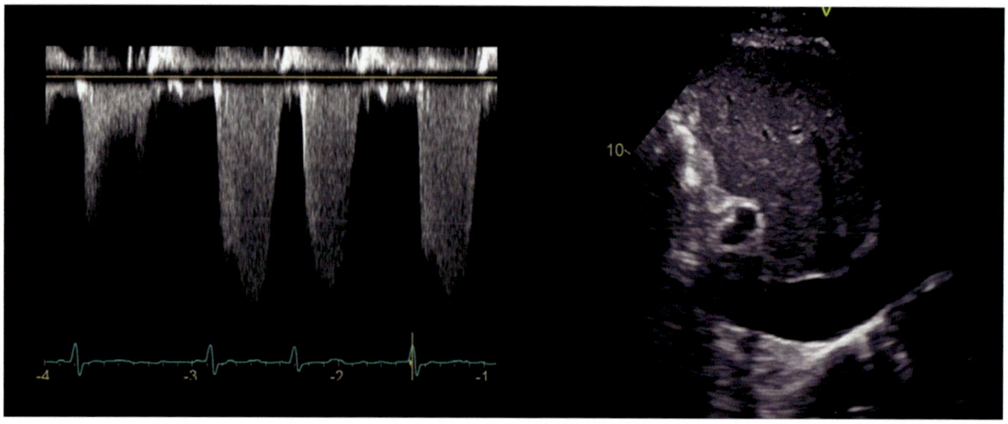

Figure 23.8 Right ventricular systolic pressures were elevated as noted by increased tricuspid valve regurgitant velocity as assessed by continuous-wave Doppler (A) and increased right atrial pressure as noted by dilated IVC (B).

rib fractures or skin lesions are more likely to cause a false-positive H/CL ratio.

CASE 3

An 85-year-old female with a history of difficult-to-manage HF with preserved EF (HFpEF) for the past year and stage 2 chronic renal disease presented with a week-long history of progressive exertional dyspnea, nocturnal cough, orthopnea, and bilateral lower extremity swelling. On physical examination the patient was noted to be tachypneic and tachycardiac with decreased breath sounds bilaterally, neck vein distention, and 2+ pitting lower extremity edema. Clinical examination and history were thereby consistent with the Framingham criteria for the diagnosis of HF.[14]

Laboratory studies were notable for decreased renal function (creatinine 2.1 mg/dL, glomerular filtration rate 23 mL/min/BSA), hyperkalemia (5.4 mmol/L), and hypermagnesemia (2.5 mg/dL). Resting 12-lead ECG demonstrated sinus rhythm with low-voltage QRS and septal q-waves (Figure 23.11). Transthoracic echocardiogram revealed mild-moderate concentric hypertrophy with abnormal longitudinal peak systolic strain (−10%). Cardiac MRI was notable for concentric hypertrophy with maximal thickness measuring 16 mm and no regional wall-motion abnormalities (▶ Video 23.4). There was difficulty nulling the blood pool,

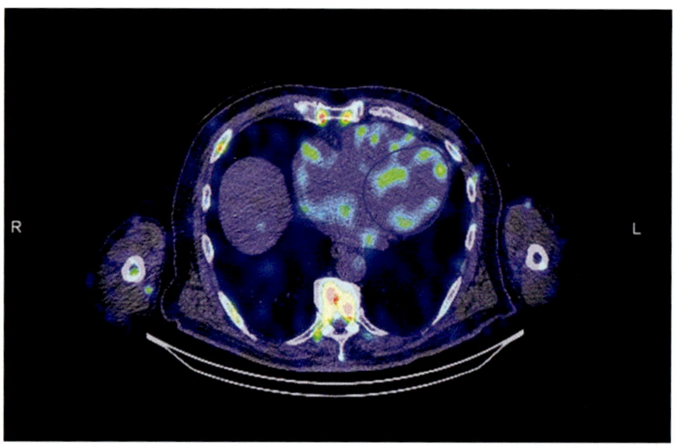

Figure 23.9 Hybrid SPECT/CT axial slice demonstrates myocardial PYP uptake. When there are discrepant results between the SPECT/CT scan and the planar scan (figure 6), the SPECT/CT results take priority. Imaging obtained at three hours.

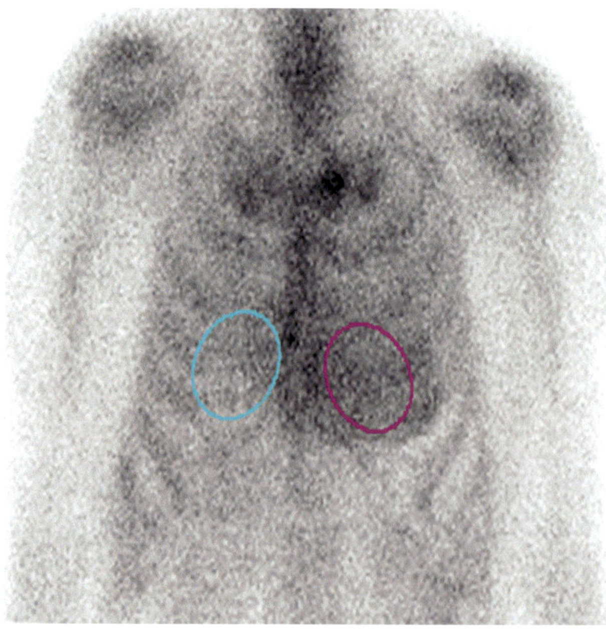

Figure 23.10 99mTc-PYP cardiac scintigraphy H/CL ratio was negative (1.24). However, note that the contralateral region of interest (blue circle) included an area of focal PYP uptake resulting in a false-negative H/CL ratio. Imaging obtained at three hours.

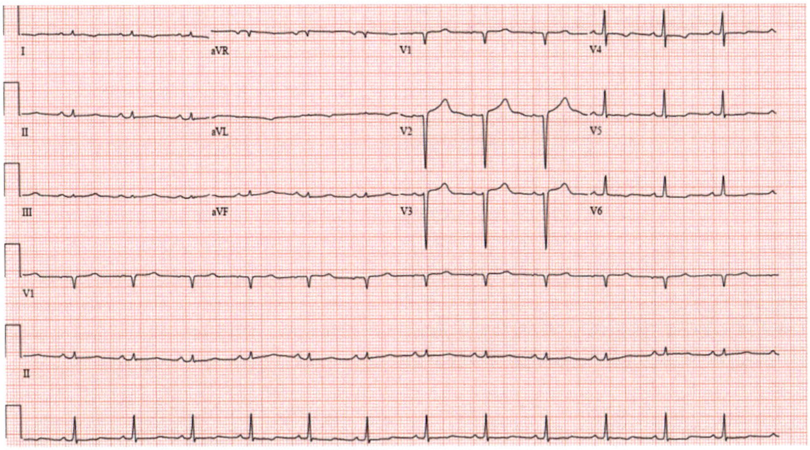

Figure 23.11 Resting twelve-lead ECG demonstrates sinus rhythm with anteroseptal q waves and low voltage.

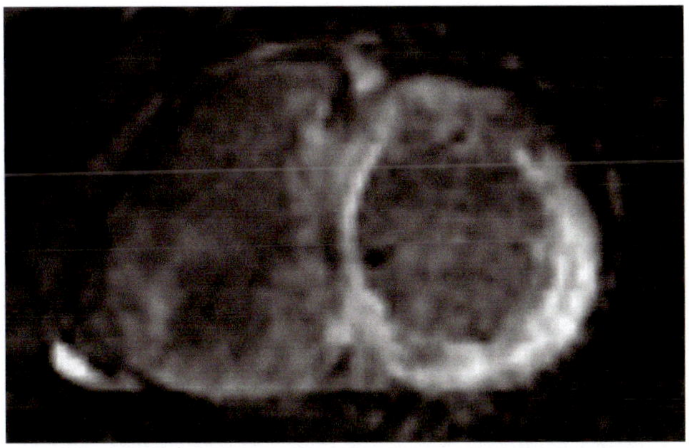

Figure 23.12. Cardiac magnetic resonance imaging (MRI) delayed enhancement (DE) assessment revealed diffuse circumferential subendocardial abnormal DE. When coupled with abnormal nulling kinetics, the MRI findings were highly suggestive of cardiac sarcoidosis.

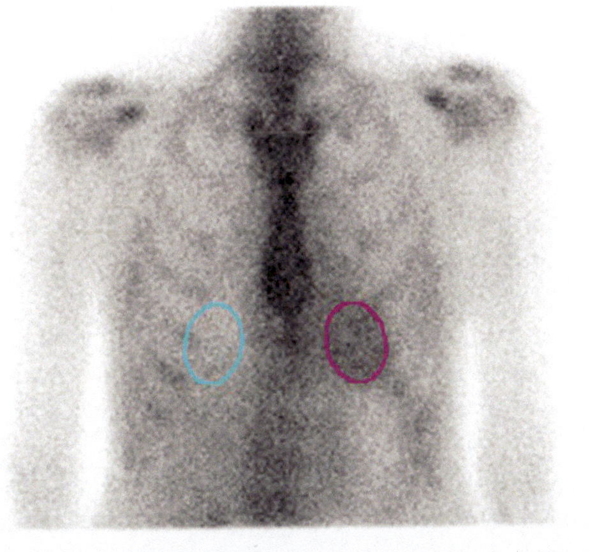

Figure 23.13 99m Technetium-pyrophosphate SPECT/CT three-hour planar image heart to contralateral ratio is positive (>1.3). Imaging obtained at three hours.

and delayed enhancement (DE) imaging demonstrated diffuse circumferential subendocardial abnormal DE throughout both ventricles (Figure 23.12). Pooled sensitivity and specificity of cardiac MRI for the detection of cardiac amyloidosis is 85% and 92% respectively[15] but is not able to reliably discern between ATTR and AL amyloid.

^{99m}Tc-PYP cardiac scintigraphy H/CL ratio was positive (1.6, positive ≥ 1.3) (Figure 23.13) with grade 2 uptake. SPECT/CT findings were congruent with the planar results (Figure 23.14). Additional laboratory studies revealed an elevated monoclonal protein, and subsequent fat aspirate with mass spectroscopy demonstrated AL amyloidosis. Despite aggressive treatment for advanced HF, the patient passed away and autopsy confirmed AL CA.

The current case demonstrates that ^{99m}Tc-PYP is not entirely specific for ATTR amyloidosis, and upwards of 20% of AL patients may have ^{99m}Tc-PYP uptake, and even grade 3 uptake may be present in AL CA.[16] It is therefore critical that ^{99m}Tc-PYP studies be interpreted and reported in the context of serologic protein studies and the appropriate clinical context. Finally, this patient scenario reveals that the diagnosis of ATTR CA is often delayed, and it is therefore imperative that the clinician maintain an appropriate level of suspicion when a patient presents with unexplained HFpEF.[17]

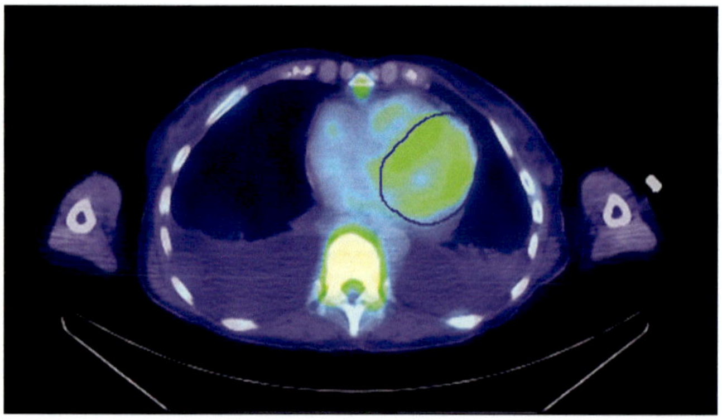

Figure 23.14 Hybrid SPECT/CT axial slice demonstrated myocardial uptake of 99m Technetium-pyrophosphate and confirms the positive planar and 3D scores consistent with ATTR cardiac amyloidosis in the right clinical setting (specifically in the absence of a positive serum monoclonal protein assessment). Imaging obtained at three hours.

QUESTION

3. Which of the following has been reported as a possible cause of myocardial ^{99m}Tc-PYP uptake? Choose the best answer.
   a. Cardiac device
   b. Hydroxychloroquine toxicity
   c. Hypertrophic cardiomyopathy
   d. Stable coronary artery disease

ANSWER

3b. Any object such as a cardiac device anterior to the myocardium can attenuate ^{99m}Tc-PYP uptake but should not cause uptake in the myocardium. Hypertrophic cardiomyopathy and stable coronary artery disease by themselves should not cause myocardial ^{99m}Tc-PYP uptake; however, unstable angina and myocardial infarction can cause myocardial ^{99m}Tc-PYP uptake. Hydroxychloroquine-mediated cardiotoxicity has been reported as a cause of myocardial ^{99m}Tc-PYP uptake.[18]

REFERENCES

1. Grogan M, Scott CG, Kyle RA, et al. Natural history of wild-type transthyretin cardiac amyloidosis and risk stratification using a novel staging system. *J Am Coll Cardiol.* 2016;68:1014–1020.
2. Gillmore JD, Damy T, Fontana M, et al. A new staging system for cardiac transthyretin amyloidosis. *Eur Heart J.* 2018;39:2799–2806.
3. Cyrille NB, Goldsmith J, Alvarez J, Maurer MS. Prevalence and prognostic significance of low QRS voltage among the three main types of cardiac amyloidosis. *Am J Cardiol.* 2014;114:1089–1093.
4. Phelan D, Collier P, Thavendiranathan P, et al. Relative apical sparing of longitudinal strain using two-dimensional speckle-tracking echocardiography is both sensitive and specific for the diagnosis of cardiac amyloidosis. *Heart.* 2012;98:1442–1448.
5. Dorbala S, Ando Y, Bokhari S, et al. ASNC/AHA/ASE/EANM/HFSA/ISA/SCMR/SNMMI expert consensus recommendations for multimodality imaging in cardiac amyloidosis: Part 1 of 2: Evidence base and standardized methods of imaging. *J Nucl Cardiol.* 2019;26:2065–2123.
6. Castano A, Haq M, Narotsky DL, et al. Multicenter study of planar technetium 99m pyrophosphate cardiac imaging: Predicting survival for patients with ATTR cardiac amyloidosis. *JAMA Cardiol.* 2016;1:880–889.
7. Fine NM, Arruda-Olson AM, Dispenzieri A, et al. Yield of noncardiac biopsy for the diagnosis of transthyretin cardiac amyloidosis. *Am J Cardiol.* 2014;113:1723–1727.
8. Varga C, Dorbala S, Lousada I, et al. The diagnostic challenges of cardiac amyloidosis: A practical approach to the two main types. *Blood Rev.* 2021;45:100720.
9. Donnellan E, Wazni OM, Hanna M, et al. Atrial fibrillation in transthyretin cardiac amyloidosis: Predictors, prevalence, and efficacy of rhythm control strategies. *JACC Clin Electrophysiol.* 2020;6:1118–1127.
10. El-Am EA, Dispenzieri A, Melduni RM, et al. Direct current cardioversion of atrial arrhythmias in adults with cardiac amyloidosis. *J Am Coll Cardiol.* 2019;73:589–597.
11. Geller HI, Singh A, Alexander KM, et al. Association between ruptured distal biceps tendon and wild-type transthyretin cardiac amyloidosis. *JAMA.* 2017;318:962–963.
12. Cirulis MM, Emerson LL, Bull DA, et al. Pulmonary arterial hypertension in primary amyloidosis. *Pulm Circ.* 2016;6:244–248.
13. Singh V, Falk R, Di Carli MF, et al. State-of-the-art radionuclide imaging in cardiac transthyretin amyloidosis. *J Nucl Cardiol.* 2019;26:158–173.
14. McKee PA, Castelli WP, McNamara PM, Kannel WB. The natural history of congestive heart failure: The Framingham study. *N Engl J Med.* 1971;285:1441–1446.
15. Zhao L, Tian Z, Fang Q. Diagnostic accuracy of cardiovascular magnetic resonance for patients with suspected cardiac amyloidosis: A systematic review and meta-analysis. *BMC Cardiovasc Disord.* 2016;16:129.
16. Gillmore JD, Maurer MS, Falk RH, et al. Nonbiopsy diagnosis of cardiac transthyretin amyloidosis. *Circulation.* 2016;133:2404–2412.
17. Ladefoged B, Dybro A, Povlsen JA, et al. Diagnostic delay in wild-type transthyretin cardiac amyloidosis: A clinical challenge. *Int J Cardiol.* 2020;304:138–143.
18. Chang ICY, Bois JP, Bois MC, et al. Hydroxychloroquine-mediated cardiotoxicity with a false-positive (99m)Technetium-labeled pyrophosphate scan for transthyretin-related cardiac amyloidosis. *Circ Cardiovasc Imaging.* 2018;11(1):e007059.

24.

IMAGING INFECTION OF VALVES AND DEVICES

Thomas H. Schindler, Soraya El Ghannudi, and Alessio Imperiale

CASE 1

A 34-year-old man presented at the emergency department with acute and ongoing thoracic chest pain. Electrocardiogram demonstrated sinus rhythm at 65 bpm, normal axis and PQ interval, normal R/S transition and repolarization, and normal serial troponin plasma levels. Given ongoing and intermittent stabbing chest pain, contrast chest CT was performed subsequently that identified an acute type A aortic dissection. The patient underwent immediate surgical repair. Following surgery, he developed severe aortic regurgitation and root dilatation that necessitated a second surgery with a bioprosthetic aortic valve and root and a bypass graft to the right coronary artery and a Cabrol graft to the left coronary artery. Postoperatively, he developed sternal osteomyelitis with abscess formation requiring surgical revision and antibiotic treatment with vancomycin and ceftriaxone. During the course of treatment, the patient developed chills and fever. Subsequent echocardiography was technically limited but signified normal right and left ventricular function. The bioprosthetic aortic valve could not be well visualized. The graft of the aortic root appeared to be thickened. The peak gradient across the aortic bioprosthetic valve was 36 mmHg, which was slightly higher than seen on prior echocardiograms. The function of the bioprosthetic aortic valve was otherwise normal. The additionally performed TEE, however, was concerning for infection of the aortic graft, while no vegetations were noted on the bioprosthetic aortic valve. ^{18}F-FDG PET was then conducted that showed the development of a markedly FDG-avid sinus tract (fistula) between the sternal notch and the anterior mediastinum extending inferiorly to the level of the aortic arch with new, markedly FDG-avid soft tissue stranding anterior to the manubrium consistent with worsening graft and sternal infection (Figure 24.1A). In addition, persistent intense FDG activity was noted in the region of the graft in the aortic arch (Figure 24.1B) and prosthetic aortic valve, consistent with infection (Figure 24.1C). Given these findings, the patient underwent urgent surgical revision of sternal osteomyelitis and replacement of the infected graft and bioprosthetic aortic valve.

QUESTION

1. ^{18}F-FDG PET/CT for evaluation of prosthetic valve endocarditis is indicated:
   a. To confirm vegetations and/or abscess formation described by TTE or TEE
   b. To confirm surrounding abscess formation detected by contrast CTA
   c. To evaluate further when the findings of TTE and/or TEE are equivocal
   d. To routinely evaluate prosthetic valve inflammation or infection 6 months after implantation

ANSWER

1c. Answer c is correct, as clinical evaluation in conjunction with TTE and/or TEE is the mainstay in the evaluation in patients with suspicion for NVE and PVE. Given the prosthetic valve–induced shadowing on echocardiography, equivocal findings may arise that require further evaluation with contrast CTA and/or ^{18}F-FDG PET/CT for the detection of PVE. Answers a and b are not correct as positive findings for PVE on echocardiography and/or CTA are sufficient for the diagnosis and they do not need to be confirmed by ^{18}F-FDG PET/CT. Answer d is also incorrect as there is no clinical indication for routine follow-up investigation of the prosthetic valve with ^{18}F-FDG PET/CT.

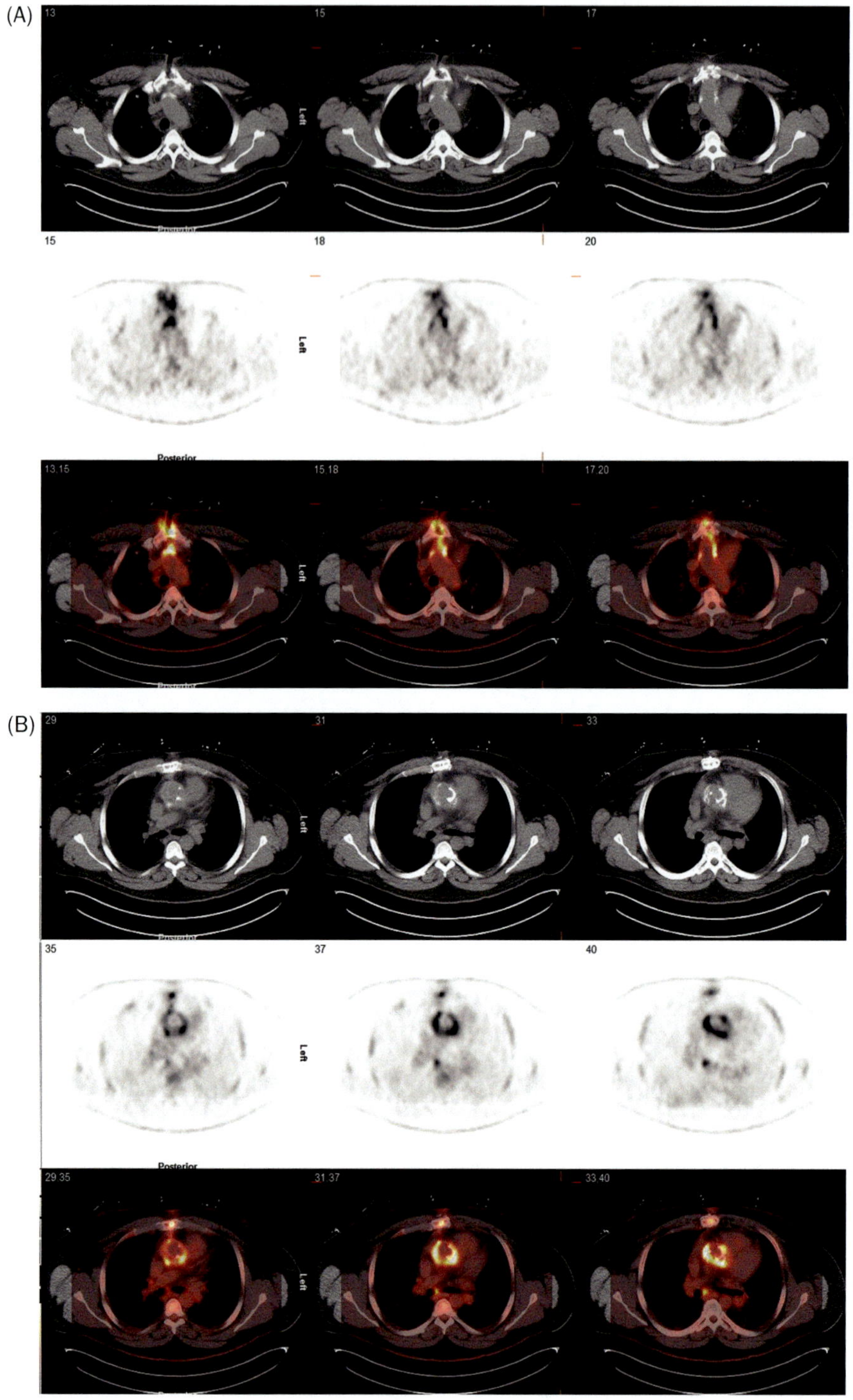

Figure 24.1. Case 1. (A) ^{18}F-FDG PET/CT demonstrates abnormal FDG uptake in the subcutaneous soft tissue around the manubrium, in the manubrium, and further inferiorly to the level of the aortic arch on axial images (middle panel, ^{18}F-FDG PET only; lower panel with CT fusion for ^{18}F-FDG PET/CT display). Thus, between the infected sternal notch and anterior mediastinum, an infected fistula or sinus tract has developed. CT (upper panel) signifies the new tissue formation of the sinus tract stranding from the sternal notch to the anterior mediastinum. Postsurgical changes of median sternotomy are evident. (B) ^{18}F-FDG PET/CT of the aortic arch portion shows heterogenous and intense FDG uptake around the graft and arterial wall on axial images denoting the extension of the sternal infection to the graft in the aortic arch (middle panel, ^{18}F-FDG PET only; lower panel with CT fusion for ^{18}F-FDG PET/CT display). The abnormal FDG uptake in the infected sinus tract is still mildly visible on the left image. CT (upper panel) demonstrates part of the sinus tract in front of the aorta (left and middle image) with postsurgical changes of median sternotomy. (C) ^{18}F-FDG PET/CT depicts heterogenous and intense FDG uptake around the prosthetic aortic valve on axial images that signifies also an infected aortic prosthetic valve (middle panel, ^{18}F-FDG PET only; lower panel with CT fusion for ^{18}F-FDG PET/CT display). CT (upper panel) demonstrates localization of the infected prosthetic aortic valve.

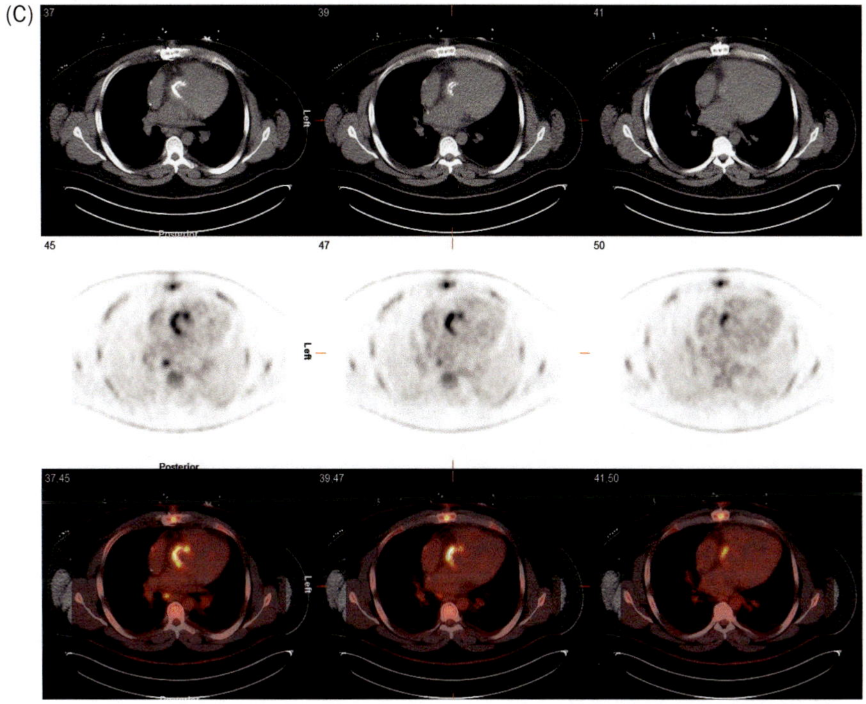

Figure 24.1. Continued

CASE 2

A 48-year-old heroin-addicted woman presented in May 2017 with chronic cutaneous lesions on both forearms and contiguous osteitis. Between November 2012 and January 2013, the patient's history included multiple episodes of aortic IE complicated by purulent meningitis, splenic infarction, and aortic valve destruction needing several lines of antibiotics. In May 2013, the patient presented with a new episode of *Staphylococcus aureus* endocarditis associated with acute heart failure treated emergently by aortic valve replacement with pulmonary valve (ROSS intervention). At the same time, the pulmonary valve was replaced by a bioprosthesis (Contegra tube). The patient started antibiotic therapy (cloxacillin and gentamicin, later replaced by rifampin and ofloxacin). In November 2013, the patient had a fourth episode of IE (*Enteroccocus faecalis* and *Candida tropicalis*) complicated by infectious pulmonary trunk thrombosis and pulmonary septic emboli, requiring pulmonary valve replacement by a biologic valve (homograft and pericardial patch). In December 2013, she underwent aortic valve replacement using a mechanical valve due to aortic autograft dysfunction with major valvular insufficiency (Figure 24.2). Afterwards, the patient refused any kind of complementary investigation and stopped the clinical follow-up for several years. In May 2017, she was hospitalized for fever (39°C), biologic inflammatory syndrome (increased C-reactive protein [CRP]: 104 mg/L, leukocytes: 8.27/mm^3), and recurrent *E. faecalis* bacteremia. On clinical examination, there was discrete edema of the lower limbs with preserved peripheral pulses, without other signs of heart failure. Rest electrocardiogram (ECG) and standard chest radiograph were normal (see Figure 24.2). No evidence of endocarditis was obtained by both TTE and TEE. TEE showed good functioning of the aortic prosthesis and a moderate dysfunction of the homograft pulmonary biologic valve without valvular vegetations. Left ventricular ejection fraction was 67%.

To exclude the presence of IE, she underwent ^{18}F-FDG PET/CT a few days later, revealing a heterogeneous and multifocal glucose hypermetabolism at the periphery of the pulmonary biologic valve (Figure 24.2C), also evident on non–attenuation-corrected PET images (Figure 24.3).

In contrast, no significant abnormalities of ^{18}F-FDG uptake were detected around the mechanical aortic valve (Figure 24.4).

Moreover, an area of moderate but pathologic ^{18}F-FDG uptake was seen corresponding to a condensation zone at the lower lobe of the right lung, along the vascular tree (Figure 24.5).

Overall, ^{18}F-FDG PET/CT suggested the diagnosis of IE of the pulmonary biologic prosthesis with probable

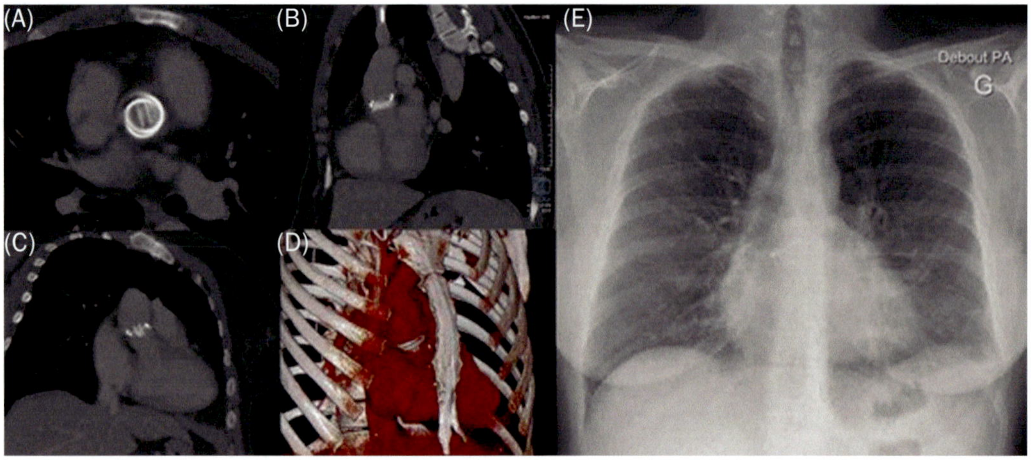

Figure 24.2. Case 2. Gated cardiac CTA showing the aortic mechanical valve without sign of infectious complication: multiplanar reconstruction (MPR), axial (A), sagittal (B), coronal (C), and 3D rendering (D). Normal chest radiograph (anterior projection) showing no parenchymal abnormalities (E).

embolism in the right lower pulmonary lobe, without evidence for endocarditis on the mechanical aortic valve. Novel TEE performed about 7 days after PET/CT showed strong suspicion for bacterial vegetation of the pulmonary homograft with valvular functional dysfunction (Figure 24.6).

Accordingly, the final diagnosis was endocarditis that developed on the pulmonary biologic prosthesis complicated by an asymptomatic right lower lobe pulmonary septic embolus. Chronic ulcerated and fibrinous cutaneous wounds of both forearms were considered the origin for the *E. faecalis* bacteremia and valvular infection. The patient was started on intravenous antibiotic therapy including ceftriaxone (4 g/day) and amoxicillin (12 g/day) for 6 weeks with a favorable response (negative blood cultures, stable ultrasound findings, complete regression of inflammatory syndrome and fever) without further surgical intervention. The patient has had no further episodes of IE during regular monitoring for 15 months.

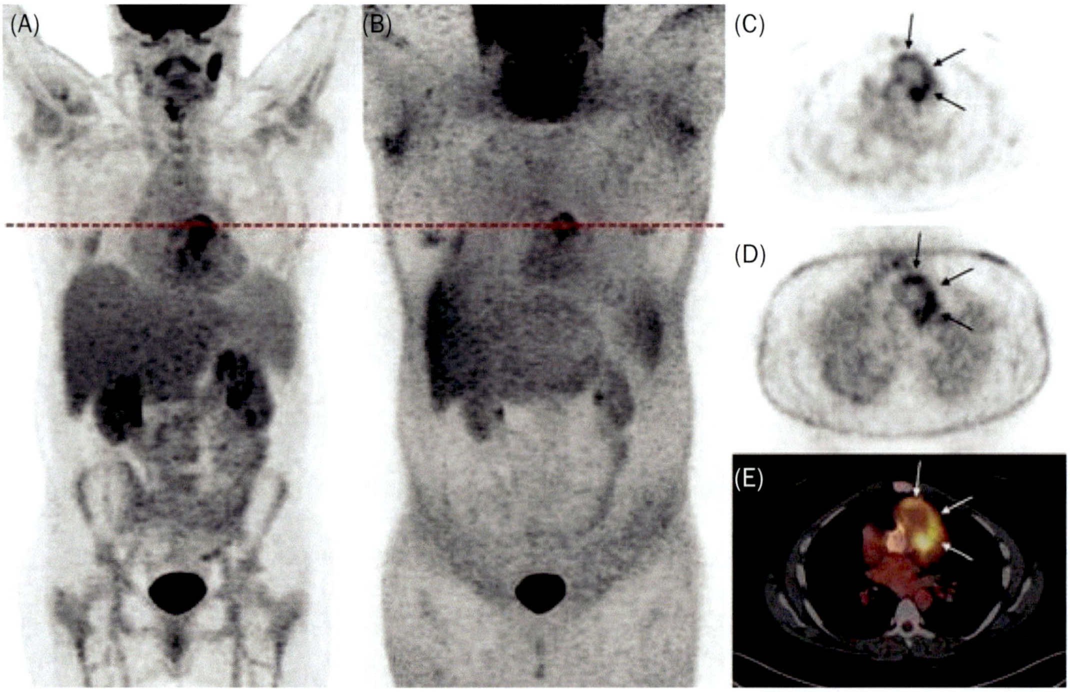

Figure 24.3. Case 2. Attenuation-corrected PET study (A, C) showing pathologic ^{18}F-FDG uptake (arrows) at the periphery of the pulmonary biological valve (PET/CT, E), persisting on non–attenuation-corrected PET images (B, D).

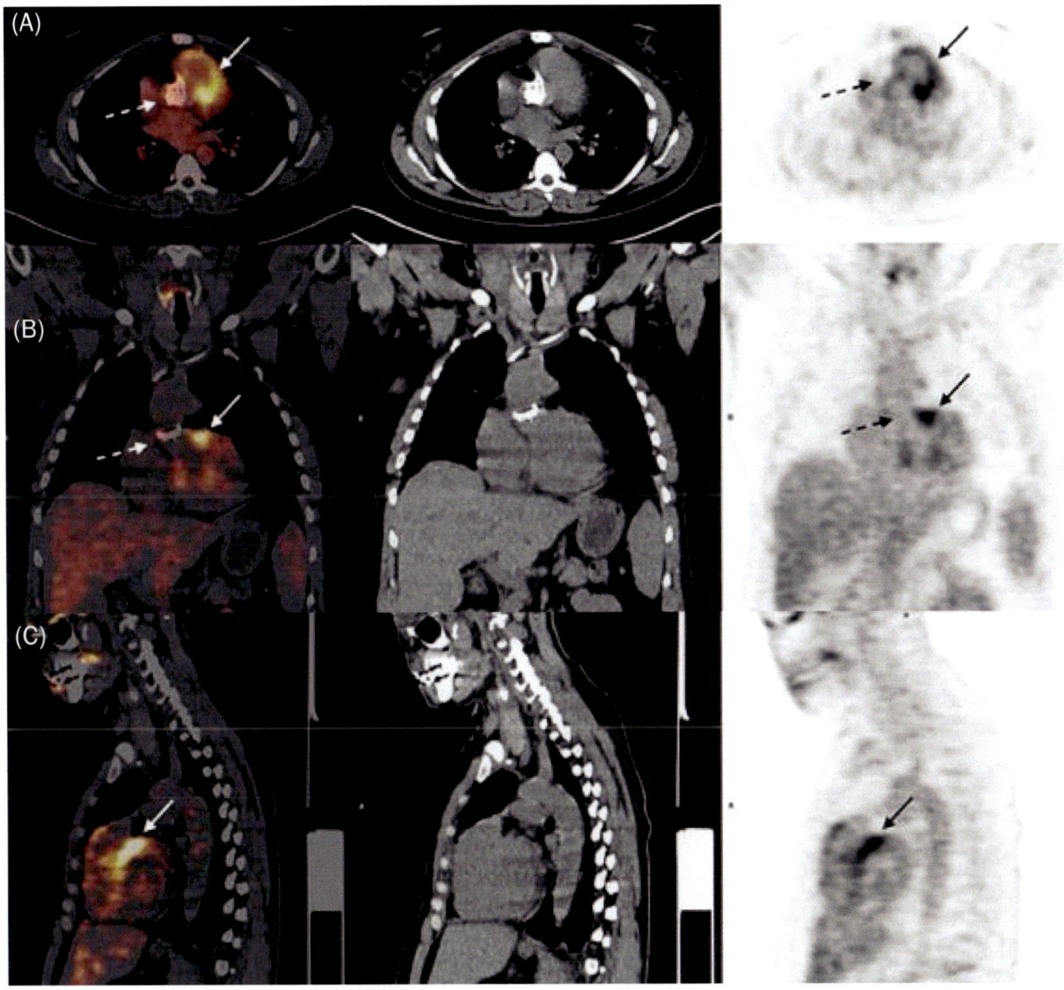

Figure 24.4. Case 2. Axial (A), coronal (B), and sagittal (C) PET/CT, CT, and PET images showing a pathologic ^{18}F-FDG uptake peripheral to homograft pulmonary valve (arrows). No significant ^{18}F-FDG uptake abnormalities were detected around the mechanical aortic valve (dotted arrows).

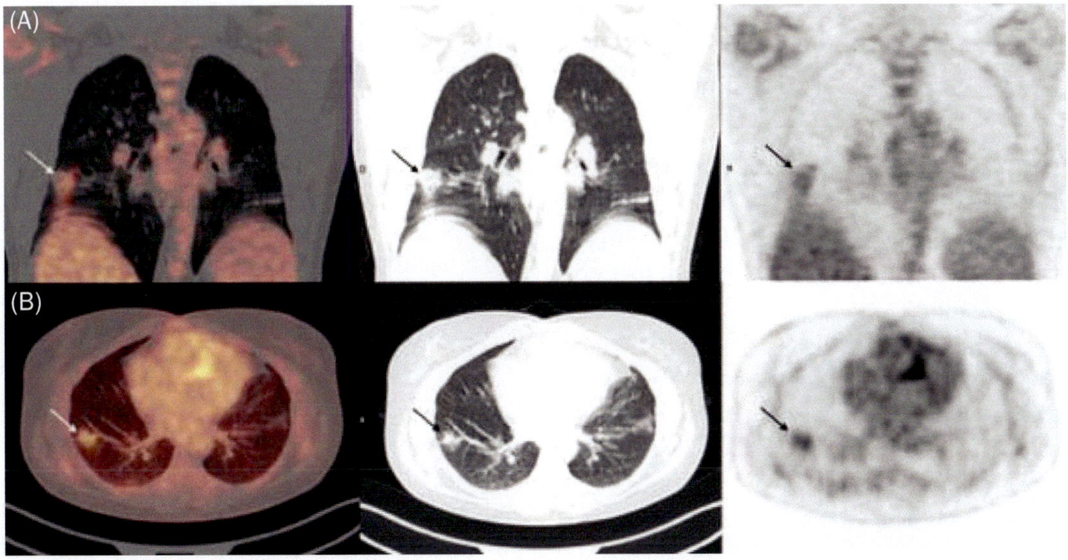

Figure 24.5. Case 2. Coronal (A) and axial (B) PET/CT, CT, and PET images showing a condensation zone at a right posterior lateral lung, with moderately increased ^{18}F-FDG uptake (arrows) suggesting septic embolism in the right lower pulmonary lobe.

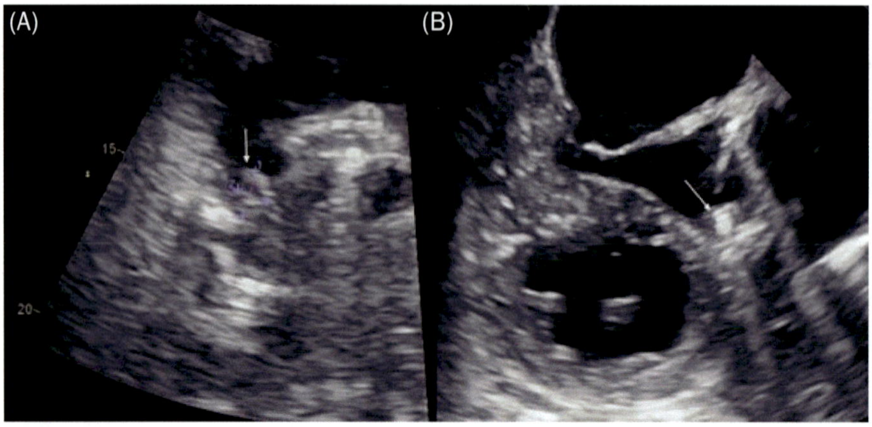

Figure 24.6. Case 2. TTE and TEE showed a small mobile mass on pulmonary valve homograft highly suspicious for vegetation (arrows).

QUESTION

2. Four months after implantation of an aortic prosthetic valve, there is clinical suspicion for an infection of the aortic prosthetic valve, and ^{18}F-FDG PET/CT images demonstrate mild-to-moderate intense and homogenous FDG uptake surrounding the prosthetic valve in aortic position. Such findings on ^{18}F-FDG PET/CT:
   a. Are diagnostic for PVE
   b. No confirmation of FDG-uptake on non–attenuation-corrected ^{18}F-FDG PET is needed.
   c. Are equivocal, as they could reflect implantation-caused sterile inflammation
   d. Additional quantification of SUV max and mean should be performed for definite diagnosis of PVE.

ANSWER

2c. Answer c is correct, as implantation-induced sterile inflammation is commonly seen up to 6 months postoperatively. In newer models of bioprosthetic or prosthetic valves, the concurrent sterile inflammation may even last longer than 12 months. Such postinterventional sterile inflammation causes homogenous FDG uptake around the prosthetic valve and is unlikely to reflect PVE unless there is a high clinical suspicion and very intense FDG uptake. Thus, such findings are equivocal or rather reflect implantation-caused sterile inflammation. This also means that answer a is not correct. Answer b is also not correct, as any abnormal FDG uptake around the prosthetic valve needs to be confirmed by non–attenuation-corrected ^{18}F-FDG PET. This is because the FDG signal in proximity to high-density regions such as a metal device or prosthetic valve may be erroneously elevated owing to an attenuation overcorrection based on the CT-captured metal density. With regards to answer d, the quantification of the FDG signal with SUVs is not much help, as several investigations have outlined.

CASE 3

A 68-year-old man with a prior history of aortic dissection treated with mechanic aortic valve replacement and Bentall surgery 11 years ago was referred for routine follow-up. He had multiple cardiovascular risk factors, including diabetes mellitus, arterial hypertension, and hypercholesterolemia. Five years earlier, the patient had had an ischemic cerebral attack with secondary hematoma developing while receiving oral anticoagulant treatment. On physical examination, the patient appeared physically sick but without fever (37C°). He was hemodynamically stable without clinical signs of heart failure. Electrocardiogram showed first-degree atrioventricular block and inverted T waves in anterior leads. He had a moderate increase in CRP (35 mg/L), fibrinogen (6.8 g/L), and brain natriuretic peptide (BNP) (108 ng/L), but the total leukocyte count was normal (7×10^9/L). Multiple blood cultures were positive for *E. faecalis*. TTE showed no vegetation or mechanic aortic valve dysfunction. However, it revealed a peri-aortic prosthetic collection extending to the lateral and posterior part of the aortic annulus, suggesting a periprosthetic abscess. TEE confirmed the TTE findings, also disclosing preserved function of the mechanic aortic valve (Figure 24.7).

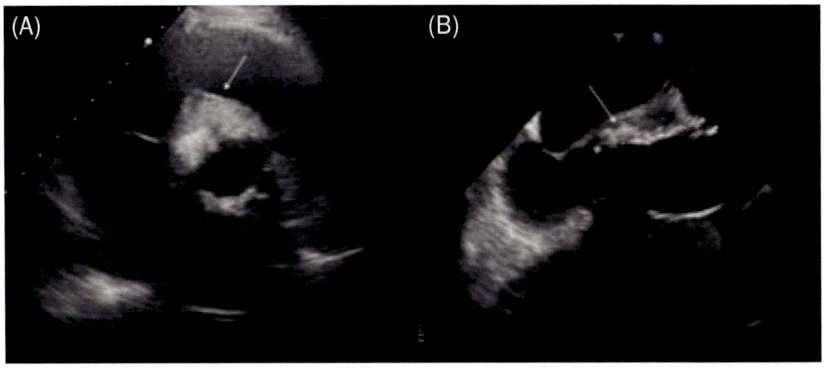

Figure 24.7. Case 3. (A) TTE showing peri-aortic prosthetic collection (arrow). (B) TEE showing peri-aortic prosthetic collection extending to the lateral and posterior part of the aortic annulus (arrow).

According to Duke criteria (ESC 2015), the diagnosis of IE of the mechanic prosthetic aortic valve and a peri-prosthetic abscess of the Bentall tube was made. Thoracoabdominal CTA did not reveal any septic embolization, and the patient started treatment with ceftriaxone (4 g/day) and amoxicillin (12 g/day) intravenously; oral anticoagulant medication was continued as part of his usual treatment. Cardiac surgery was planned but the patient presented 1 month later with dysarthria and right hemiparesis. Cerebral MRI revealed a huge left thalamic hematoma without acute ischemic cerebral lesions or mycotic abscess. Cardiac surgery was deferred and intravenous anticoagulation was started for 3 weeks. At the 1-month follow-up, TTE and TEE showed moderate increase of peri-aortic and aortic annular abscess size. Moreover, an aorto-mitral trigone fistula was revealed on TEE color Doppler investigation (Figure 24.8).

Gated cardiac CTA confirmed the increasing size of the peri-prosthetic abscess in addition to an infectious peri-aortic annular pseudo-aneurysm (Figure 24.9).

Afterwards, the patient refused cardiac surgery and the antibiotic treatment was continued for an additional 3 months, with good biologic response (CRP 4.4 ng/L, fibrinogen 4.5 g/L). The patient is still regularly monitored without major complications.

QUESTION

3. In patients with suspicion for PVE, contrast CTA for the identification and characterization of peri-prosthetic abscess formation is indicated when:
   a. TEE has ruled out peri-prosthetic abscess formation
   b. TEE is equivocal for peri-prosthetic abscess formation
   c. TEE confirms the presence of peri-prosthetic abscess
   d. ^{18}F-FDG PET/CT is without abnormal FDG uptake and there are normal findings on the CT scan for attenuation correction

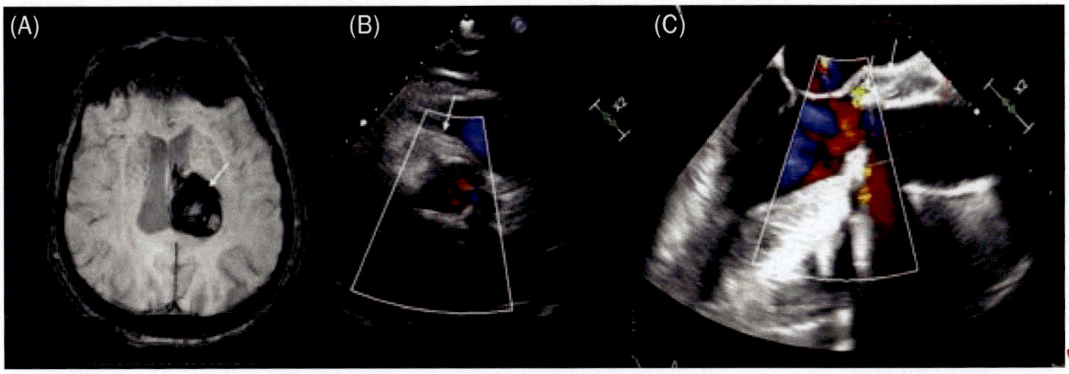

Figure 24.8. Case 3. (A) Spontaneous huge left thalamic hematoma under anticoagulant treatment shown by cerebral MRI. (B) Increased size of peri-aortic and aortic annular abscess revealed at 1-month follow-up TTE. (C) Peri-aortic and aortic annular abscess and aorto-mitral trigone fistula revealed by TEE color Doppler study.

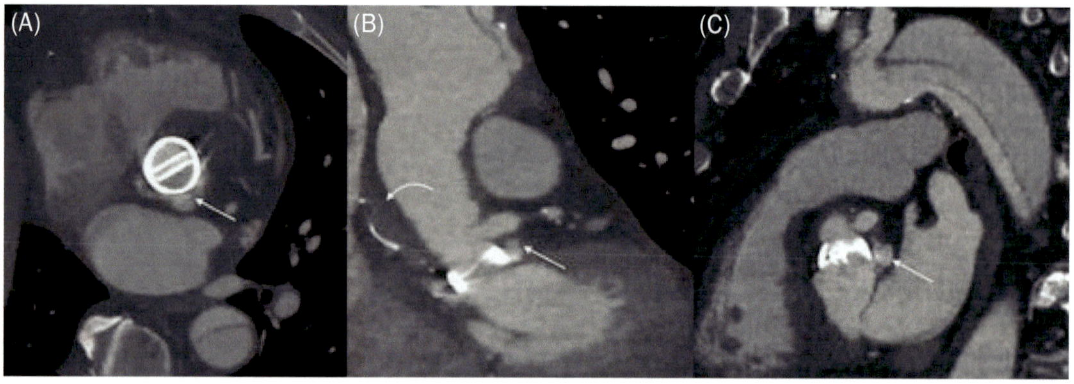

Figure 24.9. Case 3. (A) Axial view gated cardiac CTA multiplanar reconstruction (MPR) showing that a peri-aortic abscess up to 15 mm in width had developed at the posterior and left lateral side of the aortic prosthetic tube and at the aortic annulus of the mechanic valve (arrow). (B) CTA coronal and (C) sagittal MPR reconstructions showing peri-Bentall tube abscess 7 cm in height (arrows) and a pseudo-aneurysm due to a fistulous abscess into the left ventricle just below the insertion of the aortic mechanic valve (curved arrow in B).

ANSWER

3b. Given the prosthesis-induced shadowing on echocardiography, even TEE may be nondiagnostic or equivocal for peri-prosthetic abscess formation. If this is the case, contrast CTA is recommended for definite evaluation. Thus, answer b is correct. If TEE can rule out or confirms the presence of peri-prosthetic abscess formation, CT angiography is not needed (answers a and c are incorrect). Answer d is also incorrect, as ^{18}F-FDG PET/CT without abnormal FDG uptake around the prosthesis and normal findings on the noncontrast CT scan for attenuation correction render the presence of a peri-prosthetic abscess very unlikely.

25.

IMAGING CARDIAC AND VASCULAR INFLAMMATION

Sina Tavakoli and Mehran M. Sadeghi

QUESTION

1. Which one of the following tracers is typically used for detection of vessel wall inflammation in aortitis?
   a. ^{18}F-FDG
   b. ^{68}Ga-DOTATATE
   c. ^{18}F-NaF
   d. ^{82}Rb

ANSWER

1a. ^{18}F-FDG is taken up by metabolically active cells, such as macrophages, or other tissue-resident cells (e.g., smooth muscle cells), in the inflamed vessel wall. The increase in glucose utilization in these cells may be detected by ^{18}F-FDG PET (Figure 25.1). As a glucose analog, ^{18}F-FDG is taken up by the cells through glucose transporters, including glucose transporter 1 (GLUT1). Once inside the cell, ^{18}F-FDG undergoes glucokinase-mediated phosphorylation to ^{18}F-FDG-6-phosphate. Rather than processing along the glycolytic pathway like glucose-6 phosphate, FDG-6-phosphate is trapped within the cell, where it accumulates and may be imaged. Ultimately, ^{18}F decays to ^{18}O with a half-life of 110 minutes, resulting in ordinary glucose-6-phosphate, which is processed normally.

^{18}F-FDG is commonly used to assess cardiac viability, detect the foci of infection, and evaluate tumors, among other applications. However, its relative nonspecificity (accumulation in any site of active glycolysis, and inability to differentiate infection from inflammation) limits its more widespread application in cardiovascular medicine. Accordingly, more specific tracers are under development and may eventually complement or replace ^{18}F-FDG PET. ^{68}Ga-DOTATATE, which binds to somatostatin receptor 2, expressed by pro-inflammatory macrophages, is an alternative tracer that may be useful for imaging of inflammation. While studies have shown the uptake of this tracer in several inflammatory cardiovascular diseases, its effectiveness for imaging aortitis has not been established. ^{18}F-NaF is a tracer for imaging calcification due to its chemisorption to hydroxyapatite. ^{82}Rb is a potassium analog that is used as a tracer for myocardial perfusion imaging.

QUESTION

2. Which of the following statements is accurate regarding ^{18}F-FDG PET imaging?
   a. ^{18}F-FDG PET signal in aortic aneurysm is consistently predictive of future aneurysm expansion.
   b. The magnitude of the inflammatory ^{18}F-FDG signal early after MI may predict future deterioration of left ventricular function independent of infarct size.
   c. Macrophages are the only cells that retain ^{18}F-FDG in atherosclerotic plaques.
   d. ^{18}F-FDG uptake can accurately distinguish different macrophage subsets.

ANSWER

2b. Following MI, pro-inflammatory monocytes are recruited from the blood and spleen to the infarct region and contribute to tissue damage. These cells are then gradually replaced by patrolling monocytes and macrophages with inflammation-resolving phenotypes, which promote tissue repair over the next few weeks. Dysregulations of this highly coordinated process is a key determinant of post-infarct myocardial maladaptive remodeling. To differentiate ^{18}F-FDG uptake in the myocardium from that of recruited or resident leukocytes, myocardial glucose utilization should be suppressed, for instance by using a low-carbohydrate, high-fat diet and fasting. In

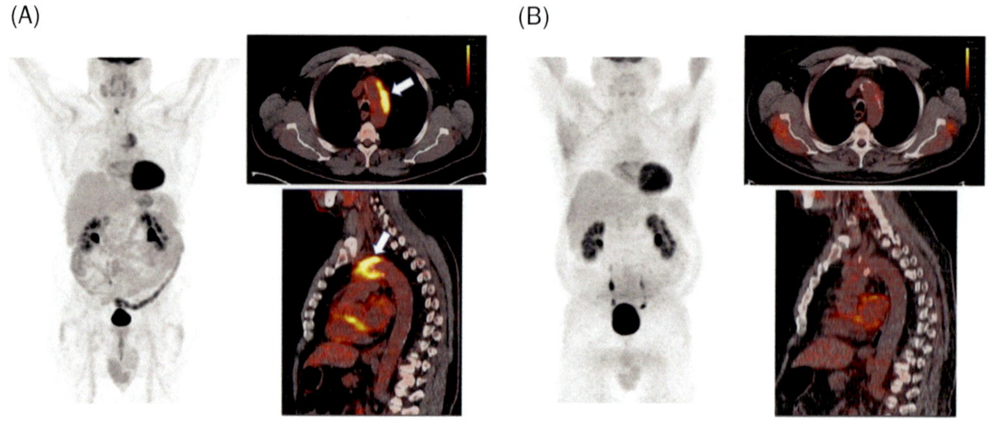

Figure 25.1. ^{18}F-FDG PET in aortitis. (A) PET/CT images of a patient with history of aortitis, demonstrating considerable uptake of ^{18}F-FDG in the aortic arch (arrows). (B) Images acquired after 2 months of treatment show markedly reduced aortic ^{18}F-FDG signal. Whole-body maximum intensity projection PET images (left panels) and selected axial (top right panels) and sagittal (bottom right panels) fused PET/CT slices are shown.

concordance with the kinetics of monocytes/macrophage accumulation, the uptake of ^{18}F-FDG in the infarcted and ischemic peri-infarct myocardium increases during the first week after infarction, and gradually decreases over the subsequent weeks. The magnitude of the ^{18}F-FDG signal early after MI strongly predicts the subsequent deterioration of global and regional left ventricular function independent of the infarct size.

^{18}F-FDG uptake in AAA has been linked to aneurysm expansion in some studies, but other studies have yielded an opposite result. In addition to macrophages, other vascular cells, such as smooth muscle cells, retain ^{18}F-FDG, and therefore the ^{18}F-FDG signal in atherosclerotic plaque does not simply reflect the presence of macrophages. While ^{18}F-FDG uptake may be higher in pro-inflammatory macrophages, this uptake is not specific to this subset of macrophages. Accordingly, ^{18}F-FDG uptake cannot accurately discriminate different activation states of macrophages.

QUESTION

3. Which of the following is a potential imaging target for assessing ongoing (micro)calcification in atherosclerotic plaque?
   a. Fibrin
   b. Phosphatidylserine
   c. Chemokine receptors
   d. Hydroxyapatite

ANSWER

3d. Hydroxyapatite is a bone constituent and a major component of (micro)calcifications in atherosclerotic plaques (Figure 25.2). Microcalcification contributes to the vulnerability of atherosclerotic plaques to rupture and may be targeted by ^{18}F-NaF. Fibrin is a target for imaging thrombosis. Chemokines regulate leukocyte trafficking, as well as

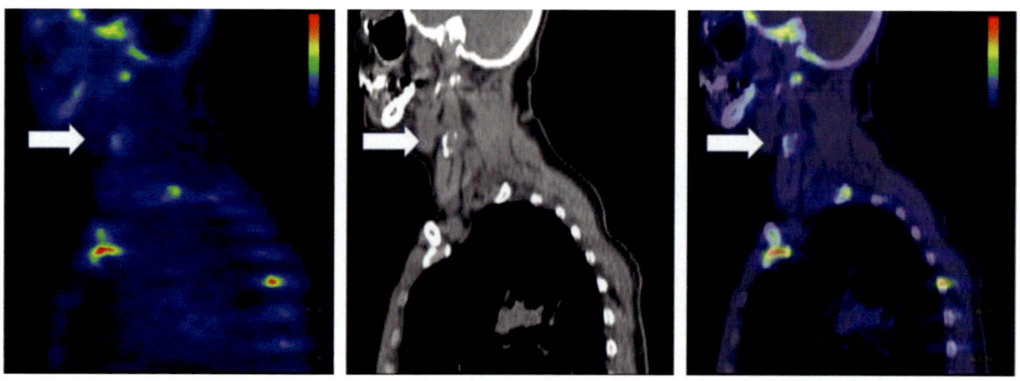

Figure 25.2. ^{18}F-NaF PET imaging of atherosclerotic calcification. Examples of ^{18}F-NaF PET (left panel), CT (middle panel), and fused PET/CT images (right panel) in a patient with calcified carotid stenosis. Arrows point to carotid bifurcation.

other aspects of leukocyte biology, including their activation in response to various inflammatory stimuli in tissues. Examples of novel tracers that target chemokine receptors include ^{64}Cu-ECL1i, ^{64}Cu-DOTA-vMIP-II, and ^{99m}Tc-labeled MCP-1 for C-C chemokine receptor 2 (CCR2) and ^{68}Ga-Pentixafor for C-X-C chemokine receptor 4 (CXCR4). Phosphatidylserine is externalized during apoptosis and may be used as target for imaging apoptosis and cell death.

26.

RADIONUCLIDE IMAGING IN HEART FAILURE

Daniel Shpilsky and Prem Soman

CASE 1

A 72-year-old man with hypertension, dyslipidemia, diabetes mellitus type 2, and CAD presented with 2 months of progressive fatigue, dyspnea, weight gain, and abdominal distension. With regards to his cardiac history, he recalled a prior MI requiring stenting but could not recall the stent location, and there were no records available. An echocardiogram was obtained that was technically difficult but suggestive of severe LV dysfunction. Given a new cardiomyopathy, a regadenoson SPECT myocardial perfusion study was pursued for evaluation of ischemia.

Tc-99m SPECT myocardial perfusion images (Figure 26.1) show an inferior attenuation artifact that is well corrected by attenuation correction (AC). AC images show only a small apical defect (arrows) that was also present on the rest images and may indicate a small infarct in the left anterior descending coronary artery territory. The rest of the LV myocardium has normal perfusion. The gated images (▶ Video 26.1) show diffuse hypokinesis with a severe reduction in global LV systolic function and akinesis corresponding to the apical defect. The normal myocardial perfusion at stress with the exception of a limited apical defect indicates that the severe LV dysfunction is most likely due to nonischemic cardiomyopathy. This patient had coexisting CAD that was not etiologically related to his cardiomyopathy.

CASE 2

A 59-year-old man with hypertension, diabetes, and end-stage renal disease on dialysis presented with 1 month of progressive dyspnea, lower extremity swelling, and sporadic chest discomfort with exertion. Presenting blood pressure was 160/92 mmHg. Physical exam was notable for inspiratory crackles, an S3 gallop, elevated jugular venous pulse to 12 cm, and 2+ pitting lower extremity edema. Clinical presentation was consistent with severe decompensated HF. He received intravenous diuresis and was started on an antihypertensive regimen. Given new-onset HF and possible angina symptoms, a regadenoson SPECT myocardial perfusion scan was ordered.

Stress and rest Tc-99m SPECT myocardial perfusion images (Figure 26.2) show normal myocardial perfusion with LV hypertrophy and remodeling. The gated images (▶ Video 26.2) show relatively preserved LV systolic function. In patients with severe left ventricular hypertrophy, quantitative programs tend to underestimate LVEF. These findings are suggestive of HF with normal EF due to hypertensive heart disease. The normal myocardial perfusion indicates a low probability of significant obstructive CAD.

CASE 3

A 57-year-old man with a history of hypertension and obesity was referred to the cardiology clinic for 5 months of exertional dyspnea and chest discomfort symptoms described as postprandial heartburn that also occasionally occurred with exertion. Examination was notable for inspiratory crackles and trace peripheral edema. A transthoracic echocardiogram was obtained by the primary care provider and was notable for a new diagnosis of dilated cardiomyopathy with LVEF of 35% to 40% and global hypokinesis. Given the diffuse wall-motion abnormalities, the atypical nature of his symptoms, and the patient's preference for noninvasive testing, an exercise Tc-99m SPECT myocardial perfusion scan was ordered by his cardiologist. The patient exercised for 6 minutes and 41 seconds and developed typical angina symptoms similar to the "heartburn" he had been experiencing, prompting termination of the test. The electrocardiogram was notable for 4-mm downsloping ST depressions in the anterolateral and inferior leads beginning 2 minutes into exercise and resolving 15 minutes into recovery. There were rare premature ventricular contractions during exercise.

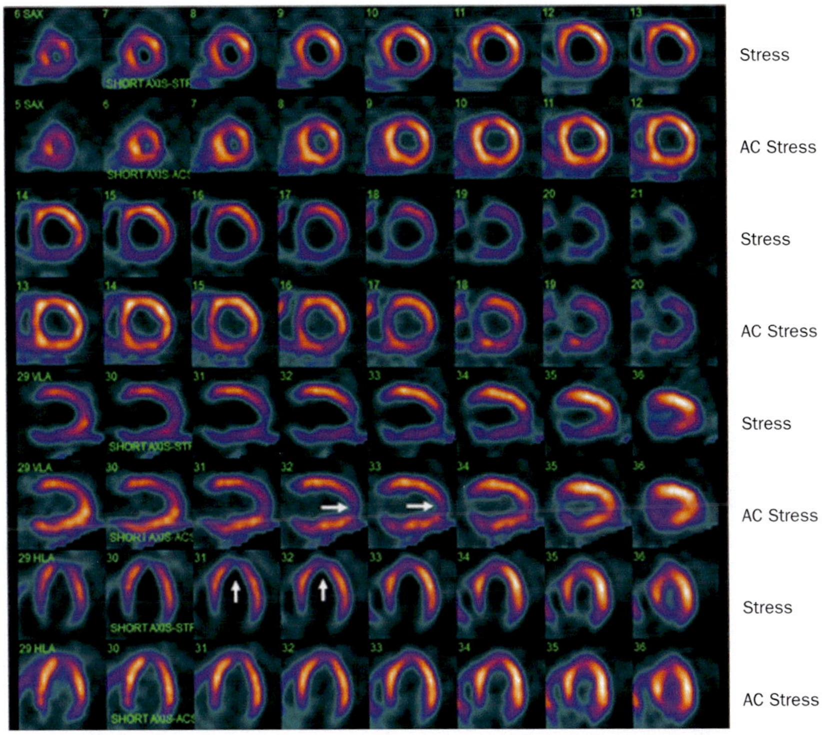

Figure 26.1. Case 1. Tc-99m SPECT myocardial perfusion images are shown (uncorrected and attenuation-corrected [AC] images, rest images not shown). SPECT shows an inferior attenuation artifact that is well corrected by AC. AC images show only a small apical defect (arrows) that was also present on the rest images and may indicate a small infarct in the left anterior descending coronary artery territory. The rest of the LV myocardium has normal perfusion.

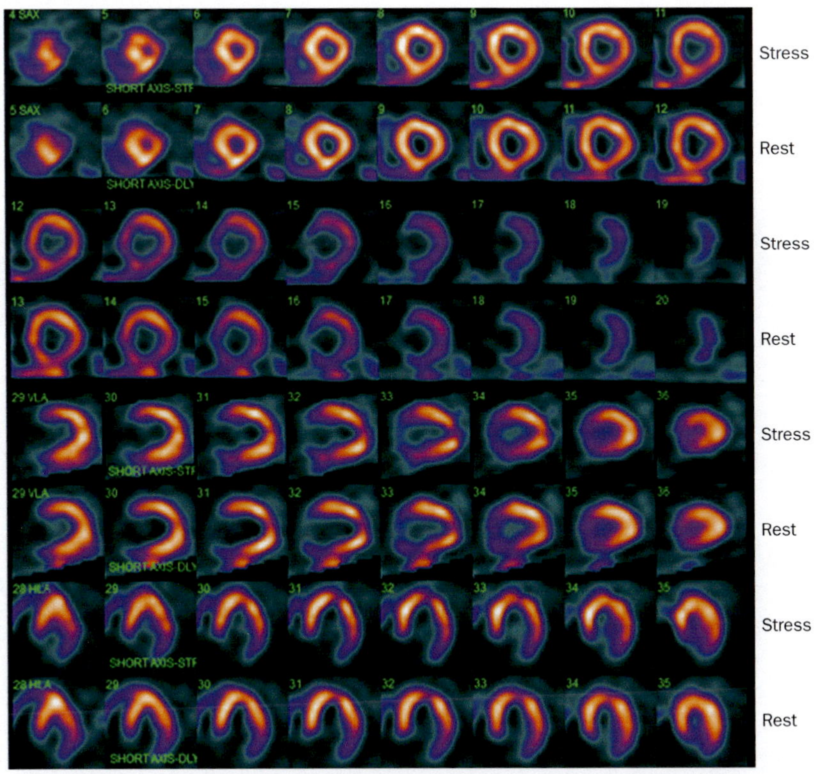

Figure 26.2. Case 2. Stress and rest Tc-99m SPECT myocardial perfusion images are shown. Images show normal myocardial perfusion with LV hypertrophy (septum is brighter than the lateral wall, cavity size is relatively small compared to LV thickness) and remodeling (LV shape is more globular than ellipsoid).

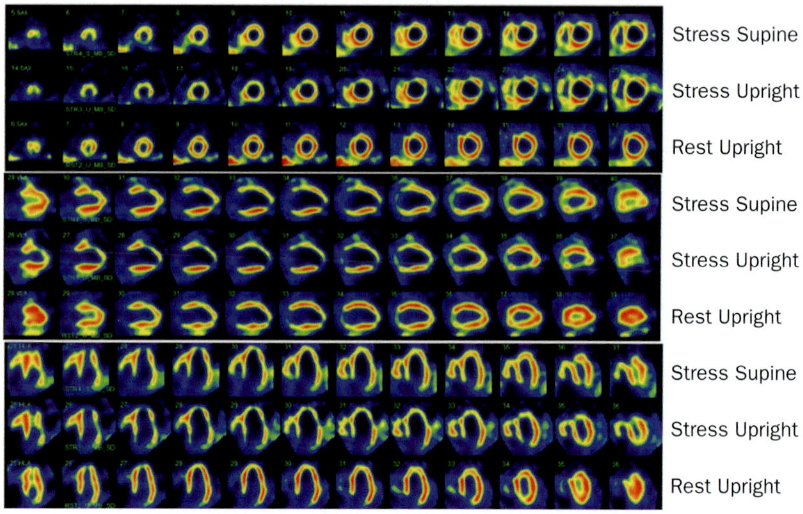

Figure 26.3. Case 3. Stress and rest Tc-99m SPECT myocardial perfusion images are shown. The LV is dilated. Transient ischemic dilatation is present as evidenced by a larger LV cavity on stress images (TID 1.25). There are increased RV counts on the stress images. Rest images demonstrate a small perfusion defect of moderate intensity involving the apical inferior wall consistent with prior infarct or severe rest ischemia. On stress images, a moderate-sized perfusion defect is noted extending from the mid anterior wall to the apex and apical inferior wall. Additionally, there is a small perfusion defect of moderate intensity involving the basal-mid inferolateral wall.

Stress and rest Tc-99m SPECT myocardial perfusion images were obtained (Figure 26.3). Images show an abnormally dilated LV. Transient ischemic dilatation (TID) is present as evidenced by a larger left LV cavity on stress images as compared to rest (TID 1.25). Increased RV counts are also noted on stress images. Rest images demonstrate a small perfusion defect of moderate intensity involving the apical inferior wall consistent with prior infarct or severe rest ischemia. On stress images, a moderate-sized perfusion defect is noted extending from the mid anterior wall to the apex and apical inferior wall. Additionally, with exercise, there is a small perfusion defect of moderate intensity involving the basal-mid inferolateral wall. On gated imaging (▶ Video 26.3), the LV systolic function is mildly reduced (EF 40%). There is global hypokinesis with more severe hypokinesis involving the anterior and inferolateral walls. Taken together, the summative findings including typical angina symptoms, early-onset ST depressions lasting into recovery, and associated perfusion defects are suggestive of HF due to an ischemic cardiomyopathy. The perfusion defects are suggestive of at least two-vessel coronary artery involvement, including a wraparound left anterior descending artery and obtuse marginal artery. Of note, the presence of TID and increased RV uptake with stress are high-risk markers suggestive of left main or high-grade triple-vessel CAD. Coronary angiography showed significant three-vessel disease.

27.

EVOLVING ROLE OF ECHOCARDIOGRAPHY, CARDIAC CT, AND CARDIAC MRI IN CAD

Arnold C. T. Ng, Victoria Delgado, and Jeroen J. Bax

CASE 1

Patient 1 is a 67-year-old female with a background of ischemic heart disease and previous coronary artery bypass grafting (saphenous vein graft to the left circumflex coronary artery and saphenous vein graft to the right coronary artery) and bioprosthetic aortic valve replacement 2 years ago for severe aortic stenosis. Other background medical history includes hypertension and dyslipidemia. She presented to the emergency department complaining of intermittent chest tightness over the last 3 weeks with associated increased exertional dyspnea. On physical examination, her pulse rate was 65 bpm regular and her blood pressure was 143/86 mmHg. Her jugular venous pulsation was elevated at 5 cm above the sternal angle, and there was a soft ejection systolic murmur on auscultation. Her chest was clear on auscultation, and there was mild bilateral pitting edema in the lower third of her shins. ECG showed sinus rhythm with nonspecific lateral T-wave changes (Figure 27.1), and the cardiac troponin I level was normal at 5 ng/L (normal <10 ng/L).

Dobutamine stress echocardiography showed normal resting LV systolic function, and no inducible ischemia at peak stress (▶ Video 27.1). However, resting images showed elevated LV filling pressures with pseudo-normalized mitral inflow pattern (transmitral E/A ratio 0.9) with an elevated septal E/e′ ratio of 17.6 (Figures 27.2 and 27.3), and elevated pulmonary pressures (estimated right ventricular systolic pressure 55 mmHg, assuming right atrial pressure 3 mmHg) (Figure 27.4). The calculated LV mass index was increased at 102 g/m^2, and the left atrial volume index was increased at 38 mL/m^2.

Using the algorithm for assessing LV filling pressures (see Figure 27.6 in the main book), the patient had evidence of grade II diastolic dysfunction with elevated left atrial pressure (three out of three positive criteria). The case demonstrated that the patient's exertional dyspnea and angina were likely secondary to increased LV mass and elevated filling pressures with resultant subendocardial ischemia, but there was no evidence of significant epicardial disease as demonstrated by the normal findings on dobutamine stress echocardiography. Treatment should be directed toward reducing the LV filling pressure by diuretic therapy.

CASE 2

Patient 2 is a 68-year-old male with a background of obesity (body mass index [BMI] 31.6 kg/m^2), type 2 diabetes, hypertension, and hypercholesterolemia. He stopped smoking 1 year ago and has a 40 pack/year smoking history. He started complaining of stable exertional angina (Canadian Cardiovascular Society [CCS] class II) 3 months ago, and his exercise tolerance had reduced to walking approximately 500 m on flat ground. On physical examination, his pulse rate was 70 bpm regular and his blood pressure was 130/75 mmHg. Cardiovascular examination was unremarkable, and his chest was clear on auscultation. ECG showed inferolateral T-wave changes (Figure 27.5).

The patient underwent an exercise stress test and was able to walk for 4 minutes and 37 seconds using the Bruce protocol, achieving a peak heart rate of 125 bpm (82% maximum predicted heart rate, 5.4 METS). The test was terminated due to dyspnea and he denied any chest discomfort at peak stress. The stress ECG showed a 1-mm upsloping ST-segment depression in the inferolateral leads at peak stress. The resting echocardiogram showed normal LV function, and there were no inducible wall-motion abnormalities immediately post-exercise. Due to the submaximal exercise stress echocardiogram, he

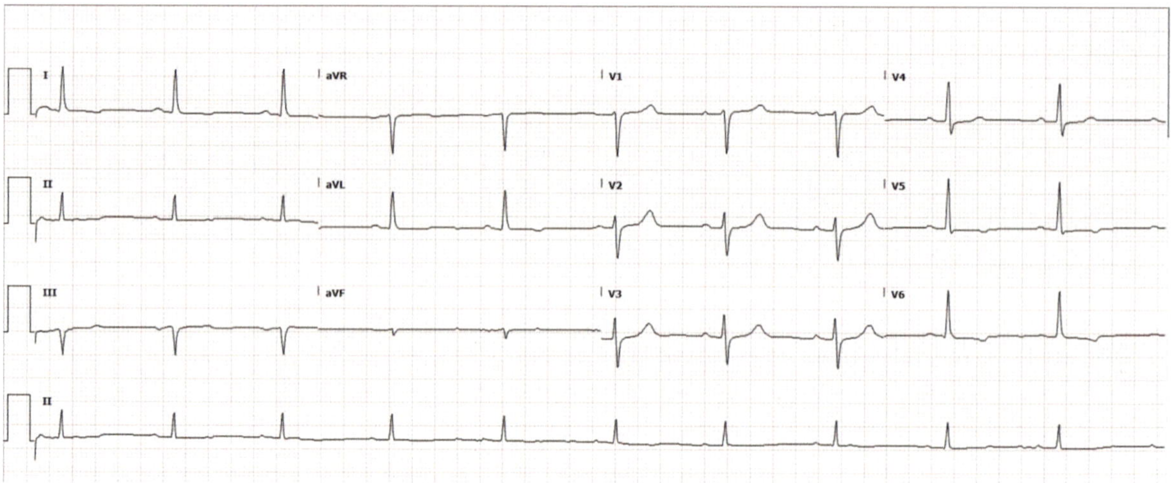

Figure 27.1. Case 1. ECG showing sinus rhythm with a heart rate of 61 bpm and nonspecific T-wave changes in leads V5 and V6.

underwent a CT coronary angiogram (Figure 27.6) with adenosine stress perfusion (Figure 27.7).

The patient eventually underwent an invasive coronary angiogram that confirmed underlying significant triple-vessel disease (Figure 27.8; ▶ Video 27.2).

CASE 3

Patient 3 is a 45-year-old man who complained of increasing exertional dyspnea over the last 3 months on a background of morbid obesity (127 kg, BMI 36.3 kg/m^2), type 2 diabetes,

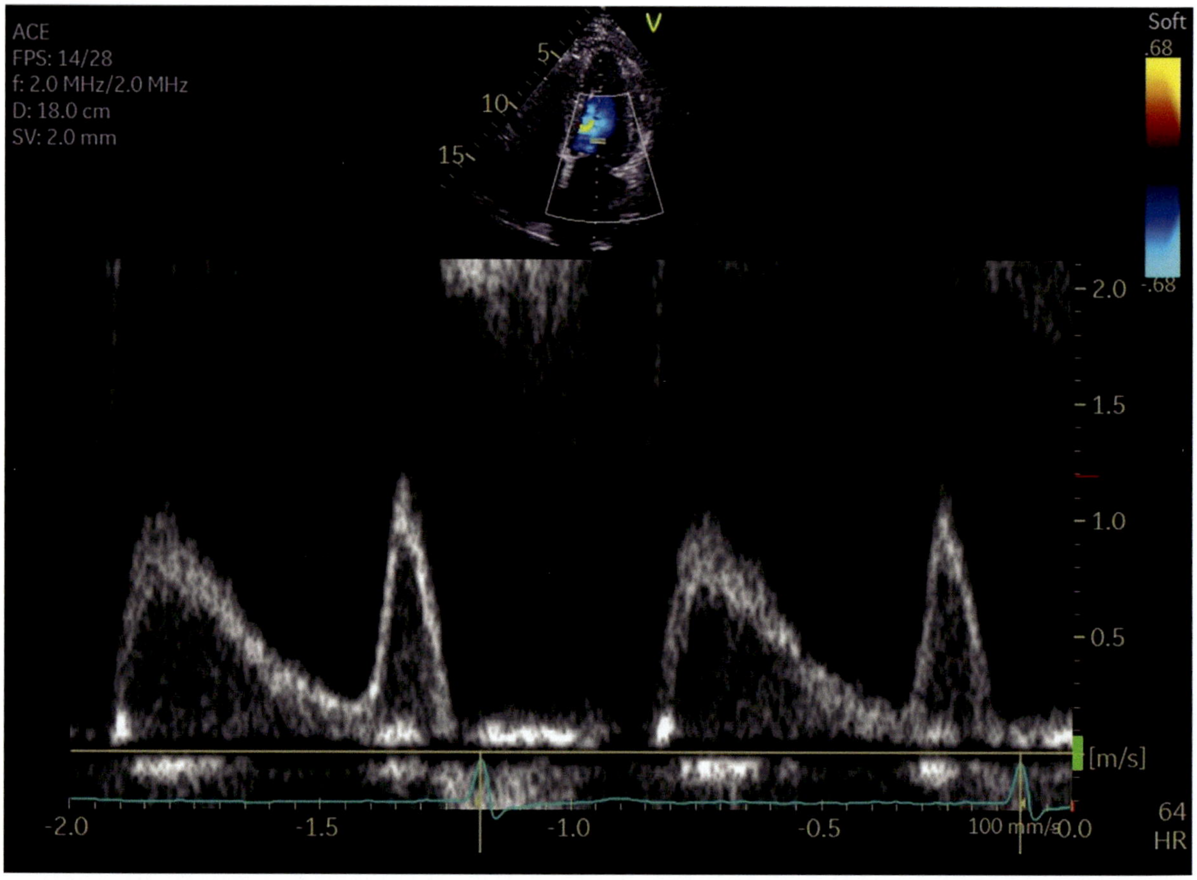

Figure 27.2. Case 1. Transmitral inflow pattern showing a pseudo-normal mitral inflow pattern with an E/A ratio of 0.95. Peak E velocity was 0.91 m/s.

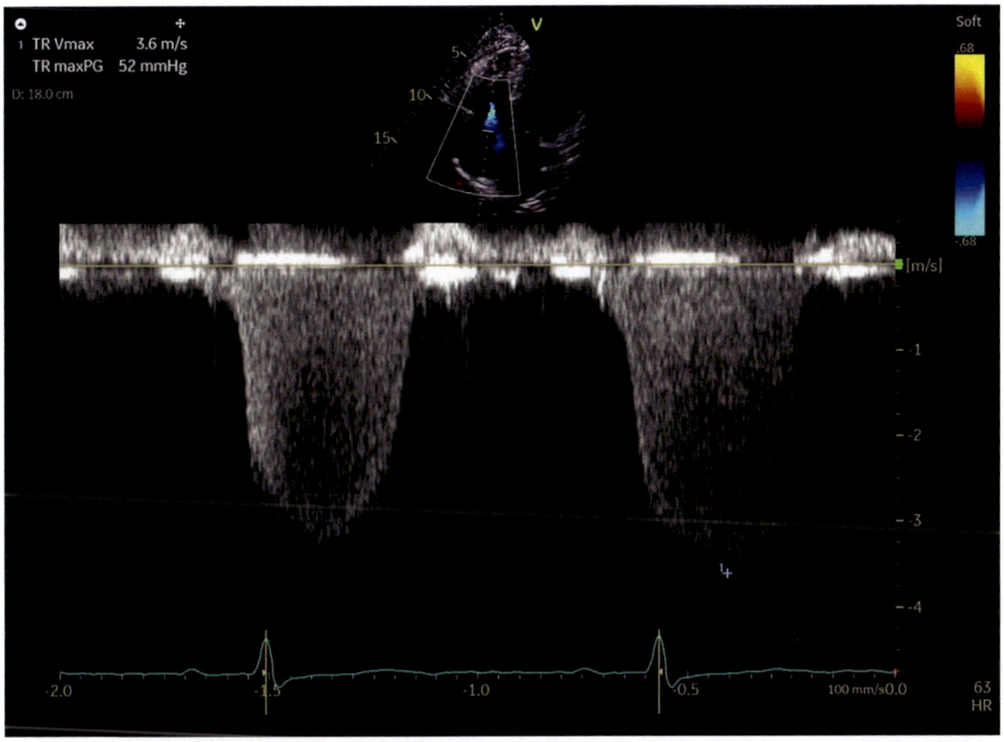

Figure 27.4. Case 1. Continuous wave Doppler of tricuspid regurgitation showing pulmonary hypertension with an estimated right ventricular systolic pressure of 55 mmHg (assuming right atrial pressure of 3 mmHg).

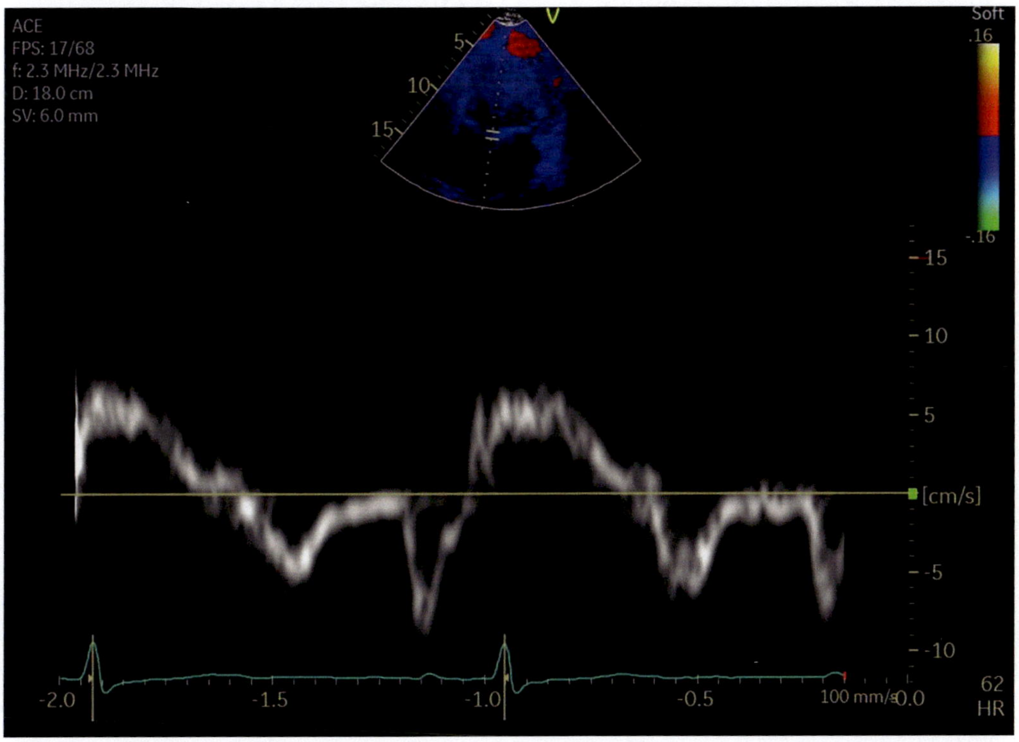

Figure 27.3. Case 1. Tissue Doppler imaging of the septal mitral annulus showing an elevated septal E/e′ ratio of 17.8. Peak septal e′ velocity was 5.1 cm/s.

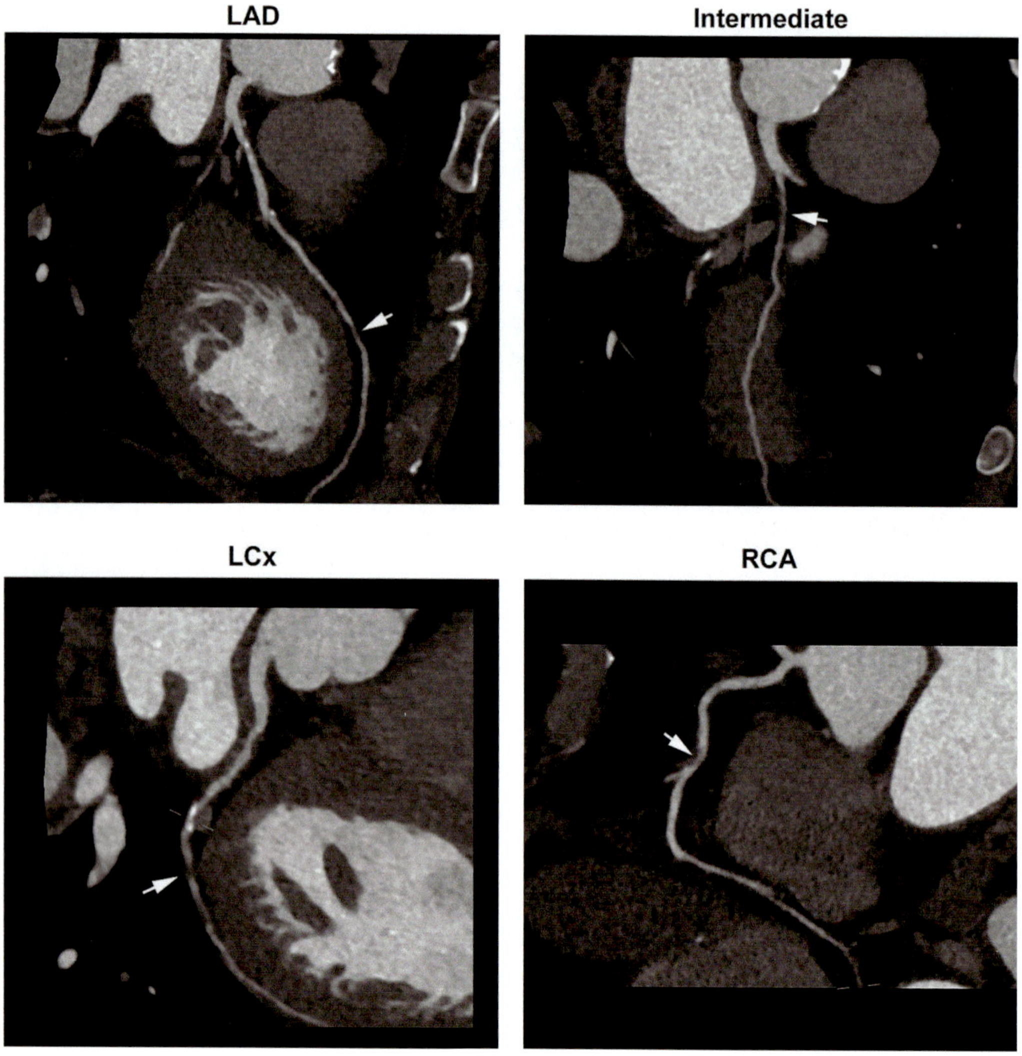

Figure 27.6. Case 2. CT coronary angiogram showing underlying coronary artery stenoses (arrows). In the LAD, there was a 50–70% stenosis in the mid segment. In the intermediate artery, there was a diffuse 50–70% stenosis in the proximal segment. In the LCx, there was a calcified plaque in the mid segment with significant blooming artifact, preventing accurate assessment of the severity of the underlying stenosis. After the calcified plaque in mid LCx, there was a focal soft plaque resulting in near-total occlusion. In the RCA, there was a 25–50% stenosis in the mid segment.

hypertension, and asthma. He also complained of daily orthopnea with associated paroxysmal nocturnal dyspnea. On physical examination, his pulse rate was 70 bpm regular and his blood pressure was 130/75 mmHg. His jugular venous pulsation was elevated at 6 cm above the sternal angle. There was a palpable parasternal heave, and the apex beat was not palpable. There were bi-basal inspiratory crackles on auscultation of his chest and mild to moderate bilateral pitting edema to his mid-shins. ECG showed sinus rhythm with right bundle branch block (Figure 27.9), and chest x-ray showed a markedly enlarged cardiac silhouette with increased perihilar bronchovascular markings (Figure 27.10).

Transthoracic echocardiogram showed a severely dilated LV and severely impaired LVEF. However, image quality was severely limited due to poor acoustic window from his morbid obesity (▶ Video 27.3). His CT coronary angiogram showed a totally occluded proximal LAD and normal left main artery, LCx, and RCA (Figure 27.11).

CMR imaging showed a severely dilated LV (indexed LV end-diastolic volume 139 mL/m^2) with severe segmental systolic dysfunction (LVEF 20%) (▶ Video 27.4). LGE imaging showed full-thickness enhancement in the akinetic anterior, anteroseptal, and apical segments (Figure 27.12). In addition, there was a small, laminated thrombus in the LV apex on LGE imaging.

QUESTION

1. A 60-year-old male with a history of hypertension and type 2 diabetes requiring insulin presented with

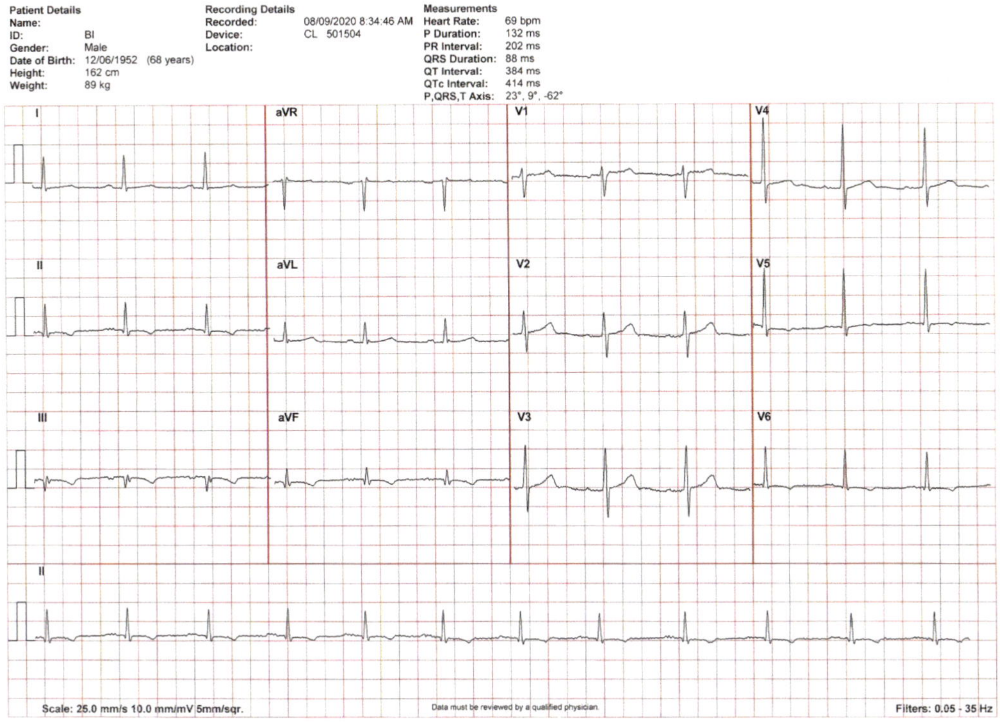

Figure 27.5. Case 2. Resting ECG showing inferior T-wave inversions in leads II, III, and aVF and nonspecific T-wave changes in leads V5 and V6.

acute chest pain and dyspnea for the last 2 hours that started while he was gardening. On examination, his pulse rate was 85 bpm regular, and blood pressure was 80/55 mmHg. He had one episode of nonsustained conscious ventricular tachycardia on telemetry while in the emergency department. ECG showed sinus rhythm with anterior Q waves (leads V1–V4) with ST-segment elevation, and inferior Q waves (leads III and aVF) (Figure 27.13).

A bedside echocardiogram showed an akinetic mid to apical septal, mid to apical anterior, basal to mid anteroseptal, and apical inferior wall (▶ Video 27.5). The most likely lesion on invasive angiography is:

a. Occluded proximal LAD
b. Occluded LCx
c. 70% lesion in RCA
d. 70% lesion in proximal LAD, 50% lesion in circumflex, 50% lesion right coronary

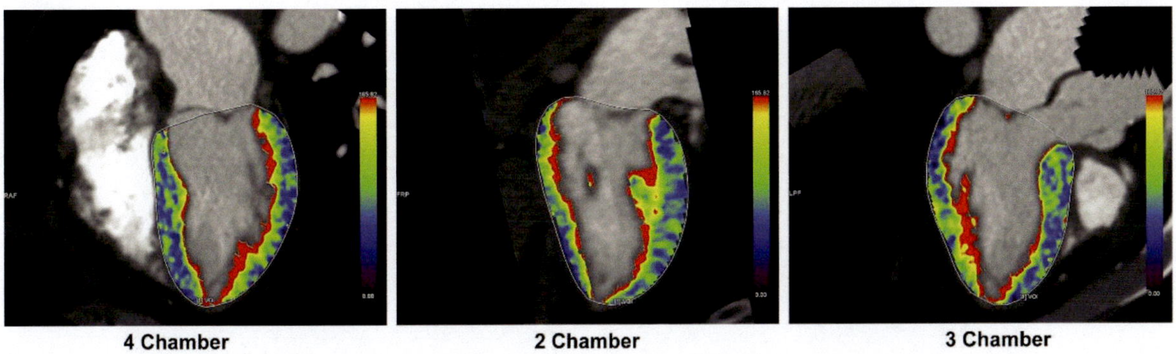

Figure 27.7. Case 2. Adenosine dynamic CT perfusion showed reduced MBF in the four-chamber view (basal to apical septal and anterolateral walls), two-chamber view (basal to mid anterior and mid to apical inferior walls), and three-chamber view (basal to mid inferolateral and anteroseptal walls). The perfusion defects indicated that the mid LAD, proximal intermediate, mid LCx, and mid RCA stenoses are hemodynamically significant. Furthermore, the "mild" disease in the mid RCA on the CT coronary angiogram (see Figure 27.6) is a possible false-negative result.

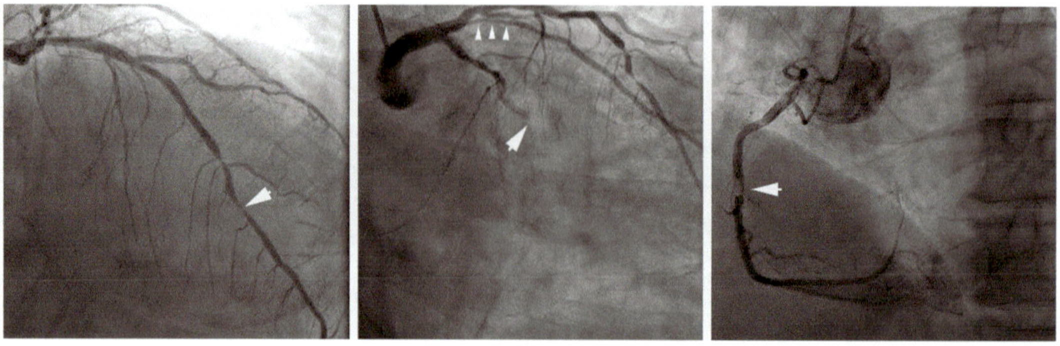

Figure 27.8. Case 2. Invasive coronary angiogram showed significant stenoses in mid LAD (left panel, arrow), proximal intermediate (middle panel, arrowheads), mid LCx (middle panel, arrow), and mid RCA (right panel, arrow). See Video 27.2.

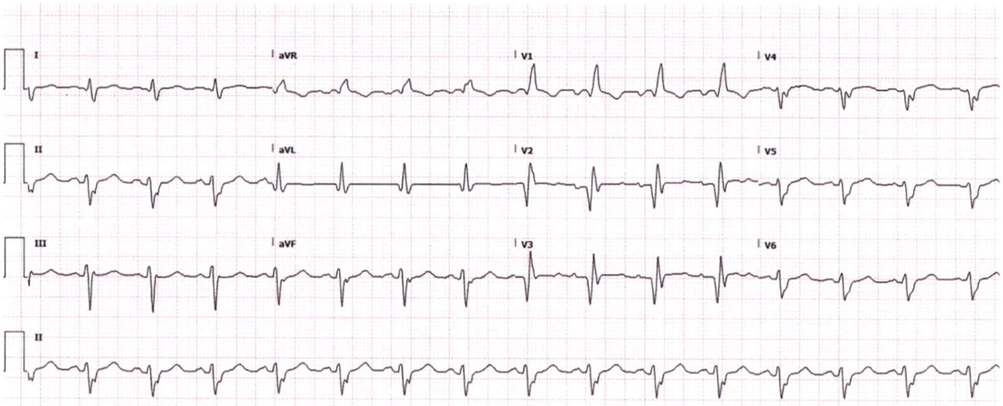

Figure 27.9. Case 3. ECG showing sinus rhythm with complete right bundle branch block.

ANSWER

1a. The ECG changes with the regional LV wall-motion changes on echocardiogram are highly suggestive of a ST-elevation myocardial infarction secondary to an occluded proximal LAD. The inferior Q waves are due to a large LAD (type III or IV) that supplies the apical inferior wall.

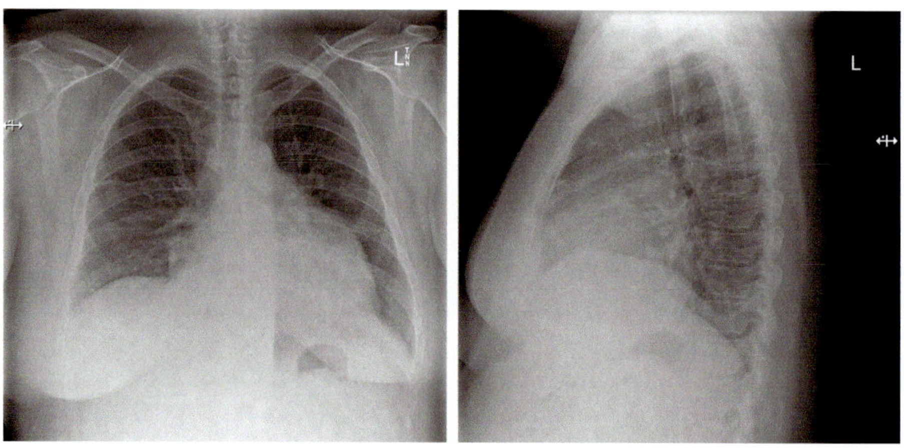

Figure 27.10. Case 3. Chest x-ray showing a markedly enlarged cardiac silhouette with a cardiothoracic ratio of 0.61. There is prominence of the perihilar bronchovascular markings as well as air space opacification in the retrocardiac lower lobes bilaterally obscuring the medial aspect of the hemidiaphragms bilaterally. Linear atelectatic bands are also seen in the mid zones bilaterally.

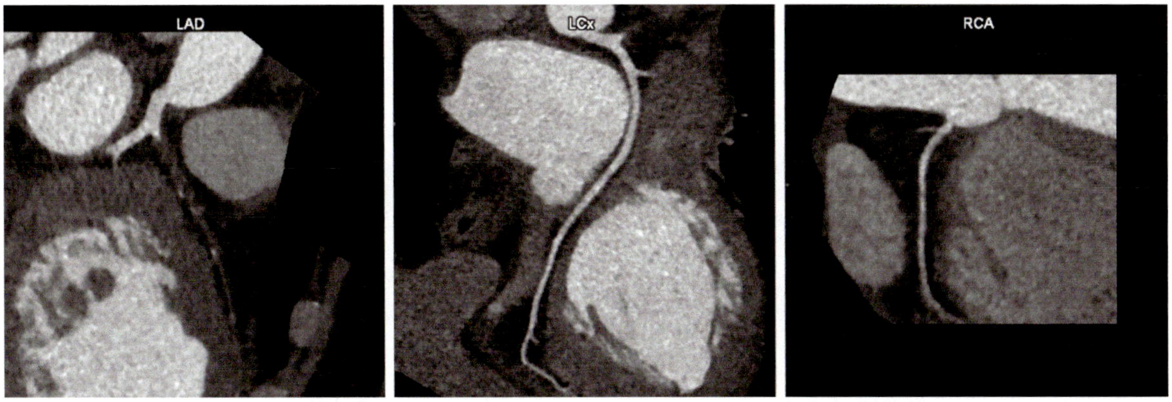

Figure 27.11. Case 3. CT coronary angiogram showing an occluded proximal LAD due to a soft atherosclerotic plaque. There were no atherosclerotic plaques seen in the left main artery, LCx, and RCA.

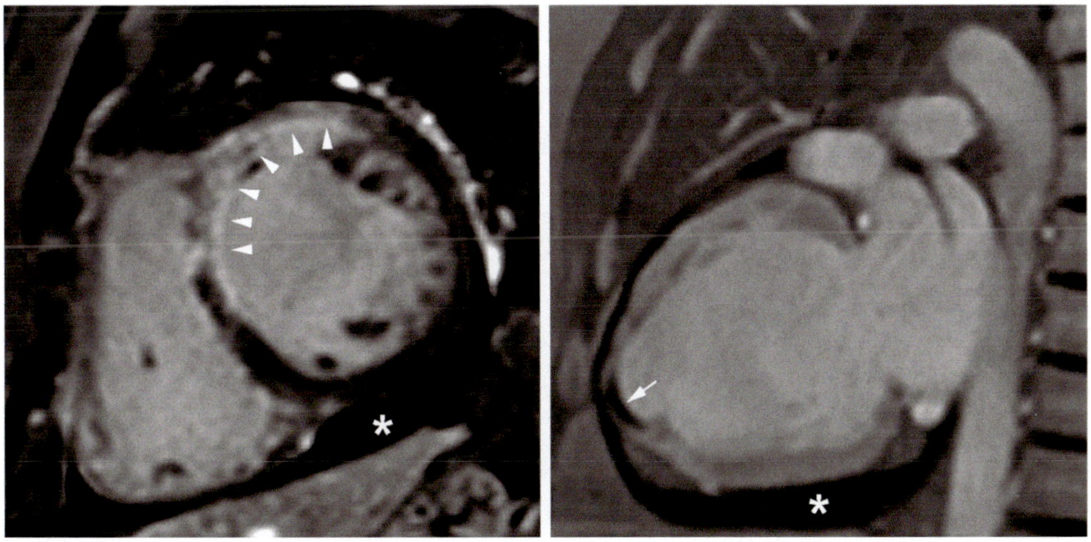

Figure 27.12. Case 3. LGE imaging showed extensive, near-full-thickness scar in the LAD territory (arrowheads) with no significant residual viability. There is a small laminated thrombus present in the LV apex (right panel, arrow), and a small pericardial effusion (*).

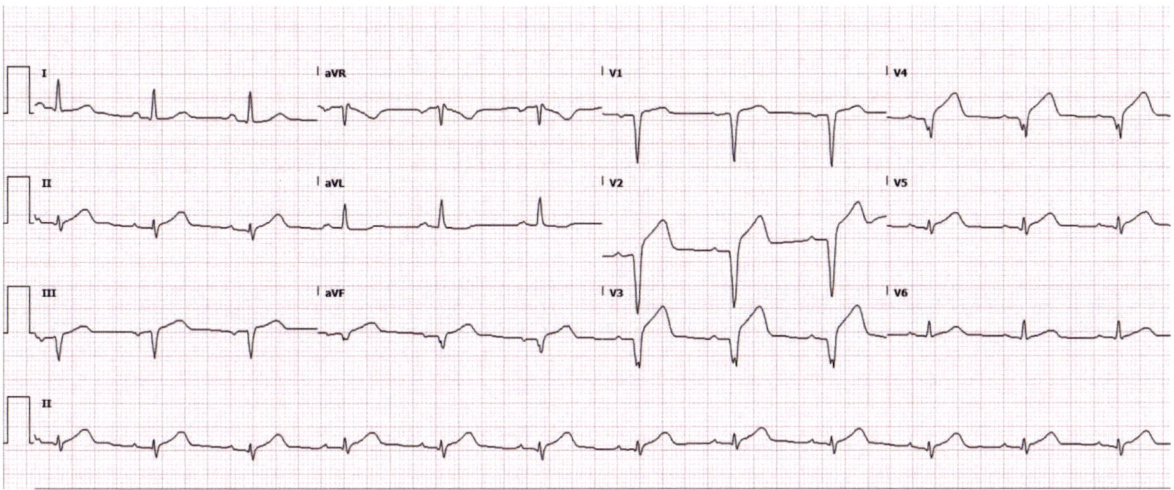

Figure 27.13. ECG showing sinus rhythm with anterior Q waves in leads V1 to V4 with associated ST-segment elevation, and inferior Q waves in leads III and aVF.

28.

HYBRID IMAGING: SPECT/CCTA, PET/MR, AND SPECT CALCIUM SCORE

WHEN AND WHY?

Philipp A. Kaufmann, Oliver Gaemperli, and Ronny R. Buechel

CASE 1

A 70-year-old female patient was referred for SPECT/CCTA hybrid imaging for the exclusion of obstructive CAD due to progressive dyspnea. Her body mass index was 21.2 kg/m^2, and she had a positive family history for cardiovascular events. CCTA was performed as the first-line test and depicted a subtotal occlusion at the bifurcation of the LAD and the first diagonal branch. Calcium score was 503 (LMA: 0, LAD: 325, LCX: 23, RCA: 155). SPECT-MPI was performed on the same day and depicted a large reversible perfusion defect in the anterior and anterolateral wall (Figure 28.1), encompassing up to 25% of the entire LV myocardium, predominantly in the area subtended by the diagonal branch (Figure 28.2, ▶ Video 28.1). Due to the extent of the perfusion defect, the patient was referred for invasive coronary angiography, which confirmed the findings (▶ Video 28.2), and subsequently revascularization was performed (▶ Video 28.3). Post-interventional SPECT-MPI confirmed successful revascularization without any evidence for residual perfusion defects (Figure 28.3).

This case demonstrates the importance of functional testing in a setting of presumed obstructive CAD as depicted by CCTA. While the latter is highly sensitive for the detection of obstructive CAD, its specificity is moderate at best, partly because CT leads to systematic overestimation of luminal narrowing due to blooming artifacts. Furthermore, functional imaging with SPECT-MPI enables perfusion assessment of the entire LV myocardium. Therefore, accurate estimation of the ischemic burden is possible, allowing identification of patients who might benefit from revascularization with regard to prognosis and/or symptoms. Finally, post-interventional functional assessment provides valuable information on the success of the revascularization process (i.e., the reduction of the ischemic burden), which has been shown to be prognostically relevant.

CASE 2

A 50-year-old male patient was referred for CCTA for the exclusion of obstructive CAD due to typical chest pain. Of note, the findings from a stress ECG and transthoracic echocardiography performed prior to referral were normal. His body mass index was 21.4 kg/m^2 and he had no known cardiovascular risk factors. CCTA depicted a single noncalcified lesion in the proximal LAD causing intermediate (70%) stenosis but otherwise normal coronaries (Figure 28.4, asterisks). The overall calcium score was zero. Due to this finding, SPECT-MPI was performed a few days later and revealed an extensive reversible perfusion defect encompassing the entire anterior and septal wall of the LV myocardium in the myocardium subtended by the LAD (Figure 28.5). Interestingly, gated SPECT acquired approximately 1 hour after physiologic stress using ergometry (Figure 28.6) revealed severe motion abnormalities in the anterior and septal wall due to ischemia and subsequent stunning. After consultation with the referring cardiologist and the local interventionalist, the patient was transferred to the chest pain unit and scheduled for urgent invasive coronary angiography (Figure 28.7). Successful revascularization of the LAD was performed early the next day.

This case again demonstrates the clinically useful diagnostic approach of hybrid SPECT/CCTA in a sequential manner, where CCTA is performed as the first-line test and SPECT as a follow-up examination in case of potentially relevant coronary lesions. Note that obstructive disease could have been missed by calcium scoring only. In this particular case, the persistent wall-motion abnormality in the area of ischemia recorded 1 hour after stress is striking and constitutes a specific sign of stunning due to ischemia. Of note, the cardiologist's sonography prior to SPECT did not show any regional wall-motion abnormalities. Finally,

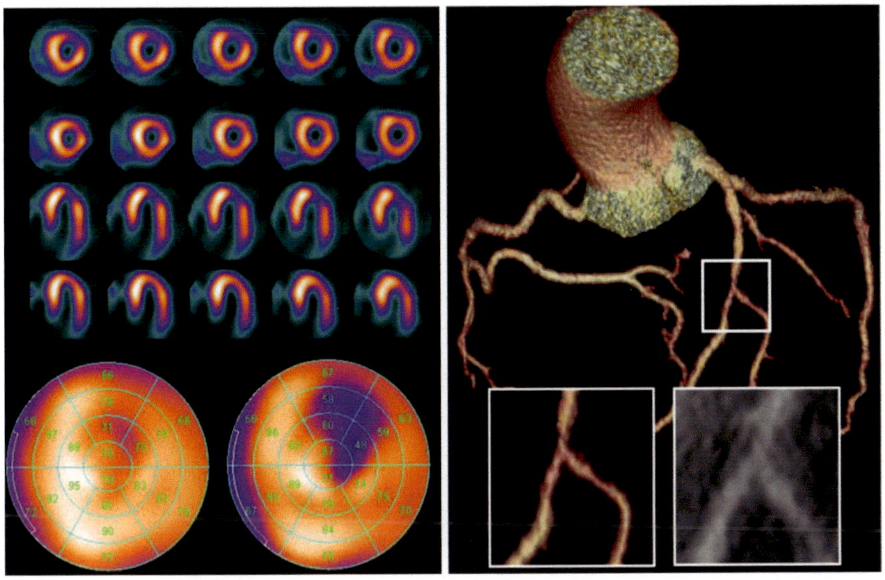

Figure 28.1 CCTA (right panel) and SPECT MPI (left panel) for Case 1.

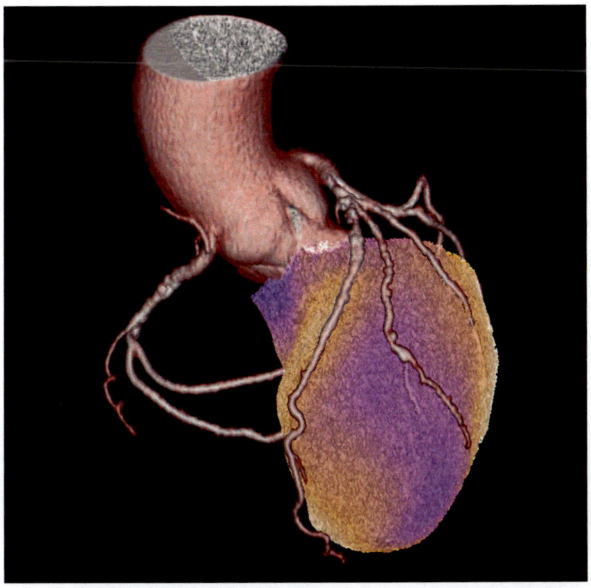

Figure 28.2 Hybrid CCTA and SPECT MPI for Case 1.

in a case of severe ischemia in a setting where symptoms are progressive, the possibility of urgent revascularization should be considered, underlining the need for close collaboration between imager and interventionalist.

CASE 3

A 70-year-old male patient was referred for SPECT/CCTA hybrid imaging for the exclusion of obstructive CAD due to atypical chest pain and a pathologic stress ECG. His body mass index was 31.3 kg/m^2, and he had known arterial hypertension and diabetes. CCTA was performed and depicted coronary lesions graded as high-grade (70–90%) in the proximal and mid-LAD, in the proximal LCX, and in the mid-RCA. Calcium score was 736 (LMA: 35, LAD: 146, LCX: 277, RCA: 278). Based on these findings, the decision was made to perform SPECT-MPI immediately afterward (Figure 28.8). No perfusion defects were noted on the stress images, hence additional rest imaging was deemed unnecessary. However, due to the diffuse nature of the obstructive disease involving all three major coronary arteries as depicted by CCTA (Figure 28.9), the suspicion of possibly balanced ischemia was raised. Consequently and due to persistent chest pain, the patient was referred for invasive coronary angiography 1 month later. The angiogram (Figure 28.10) largely confirmed the findings from CCTA, and the patient underwent coronary artery bypass surgery a few weeks later, which finally led to the relief of his symptoms.

This case emphasizes the importance of a comprehensive evaluation of all imaging and non-imaging data when performing an interpretation of any form of ischemia test. In this patient, the findings from CCTA must prompt the reader to question the existence of normally perfused reference myocardium necessary for SPECT-MPI to unmask relative perfusion defects and raise the suspicion of a false-positive test. Although CCTA may not be the preferred first-line diagnostic test for an older male patient with several cardiovascular risk factors, it proved crucially helpful as an adjunct to SPECT-MPI in this particular case because, from calcium scoring alone, potential balanced ischemia could not necessarily be expected.

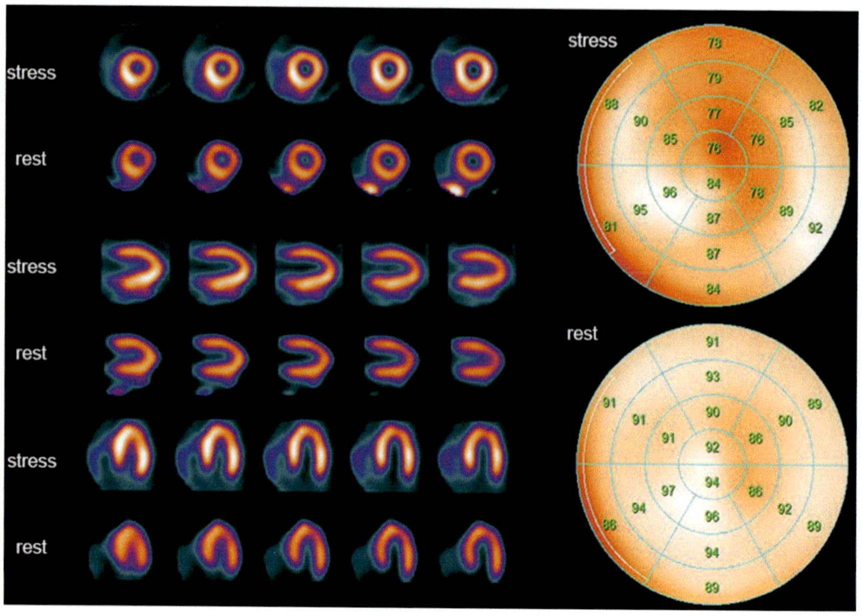

Figure 28.3 SPECT MPI post-revascularization for Case 1.

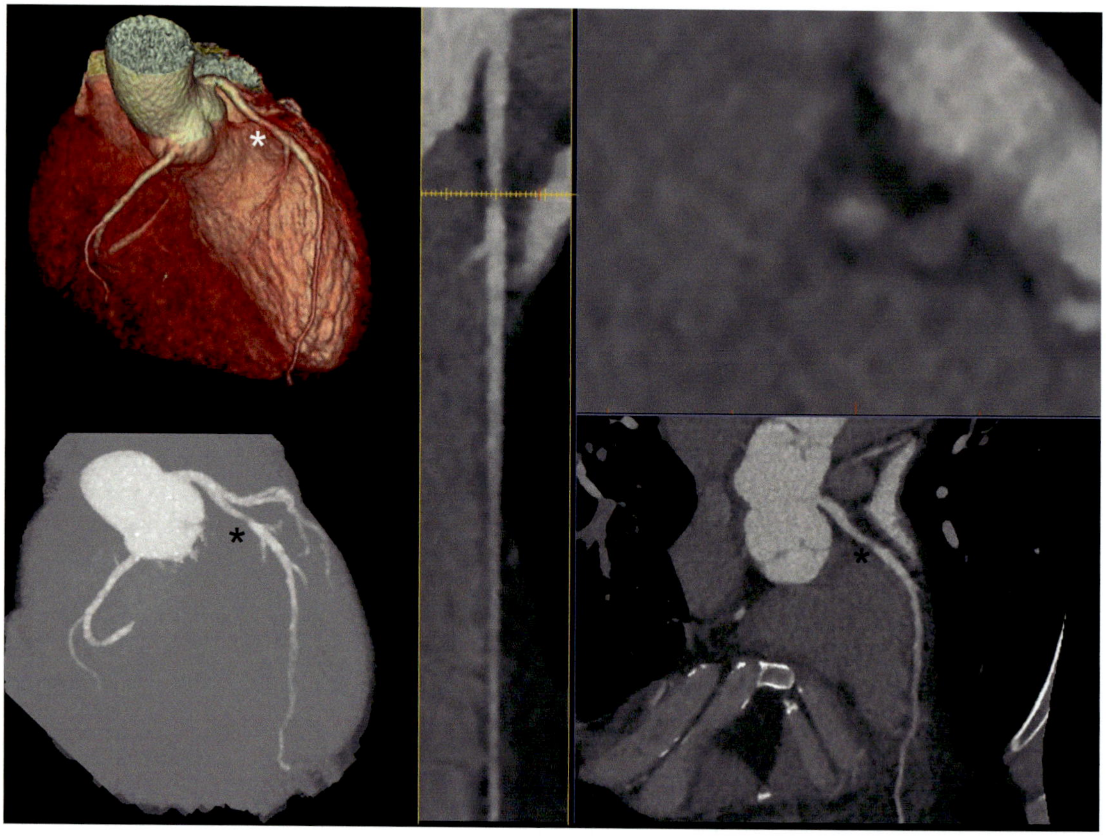

Figure 28.4 CCTA for Case 2.

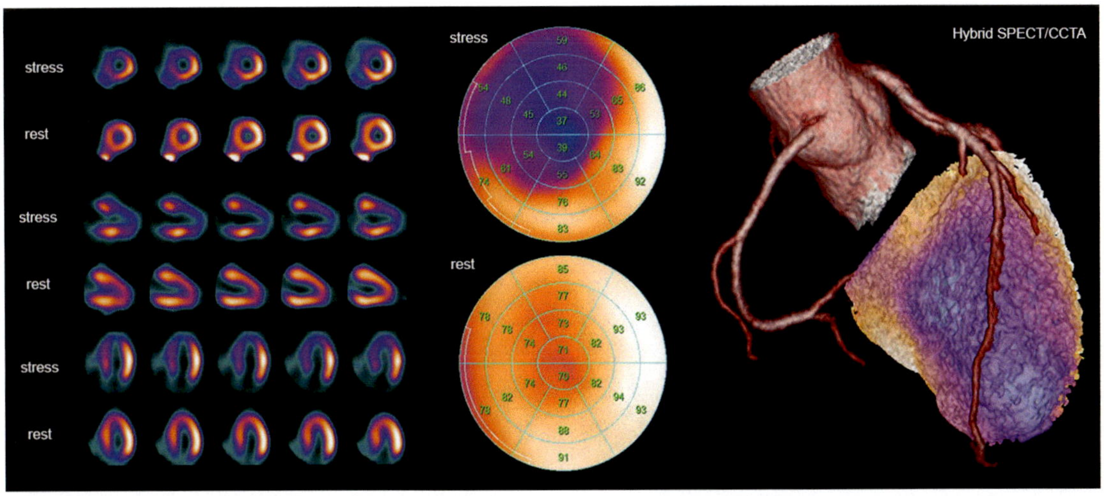

Figure 28.5 SPECT MPI for Case 2.

QUESTIONS

1. CCTA is performed in a 52-year-old male patient with atypical angina, and intermediate stenosis (50–70%) is found in the proximal left circumflex (LCX) coronary artery. Which of the following statements is correct?
   a. The patient should undergo invasive coronary angiography for revascularization.
   b. Optimal medical treatment has been shown to be associated with a better outcome than percutaneous coronary intervention in any case.
   c. A vast majority of intermediate (i.e., 50–70%) coronary stenoses are hemodynamically significant, leading to myocardial ischemia.
   d. According to current guidelines, in patients with stable angina, testing for the hemodynamic relevance of coronary stenosis is mandatory prior to potential revascularization for all coronary lesions with a luminal diameter narrowing of <90%.
   e. CCTA should not have been performed as a first-line test because of the high pretest probability of this patient.

2. Consider the following SPECT exam, which clearly demonstrates a reversible perfusion defect (i.e., ischemia) in the anterolateral wall of the LV, and the corresponding CCTA study from the same patient, which depicts intermediate stenosis (50–70%) in

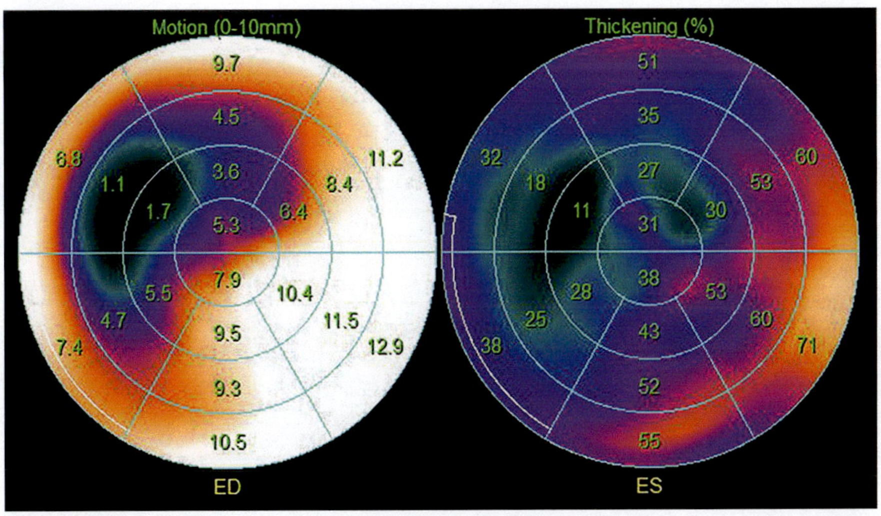

Figure 28.6 Gated SPECT MPI for Case 2.

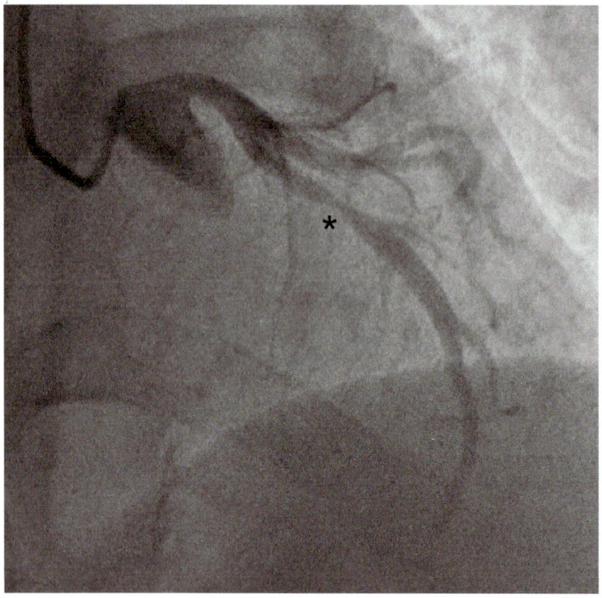

Figure 28.7 Invasive coronary angiography for Case 2.

the mid-LAD and at the origin of a second diagonal branch.

Which of the following statements is true regarding the allocation of a coronary vessel to the ischemic myocardium?

a. A side-by-side analysis of SPECT and CCTA is sufficient for identification of the culprit lesion.
b. CCTA clearly identifies the LAD artery as the culprit vessel.
c. CCTA clearly identifies the second diagonal branch as the culprit vessel.
d. Both vessels must be revascularized because CCTA depicts a stenosis.
e. Fused images are mandatory in order to identify the vessel subtending the respective myocardium.

3. CCTA tends to overestimate the severity of coronary stenosis due to which of the following?
   a. Its low spatial resolution
   b. Blooming caused by calcifications
   c. Its inherent low contrast-to-noise ratio
   d. Its inability to depict noncalcified plaques
   e. Prospective ECG triggering

ANSWERS

1. Answer 1d is correct. Please refer to the 2019 ESC guidelines for the diagnosis and management of chronic coronary syndromes. Answer a is incorrect because an intermediate stenosis is not necessarily causing ischemia. Evidence for the latter, however, is deemed mandatory for revascularization. Answer b is incorrect because optimal medical therapy may be superior in a setting with small or no ischemia but not in any case. Answer e is incorrect because the pretest probability is <50%, prompting exclusion of obstructive CAD. CCTA is optimally suited to exclude obstructive CAD because of its high sensitivity.

2. Answer 2e is correct because it has been repeatedly demonstrated that side-by-side analysis is inferior to fused analysis because of the interindividual anatomic variance, rendering the standard distribution model questionable. Answers b, c, and d are incorrect because it is impossible to deduce the hemodynamic impact of a stenosis from morphology alone.

3. Answer 3b is correct. Blooming is one of the major factors leading to systematic overestimation of stenosis severity in CCTA (also refer to Cheng et al. *JACC*

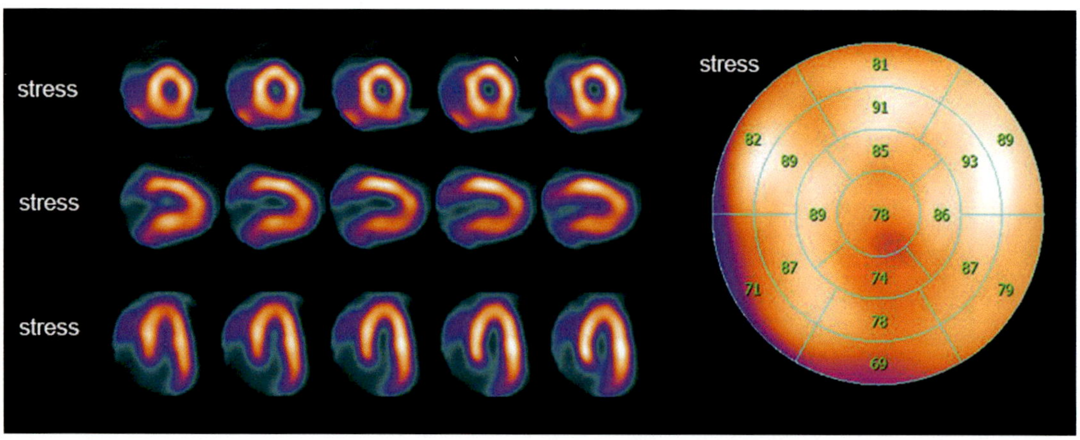

Figure 28.8 SPECT MPI for Case 3.

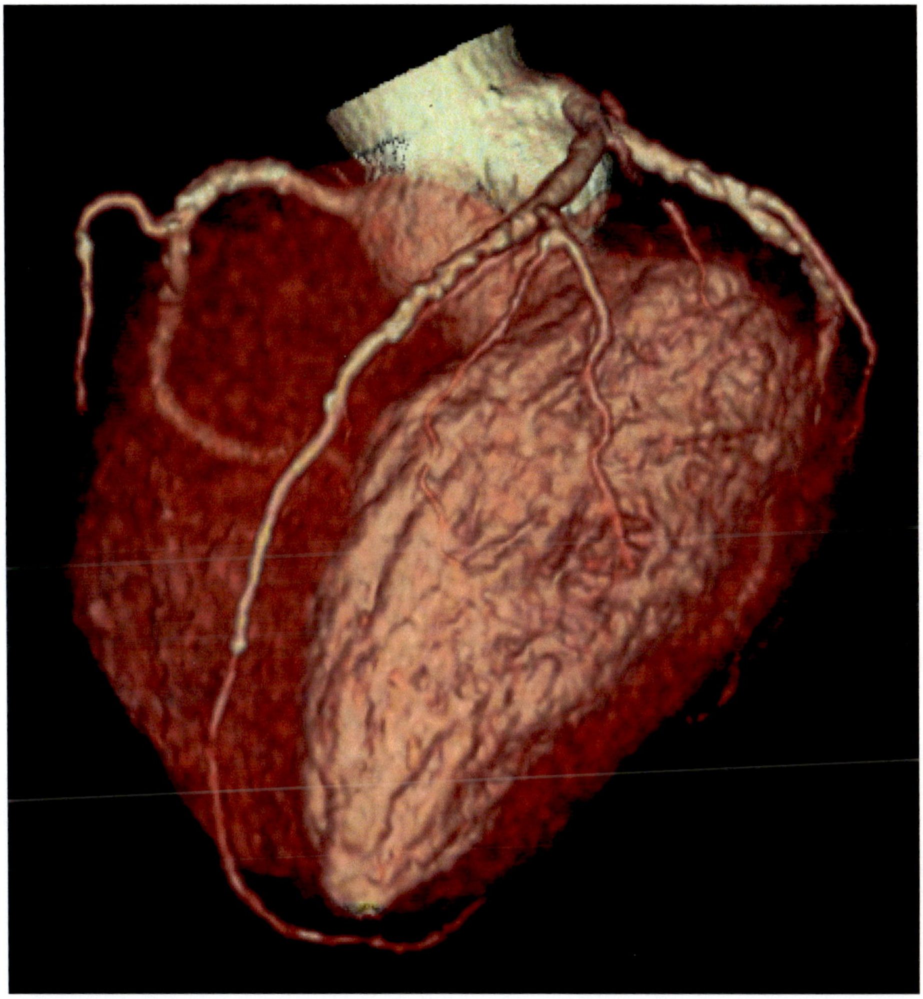

Figure 28.9 CCTA for Case 3.

Cardiovasc Imaging. 2008;1(4):460–471). Answer a is incorrect because spatial resolution in modern CT devices is very high. Answer c is incorrect because contrast-to-noise ratio is good. Answer d is incorrect because the ability to depict noncalcified lesions is, on the contrary, a valuable advantage of CCTA. Answer e is incorrect because prospective triggering is a measure of reducing radiation dose exposure.

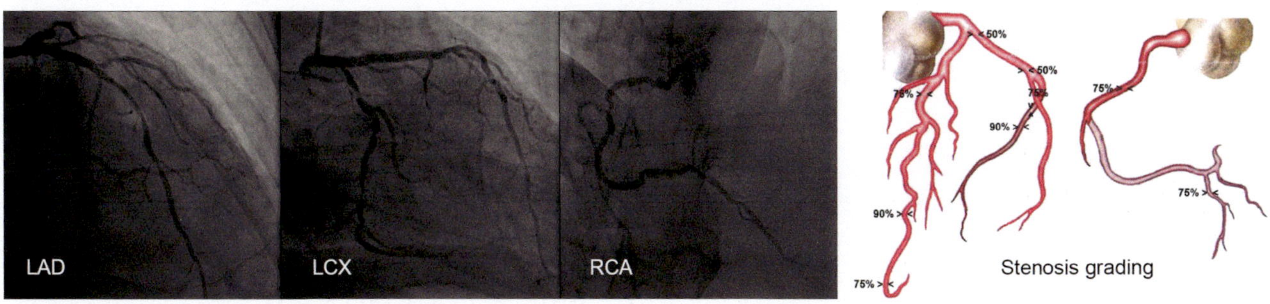

Figure 28.10 Invasive coronary angiography for Case 3.

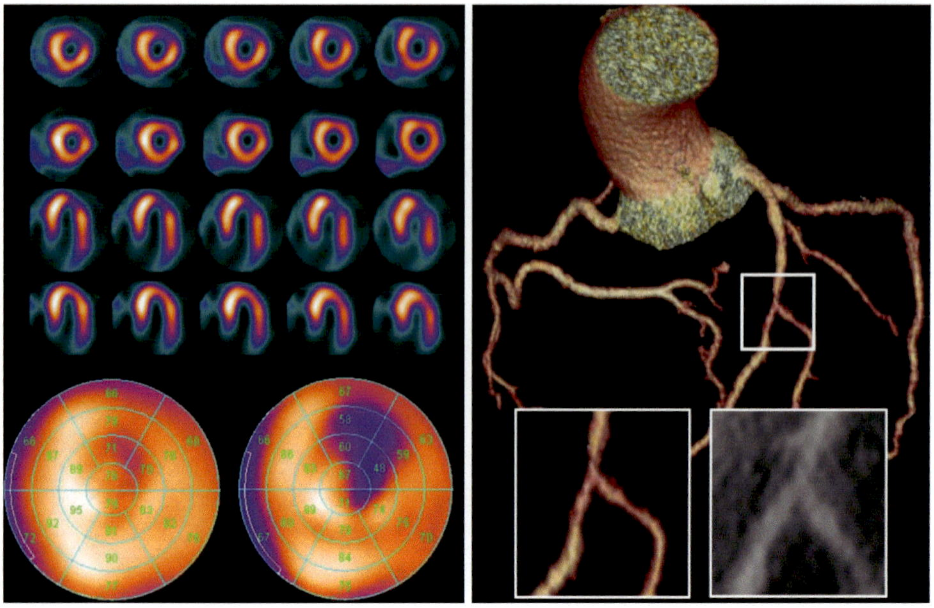

Figure 28.11 SPECT MPI (left panel) and CCTA (right panel) for Question 2.

29.

ARTIFICIAL INTELLIGENCE AND NUCLEAR IMAGING

Robert J. H. Miller and Piotr J. Slomka

CASE 1

A 57-year-old woman was referred to nuclear cardiology for an exercise rest–stress SPECT MPI. She had a history of atypical chest pain, which was described as central chest burning, that happened both with and without exertion. The pain would last for 5 to 10 minutes at a time without obvious alleviating factors. Her past medical history was significant for diabetes, hypertension, and dyslipidemia. Her pre-test probability of disease was intermediate based on Diamond-Forrester classification, and therefore exercise SPECT-MPI is considered an appropriate test (appropriate use score 7).[1] On examination, blood pressure was 128/76 mmHg and heart rate was 64 bpm. Cardiac and respiratory examination findings were unremarkable. The patient underwent exercise stress testing for 7 minutes on a Bruce protocol. Her resting ECG is shown in Figure 29.1A and peak stress ECG is shown in Figure 29.1B. The resting ECG demonstrated slight t-wave inversions through the precordial leads, with upsloping ST-segment depression at peak stress. Gated stress perfusion is shown in ▶ Video 29.1. There was moderate hypokinesis of the mid and distal anterior wall with stress. Figure 29.2 outlines the stress and rest perfusion with representative short-axis and long-axis slices and polar maps. Figure 29.3 shows deep-learning attention overlapped on the polar maps, highlighting regions in the anterior wall. The CAD-probability map is shown at the bottom and demonstrates a high probability of CAD in the LAD territory. The patient went on to have coronary angiography, which demonstrated a 90% mid-LAD lesion (▶ Video 29.2), which was subsequently stented with good improvement in the patient's symptoms.

In this case, the results of visual interpretation (summed stress score 8), quantitative analysis (stress TPD 11%), and AI interpretation all suggested a high likelihood of obstructive CAD in the LAD distribution. In this case, AI would aid clinical-decision making by increasing reader confidence in the diagnosis.

CASE 2

A 57-year-old man presented to hospital with new-onset dyspnea. He endorsed a history of progressive dyspnea over the last 3 months, currently New York Heart Association class III. He also had orthopnea and paroxysmal nocturnal dyspnea for the last 2 days. Past medical history was significant for diabetes. On examination, his blood pressure was 100/72 mmHg and heart rate was 88 bpm. He had bilateral pitting edema to mid-shin and jugular venous pressure was elevated at 8 cm above the sternal angle. He had crackles bilaterally at the bases. Cardiac examination revealed a displaced cardiac apex, S3 and 2/6 holosystolic murmur at the apex. The patient was initially treated with intravenous diuretics and started on guideline-directed medical therapy when the echocardiogram confirmed severe LV dysfunction with an LV ejection fraction of 25%.

The patient was referred for SPECT MPI to assess for the presence of significant underlying CAD with new-onset heart failure (appropriate indication, appropriate use score 8).[1] The patient exercised for 6 minutes on a Bruce protocol, with no significant ECG changes. Gated SPECT MPI images are shown in ▶ Video 29.3, which demonstrated moderately reduced LV systolic function with regional variability. Figure 29.4 outlines the stress and rest perfusion images with representative short-axis and long-axis slices and polar maps. The polar maps also demonstrate rest–stress perfusion using grayscale. In Figure 29.5, DL attention is overlapped on the polar maps and highlights regions in all coronary territories. Additionally, the per-vessel probability of CAD was elevated in each coronary territory. Invasive coronary angiography identified significant right coronary artery (▶ Video 29.4) and an ostial left main stenosis (▶ Video 29.5). The patient underwent coronary artery bypass grafting, with normalization of ventricular function at 6 months of follow-up.

In this case, visual interpretation (summed stress score 16) and quantitative analysis (TPD 23%) were both

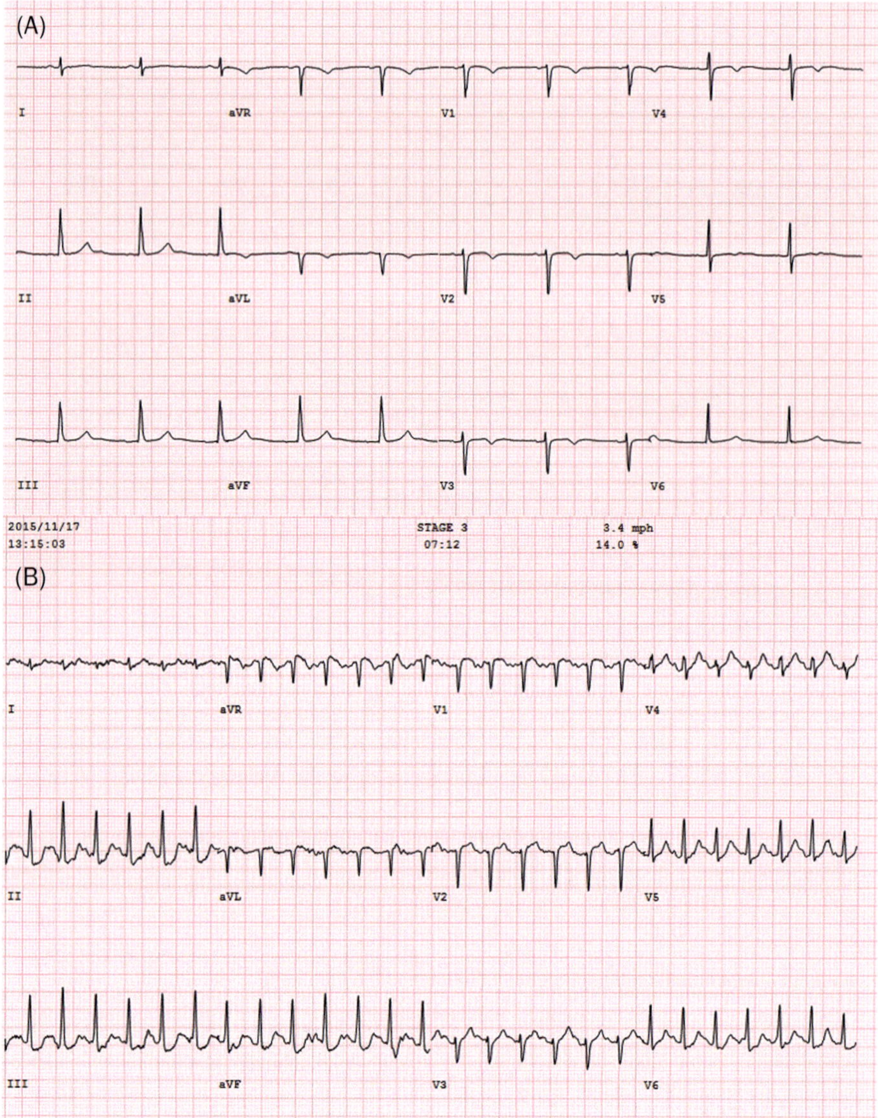

Figure 29.1. Case 1. The resting ECG (A) demonstrated slight t-wave inversions through the precordial leads, with upsloping ST-segment depression in the inferior and lateral leads at peak stress (B). There was also pseudo-normalization of the t-waves.

abnormal but may have been attributed to disease in one or two vascular territories. However, the AI prediction suggested a high risk of CAD in all coronary territories. With the result of the AI interpretation, the physician is more likely to conclude that there is a high likelihood of CAD in all vascular territories.

CASE 3

A 53-year-old woman was referred to the nuclear cardiology department for assessment regarding atypical chest pain. She described the chest pain as non-exertional and frequently brought on by emotional stress. The pain would last for 5 to 10 minutes and was described as central chest heaviness. Her past medical history was significant for dyslipidemia and a recent orthopedic injury that limited her ability to exercise. On exam, blood pressure was 130/75 mmHg and heart rate was 87 bpm. Cardiac and respiratory examination findings were unremarkable.

The patient underwent pharmacologic stress SPECT MPI to assess for ischemia in a patient with an intermediate pre-test probability who was unable to exercise (appropriate indication, appropriate use score 9).[1] The patient underwent dipyridamole pharmacologic stress with no symptoms and no ECG changes. Figure 29.6 outlines the attenuation-corrected stress and rest perfusion studies with representative short-axis and long-axis

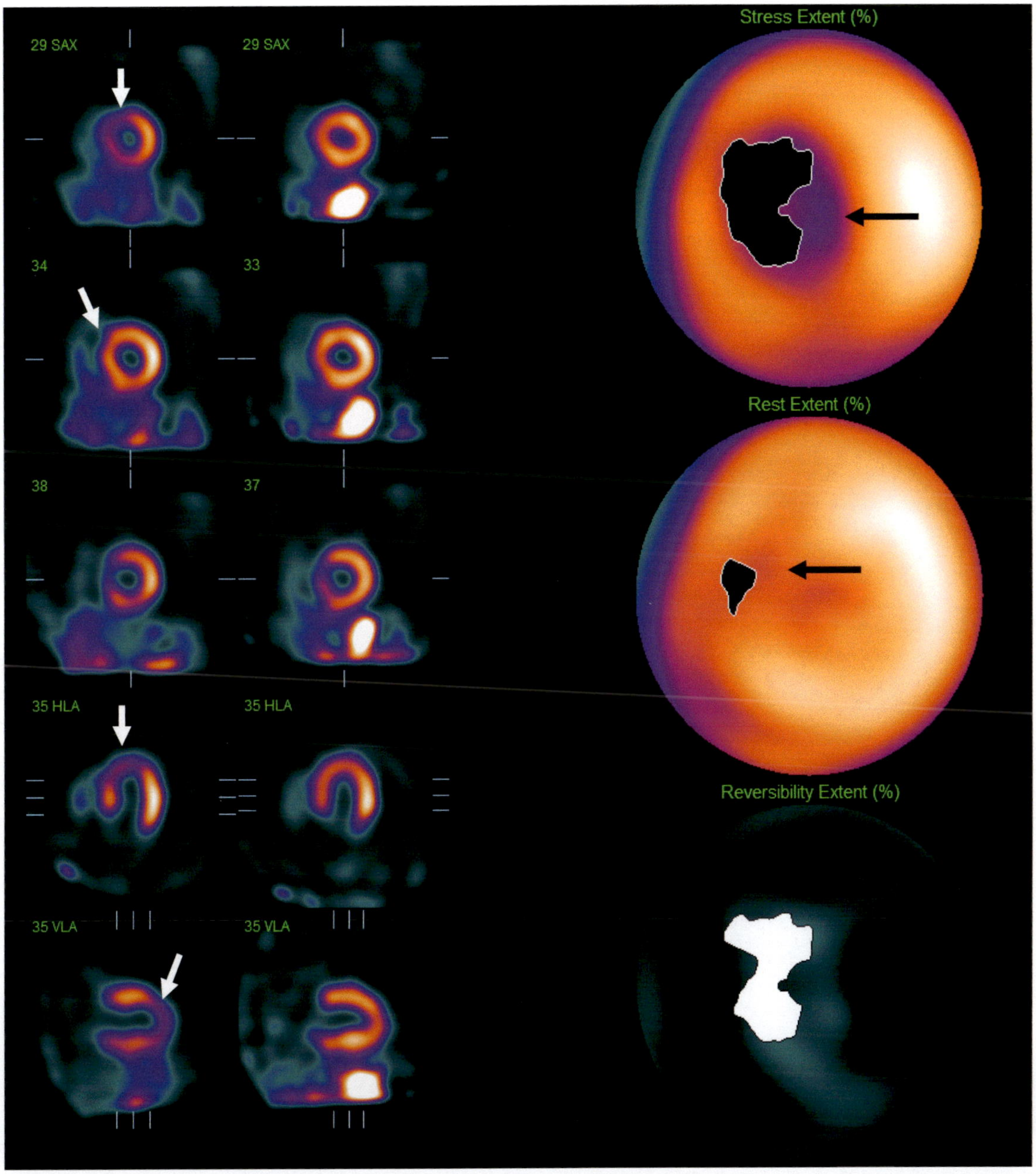

Figure 29.2. Case 1. Stress and rest perfusion results are shown on representative short-axis (SAX) and horizontal (HLA) and vertical long-axis (VLA) slices, with perfusion defects shown with white arrows. Perfusion polar maps are shown with defect extent in blackout and defects with black arrows.

slices. The study was interpreted visually as having a partially reversible perfusion abnormality in the anterior wall (white arrows). The polar maps also demonstrate rest–stress perfusion, with perfusion defects shown by black arrows. Visual interpretation (summed stress score 8) and quantitative analysis (TPD 10%) were abnormal. Results of the AI interpretation are shown in Figure 29.7. The polar maps demonstrate rest–stress perfusion using grayscale. There is no attention map due to a low probability of obstructive CAD in all vascular territories. The patient went for invasive coronary angiography, which showed no significant CAD (▶ Video 29.6).

In this case, both visual interpretation and quantitative analysis were abnormal. However, the AI prediction suggested a low likelihood of CAD in all coronary territories. The discrepant results may have prompted the physician to repeat imaging at a later time or in an alternate position to decrease gut activity in order to improve the quality of the myocardial perfusion images. This potentially could have prevented an unnecessary coronary angiogram.

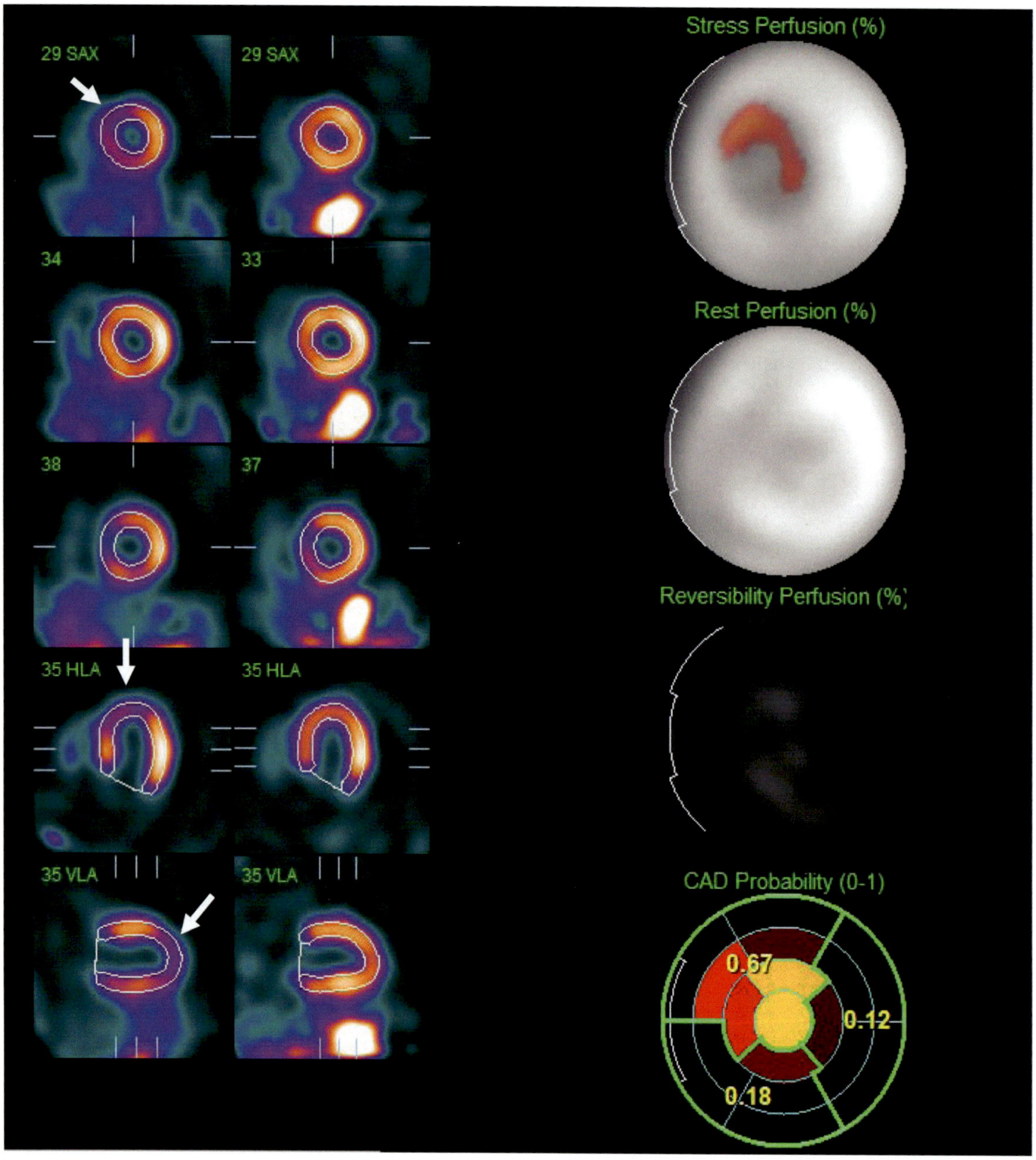

Figure 29.3. Case 1. Stress and rest perfusion results are shown on representative short-axis and long-axis slices, with white arrows pointing to perfusion defects. The polar maps also demonstrate rest–stress perfusion using a grayscale. DL attention is overlapped on the polar maps and highlights regions of the anterior wall. The CAD-probability map is shown at the bottom and demonstrates a high probability of CAD in the LAD territory.

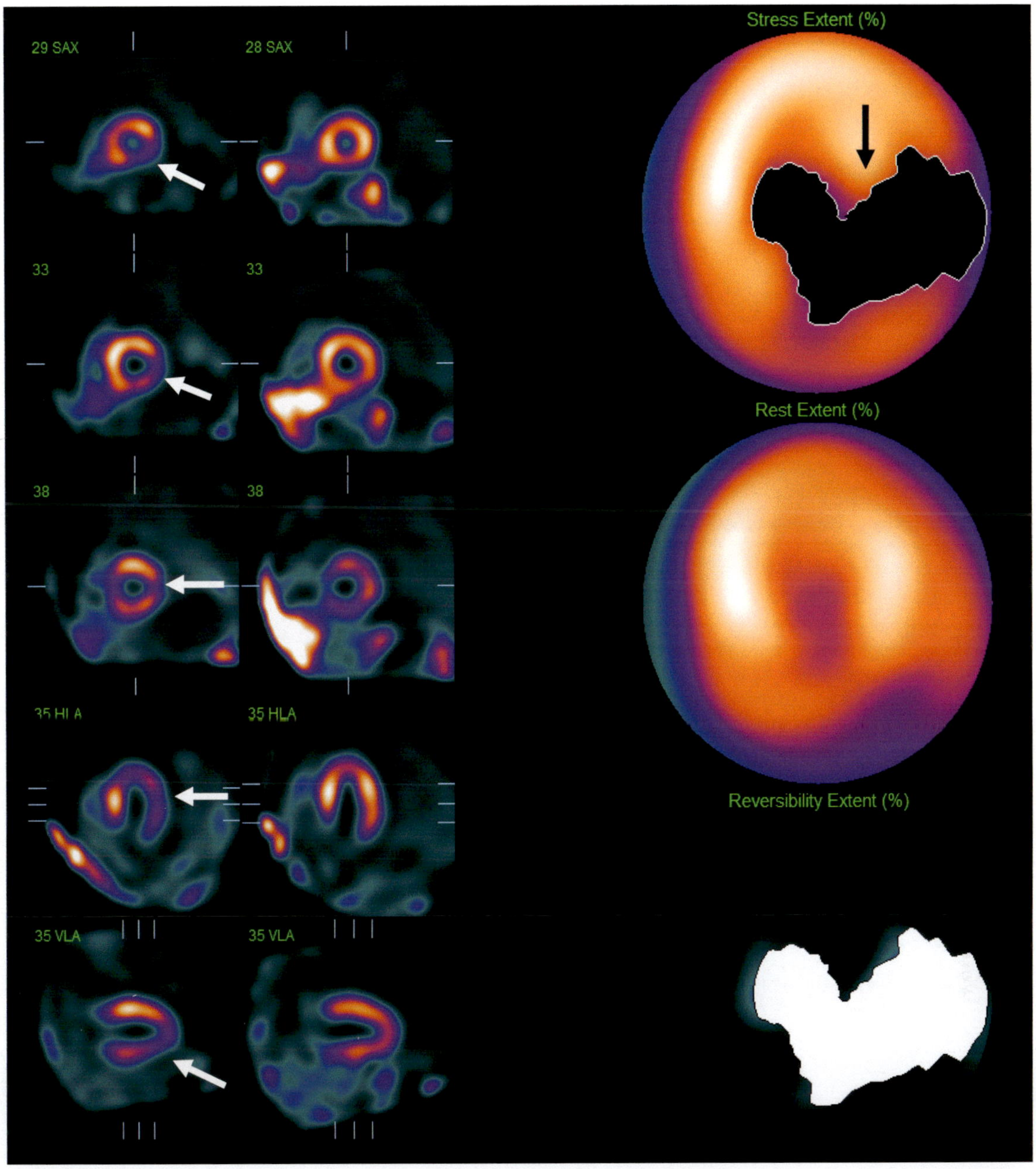

Figure 29.4. Case 2. Stress and rest perfusion results are shown on representative short-axis and long-axis slices, with perfusion defects shown by white arrows. Perfusion polar maps are shown with defect extent in blackout and defects with black arrows.

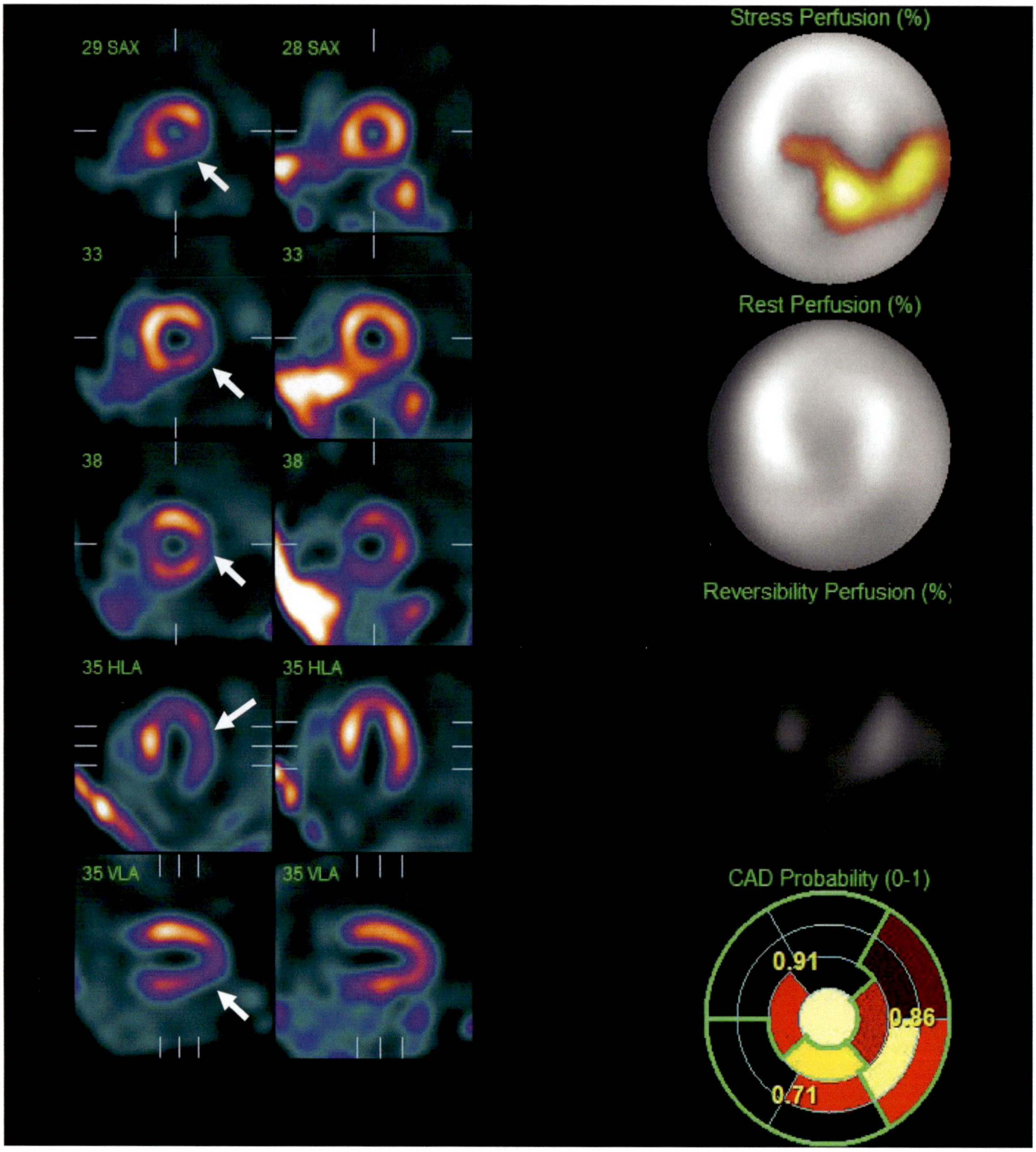

Figure 29.5. Case 2. Stress and rest perfusion results are shown on representative short-axis (SAX) and horizontal (HLA) and vertical long-axis (VLA) slices, with perfusion defects shown by white arrows. The polar maps also demonstrate rest–stress perfusion using a grayscale. DL attention is overlapped on the polar maps and highlights regions in all coronary territories. The CAD-probability map is shown at the bottom and demonstrates a high probability of CAD in all territories.

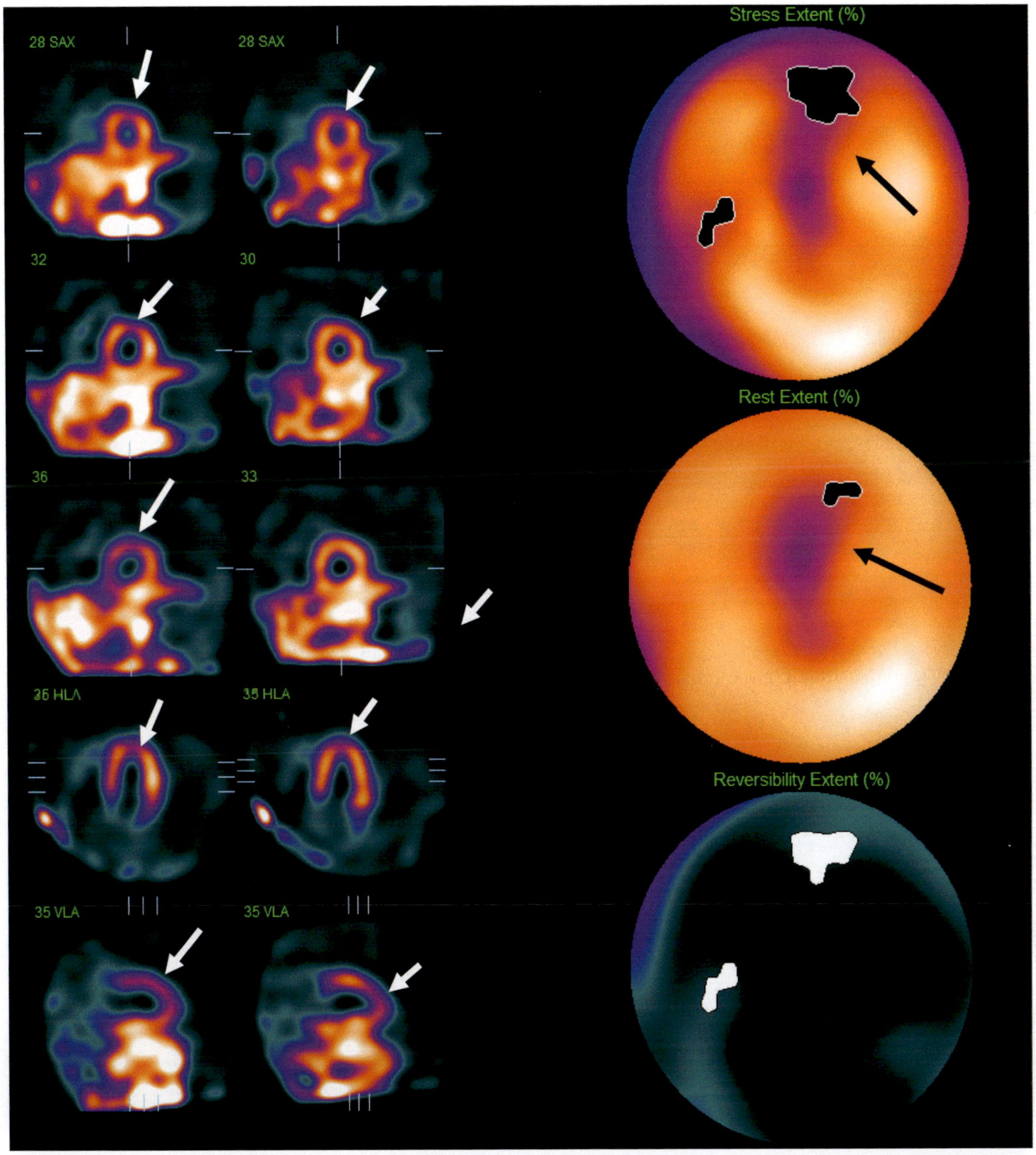

Figure 29.6. Case 3. Stress and rest attenuation-corrected perfusion results are shown by representative short-axis (SAX) and horizontal (HLA) and vertical long-axis (VLA) slices, with perfusion defects noted by white arrows. Polar maps also demonstrate stress and rest attenuation-corrected perfusion, with defects noted by black arrows.

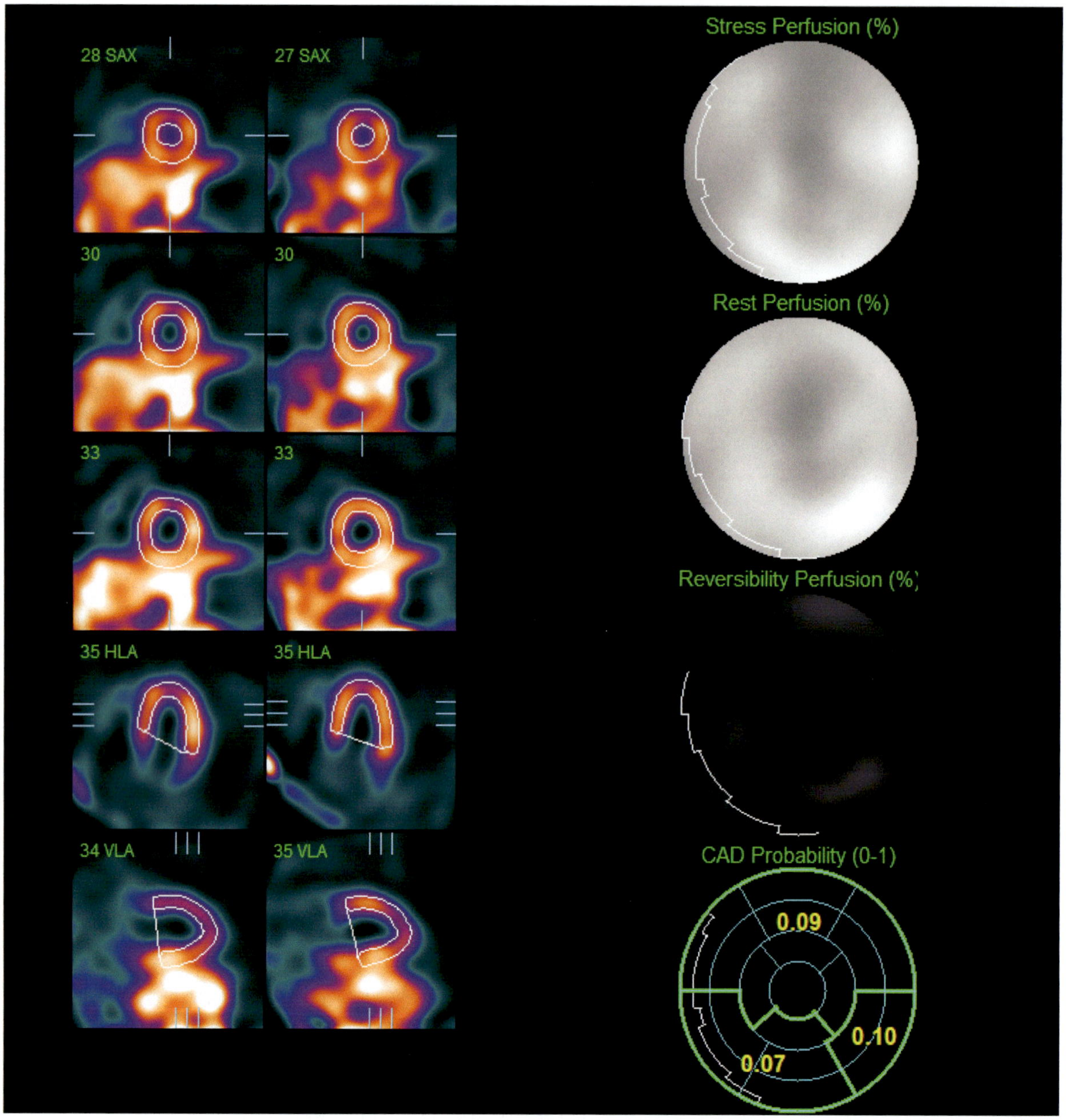

Figure 29.7. Case 3. Stress and rest perfusion results are shown on representative short-axis and long-axis slices. The polar maps also demonstrate rest–stress perfusion using a grayscale. The DL attention map is not shown due to a low probability of obstructive CAD in all territories.

REFERENCE

1. Hendel RC, Berman DS, Carli MFD, et al. ACCF/ASNC/ACR/AHA/ASE/SCCT/SCMR/SNM 2009 appropriate use criteria for cardiac radionuclide imaging. *Circulation*. 2009;119:e561–e587.

30.

NUCLEAR IMAGING IN PATIENTS WITH SERIOUS ARRHYTHMIAS

Ravi Venkatesh and Saurabh Malhotra

CASE 1

A 54-year-old man with a history of CAD and ICM presented to the emergency department with complaints of ICD shocks. His ICD was placed at another institution 1 year earlier, following non-ST-elevation MI, which was treated by percutaneous coronary intervention in the left anterior descending and left circumflex coronary arteries. At that time his LVEF was 30%. On presentation his blood pressure and heart rate were 133/88 mmHg and 56 bpm, respectively. His ECG (Figure 30.1) showed sinus bradycardia, with frequent premature ventricular contractions and prior inferior MI.

The patient was admitted to the telemetry unit for observation, with continuation of dual antiplatelet agents, beta-blocker, and angiotensin-converting enzyme inhibitor therapy. His 2D-echocardiogram revealed a preserved LVEF of 50% (improved from prior report) (▶ Video 30.1). ICD interrogation revealed five episodes of nonsustained VT, with three episodes of sustained VT, one of which (22 bpm) was terminated by ICD shock (Figure 30.2), and the others by anti-tachycardia pacing.

Rest/regadenoson stress SPECT MPI was performed to assess for ischemia as a cause of these arrhythmias (Figure 30.3). SPECT MPI showed a moderate size area of severe fixed perfusion defect in the basal and mid inferior wall, and adjacent inferolateral segments. In addition, there are two areas of focal moderate to severe fixed perfusion defects in the mid anterior wall and the distal lateral wall. The global myocardial scar burden was approximated at 24% of the LV myocardium.

The patient was discharged on medical therapy for CAD and heart failure, with the addition of amiodarone to prevent the recurrence of VT. However, 3 weeks after discharge, the patient again presented with multiple ICD shocks, despite being compliant with medical therapy. He had no symptoms or signs of decompensated heart failure. Invasive coronary angiogram was performed and representative images are shown in Figure 30.4; there are no significant stenoses.

The patient was referred for EPS with the intention of VT ablation. Based on the findings of the prior SPECT MPI, the suspect site of VT was thought to be the severe scar in the inferior wall. VT was readily induced on EPS (Figure 30.5) and was mapped to the inferior wall of the LV (Figure 30.6A), followed by ablation in that region (Figure 30.6B), resulting in termination of VT.

This case illustrates the inability of LVEF to risk stratify occurrence of VT. The patient's LVEF had recovered after ICD implantation and despite an LVEF of 50%, he continued to have drug-refractory VT. SPECT MPI not only allowed the physicians to rule out ischemia as a cause of recurrent VT but also identified the presence and location of abnormal myocardial substrate that guided definitive VT ablation.

CASE 2

A 64-year-old female with known history of CAD and prior coronary artery bypass grafting in 2013 was admitted with syncope. She has a history of ICM and received an ICD in 2015, when her LVEF was 25%. She has been on guideline-directed medical therapy for heart failure, and the most recent LVEF was reported to be 60% (▶ Video 30.2). She reports frequent "dizzy" spells, resulting in falls, but had never passed out prior to this episode. On presentation her blood pressure was 153/76 mmHg and heart rate was 66 bpm. Her ECG on presentation (Figure 30.7) showed sinus rhythm with LV hypertrophy.

Her ICD was interrogated in the ED and showed multiple episodes of nonsustained VT, with one episode of sustained VT at 180 bpm, which was terminated by anti-tachycardia pacing (Figure 30.8).

The patient was admitted to the hospital for further workup of her syncope in the setting of evidence of sustained VT. She underwent a rest/regadenoson stress SPECT MPI that showed a small, mild scar in the basal inferolateral segment and a larger reversible defect

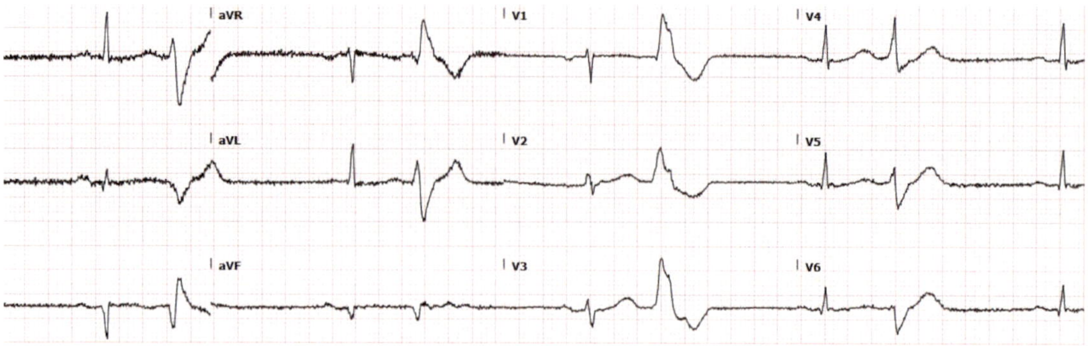

Figure 30.1. Case 1. ECG depicting sinus rhythm with frequent premature ventricular contractions.

(ischemia) in the basal to mid lateral segments and the adjacent inferior wall (Figure 30.9). Approximately 10% of the LV myocardium was considered to be at risk (summed difference score = 8). Coronary angiography showed a discrete 80% luminal stenosis in the right coronary artery just after the touchdown of the saphenous venous bypass graft (Figure 30.10a). Percutaneous coronary intervention of this lesion was performed (Figure 30.10b), with no residual stenosis and TIMI 3 flow.

This case illustrates the ability of cardiac RNI to identify arrhythmogenic substrate in a patient with CAD but normal global LV function. In this case, the arrhythmogenic substrate was a large area of myocardial ischemia due to severe stenosis in the native right coronary artery. Following percutaneous coronary intervention, the patient did not have any episodes of syncope or presyncope.

CASE 3

A 79-year-old male patient with a history of NICM secondary to alcohol abuse and primary prevention ICD, implanted 1 month ago, was seen in the cardiology clinic. The patient's last EF prior to ICD implant was 35%. He had NYHA class II heart failure symptoms, on guideline-directed medical therapy including beta-blocker, angiotensin-converting enzyme inhibitor, and spironolactone. The patient's resting ECG showed sinus rhythm and

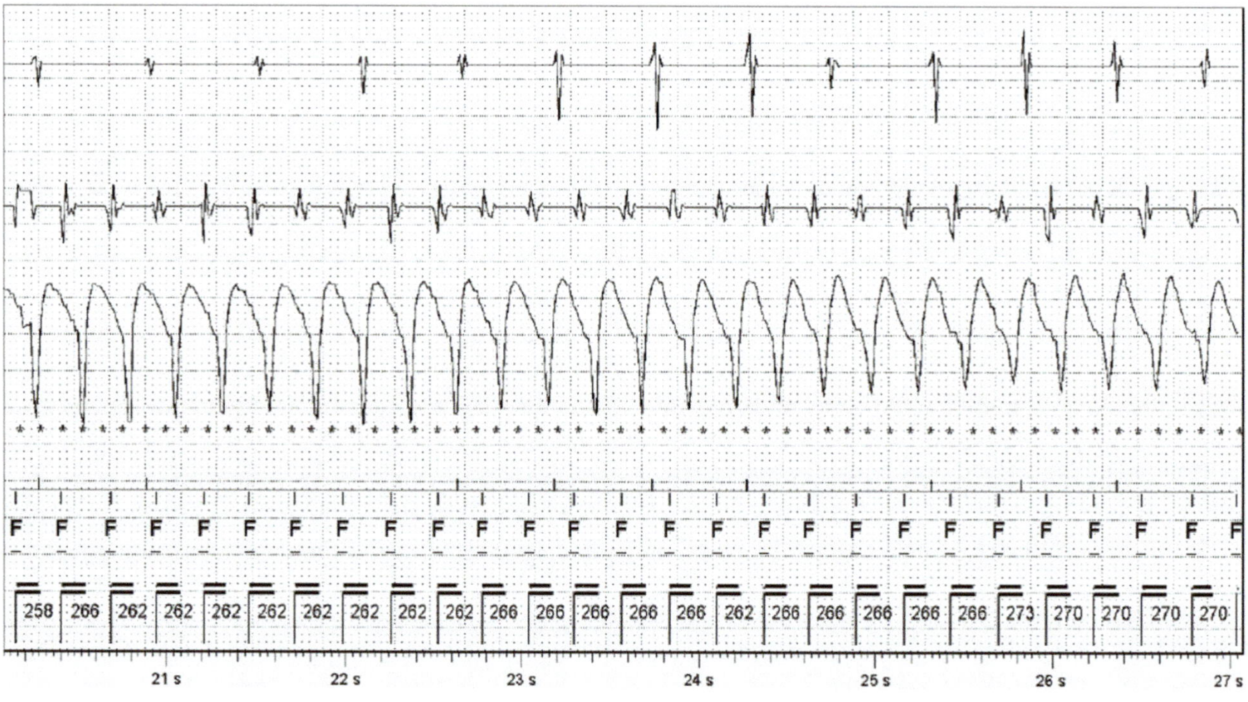

Figure 30.2. Case 1. Intracardiac ECG depicting fast ventricular tachycardia. This rhythm was ultimately terminated by ICD shock.

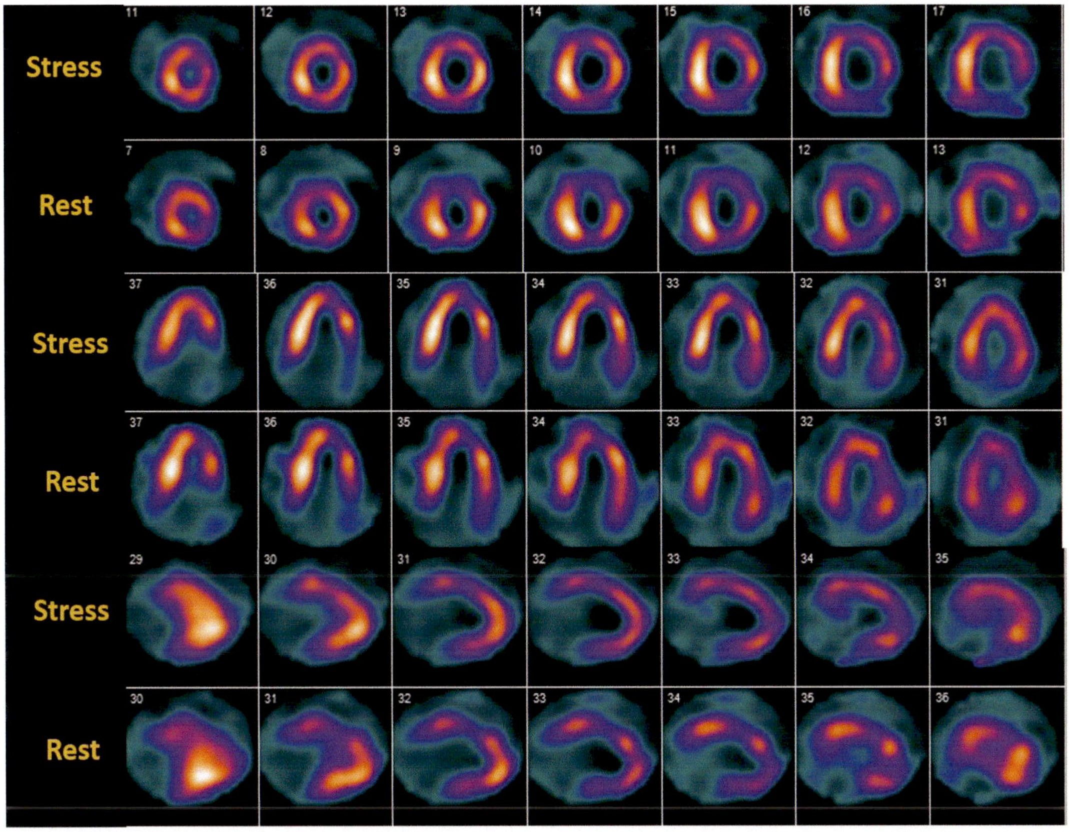

Figure 30.3. Case 1. Rest/regadenoson Stress SPECT MPI. Tomographic images at rest and post-stress depicting multiple areas of myocardial infarcts in the anterior, inferior, and lateral walls of the LV.

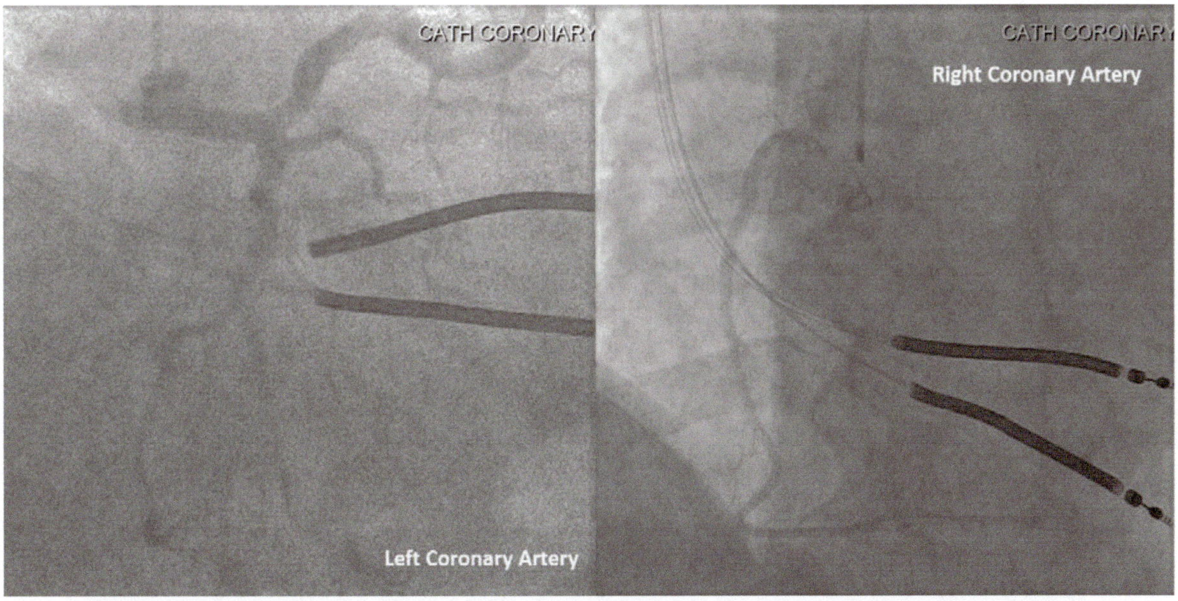

Figure 30.4. Case 1. Invasive coronary angiogram of the left and right coronary arteries showing lack of anatomically significant CAD.

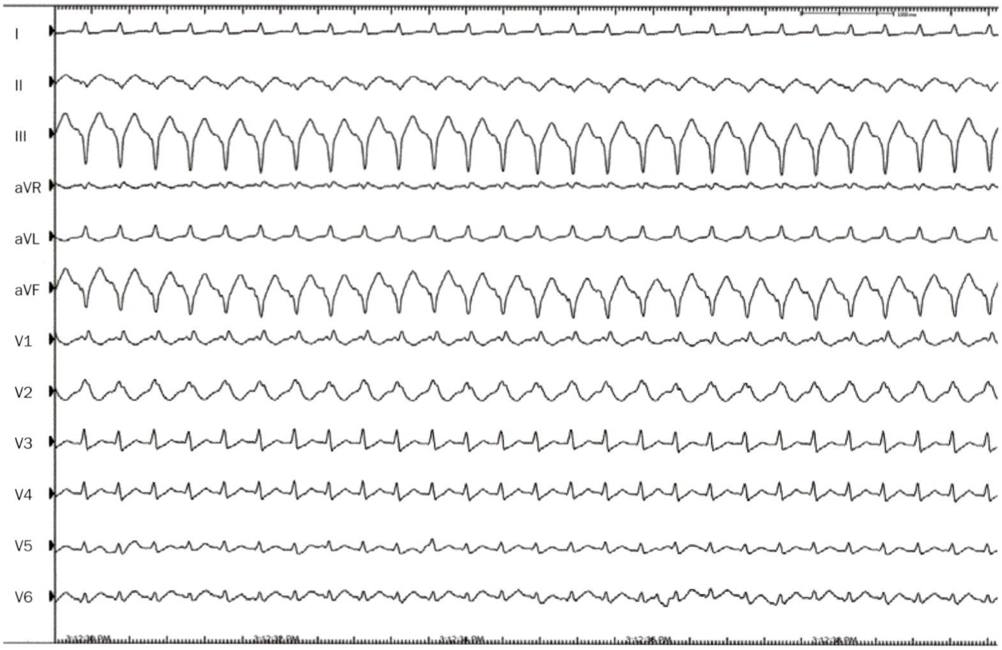

Figure 30.5. Case 1. Intracardiac electrogram obtained during EPS depicting fast ventricular tachycardia.

a right bundle branch block. His brain natriuretic peptide level was 188 ng/L. To assess prognosis from his cardiomyopathy he was referred for ^{123}I-MIBG scintigraphy.

^{123}I-MIBG scintigraphy was performed at 15 minutes (early) and at 4 hours (late) after injection of 10 mCi of Adreview (Iobenguane I-123). Planar images (Figure 30.11), show significant ^{123}I-MIBG uptake with a late HMR of 1.68. ^{123}I-MIBG SPECT was also performed at 4 hours, and tomographic data were compared to resting Tc-99m tetrofosmin scintigraphy performed a few days later (Figure 30.12). On ^{123}I-MIBG SPECT a defect score of 30 was calculated and a resting perfusion score was calculated

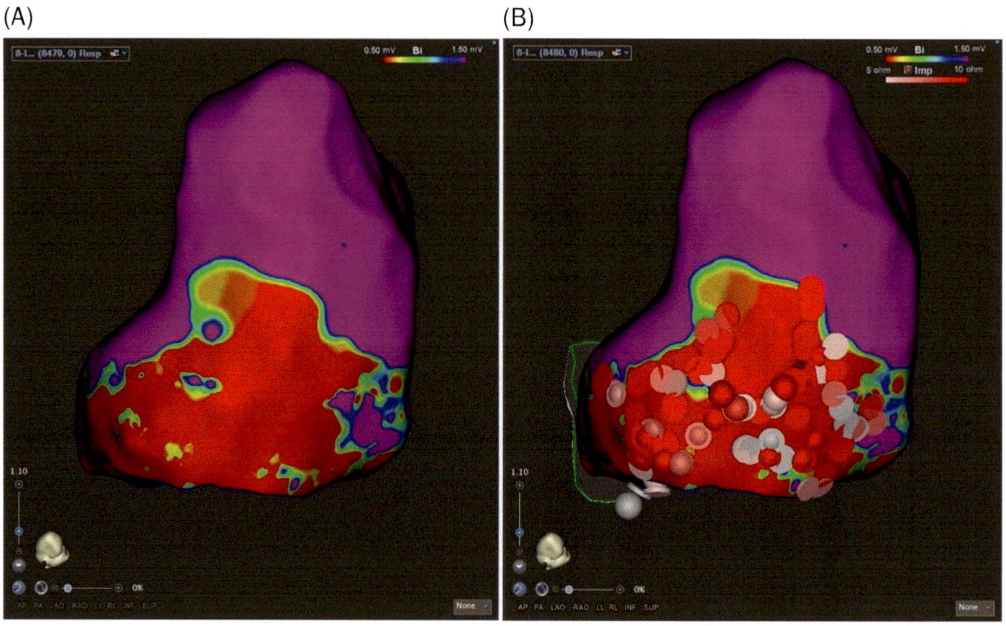

Figure 30.6. Case 1. Electroanatomic map of the LV during EPS. The map demonstrates area of low voltage with dense scar (red area, <0.5 mV) in the basal to mid inferior portion of the LV in the LAO (Left Anterior Oblique) caudal view (a), along with sites of ablation that resulted in termination of VT (b).

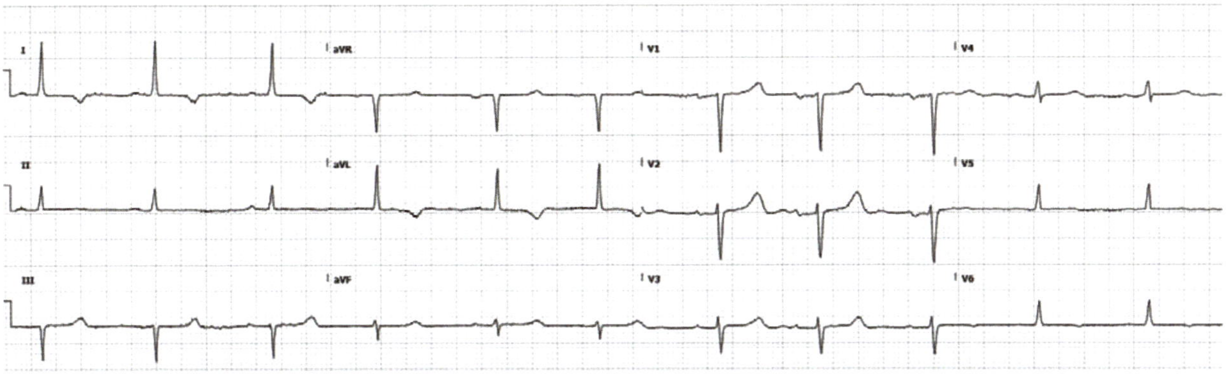

Figure 30.7. Case 2. ECG depicting sinus rhythm and LV hypertrophy.

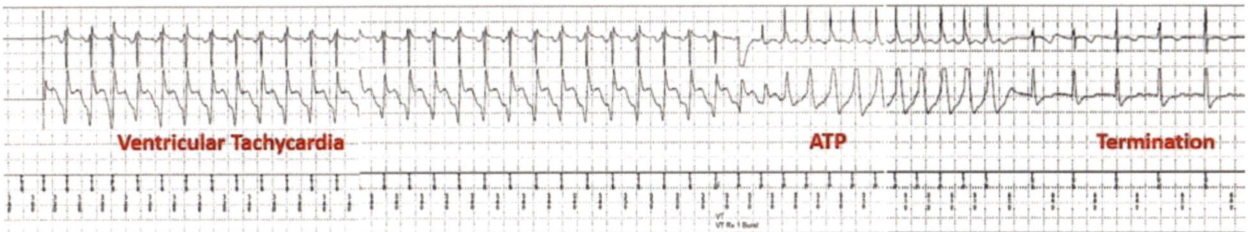

Figure 30.8. Case 2. Intracardiac electrogram obtained from ICD interrogation depicting the occurrence of ventricular tachycardia and its termination via anti-tachycardia pacing (ATP).

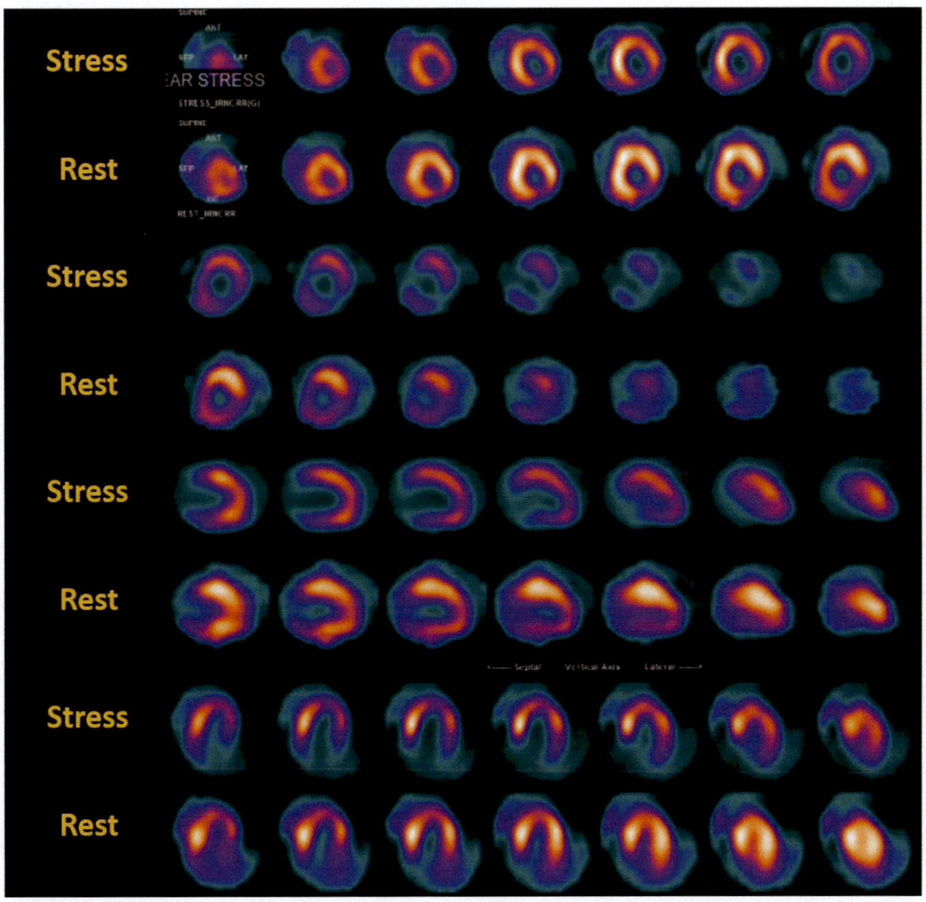

Figure 30.9. Case 2. Rest/stress myocardial perfusion SPECT with large area of ischemia in the inferior and lateral wall.

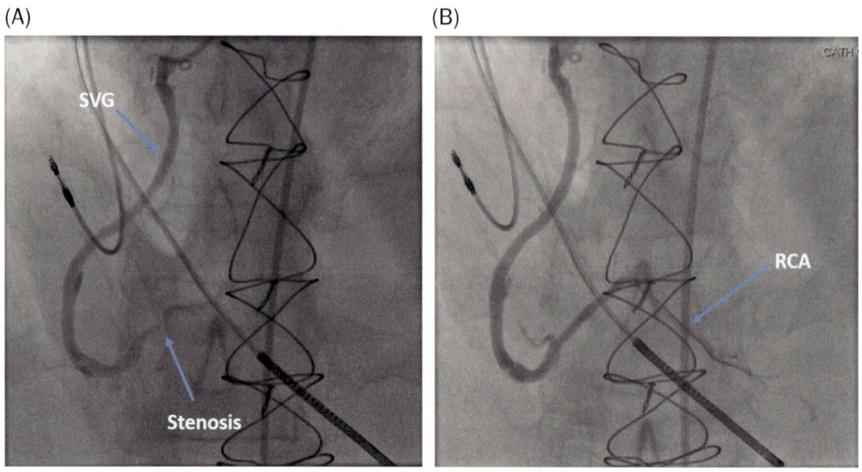

Figure 30.10. Case 2. Invasive coronary angiogram of the right coronary artery (RCA) with severe stenosis in the vessel. SVG = saphenous venous graft,

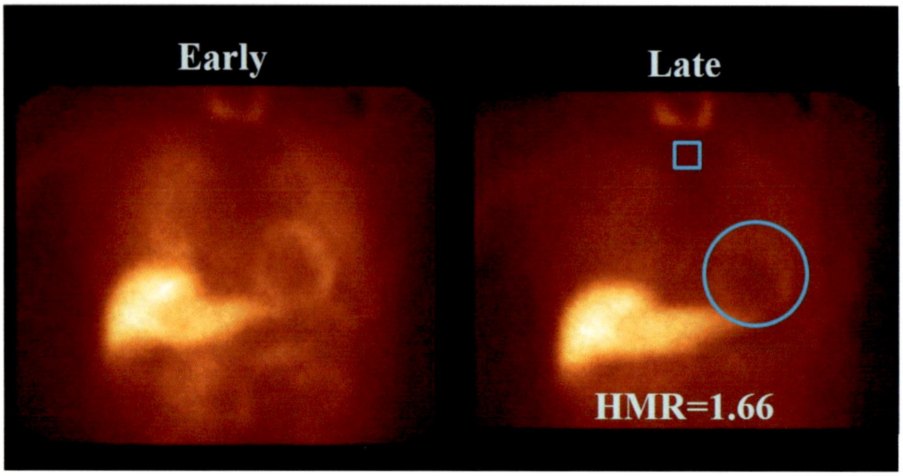

Figure 30.11. Case 3. ^{123}I-MIBG scintigraphy. Anterior planar images showing significant tracer uptake with a late HMR of 1.66, suggesting preserved sympathetic innervation. Images courtesy Mark I. Travin, MD, Montefiore Medical Center, NY.

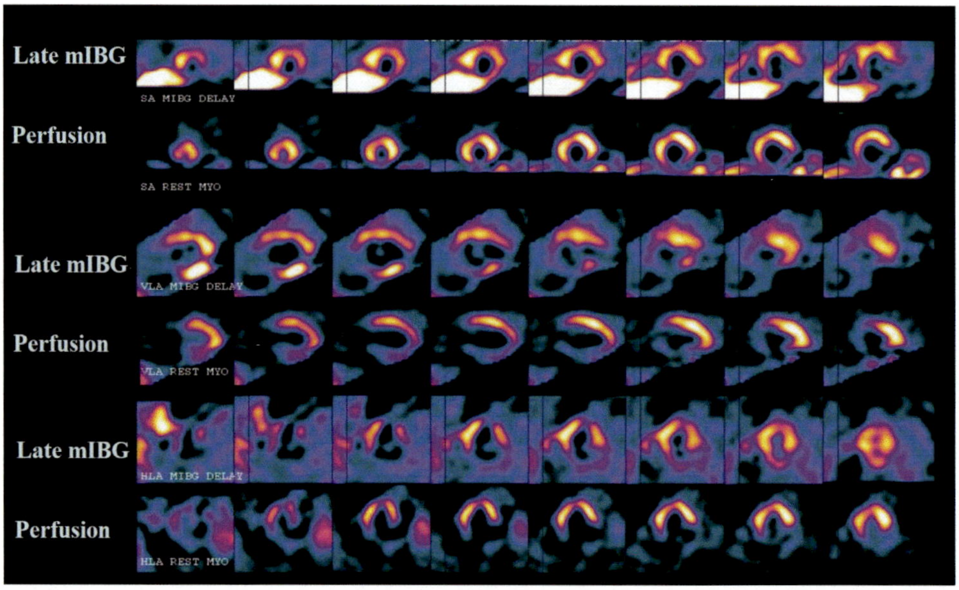

Figure 30.12. Case 3. ^{123}I-MIBG and Tc-99m tetrofosmin SPECT images. There is a small area of innervation/perfusion mismatch at the LV apex. Images courtesy Mark I. Travin, MD, Montefiore Medical Center, NY.

at 27, with a small area of innervation/perfusion mismatch at the apex. The mismatch score was calculated at 3. Over the next 5 years the patient experienced no clinical deterioration, no worsening heart failure, and no arrhythmic events on interrogation of his ICD.

This case highlights that, despite a low EF and a high infarct burden (45% of LV myocardium), preserved sympathetic innervation on planar ^{123}I-MIBG scintigraphy and a low burden of innervation/perfusion mismatch portend a favorable short-term (~2 years) prognosis in patients with heart failure. Long-term prognosis of these low-risk scintigraphic findings is not well studied thus far.

31.

THE ROLE OF NUCLEAR CARDIOLOGY IN THE MANAGEMENT OF CARDIOVASCULAR DISEASES IN PATIENTS LIVING WITH HIV

Ahmed Aljizeeri and Mouaz H. Al-Mallah

CASE 1

A 58-year-old man with HIV presented to the office complaining of episodes of burning chest pain of a few weeks' duration. He reported a history of a brief burning chest pain upon walking more than a block. The pain is sometimes relieved with rest. He did not have shortness of breath, palpitations, or lower limb swelling.

He had a PCI to his LAD 4 years ago for non-ST-elevation MI. He is also known to have hypertension and hypercholesterolemia. His medications included aspirin 81 mg once daily, metoprolol 50 mg twice daily, perindopril 5 mg once daily, and atorvastatin 40 mg once daily, in addition to antiretroviral therapy.

His clinical examination revealed a healthy-looking man in no acute distress. BP was 157/85 mmHg and heart rate was 86 bpm. The cardiac exam was normal and the lungs were clear. There was no edema.

Laboratory studies showed a hemoglobin of 14.5 g/dL and a creatinine of 1.2 g/dL. His LDL was 120 mg/dL and HDL was 35 mg/dL. The chest x-ray was normal. His ECG showed normal sinus rhythm with no acute ischemic changes (Figure 31.1). His transthoracic echocardiogram showed normal LVEF with normal wall motion without significant valvular pathology (▶ Video 31.1).

He was advised to hold his beta-blocker the day before the scheduled exercise MPI. When he presented to the stress lab, his resting BP was 187/90 mmHg. Therefore, the stress test was changed to a vasodilator stress test. He underwent regadenoson MPI with PET.

The perfusion images showed a severe perfusion defect in in the mid and distal segments of the anterior wall and apex with improvement at rest, indicating severe ischemia in the LAD territory (Figure 31.2). The stress LVEF and rest LVEF were 56% and 58% respectively. The global myocardial flow reserve (MBF) was low at 1.6 and was low in the territories of LAD (1.5) and right coronary arteries (RCA) (1.6).

He underwent coronary angiography, which showed severe in-stent stenosis in the proximal LAD and a severe stenosis of the mid RCA. He underwent PCI to the LAD and RCA (▶ Videos 31.2 and 31.3).

This is a middle-aged man with HIV and CAD presenting with atypical angina. Based on the patient's presentation, normal baseline ECG, and ability to exercise, exercise SPECT MPI was appropriately requested. However, when the patient came to his test, his BP was high, which is considered a relative contraindication to performing an exercise stress test. Therefore, a vasodilator stress test with PET MPI was alternatively performed. PET MPI is preferred over SPECT when a vasodilator is used and when PET is available.

Although the perfusion images showed ischemia in the LAD territory, PET provided additional diagnostic data regarding significant stenosis in the RCA by measuring the MBF. The PET-derived MBF and flow reserve provide added prognostic and diagnostic information to the perfusion pattern. The low global myocardial flow reserve and the low regional flow reserve in the LAD and RCA indicated a high likelihood of significant two-vessel disease in this patient.[1–4]

CASE 2

A 46-year-old man recently diagnosed with HIV presented to the emergency department with a 1-hour history of chest pain. The pain was felt as a dull ache in the middle of the chest and was not associated with other symptoms. There were no cough, shortness of breath, or palpitations He was diagnosed with HIV 6 months earlier when he visited his family physician for unusual skin lesions. He was started on ART. He was a known intravenous drug abuser but had no other pertinent medical history. His medications included ART and over-the-counter pain medications.

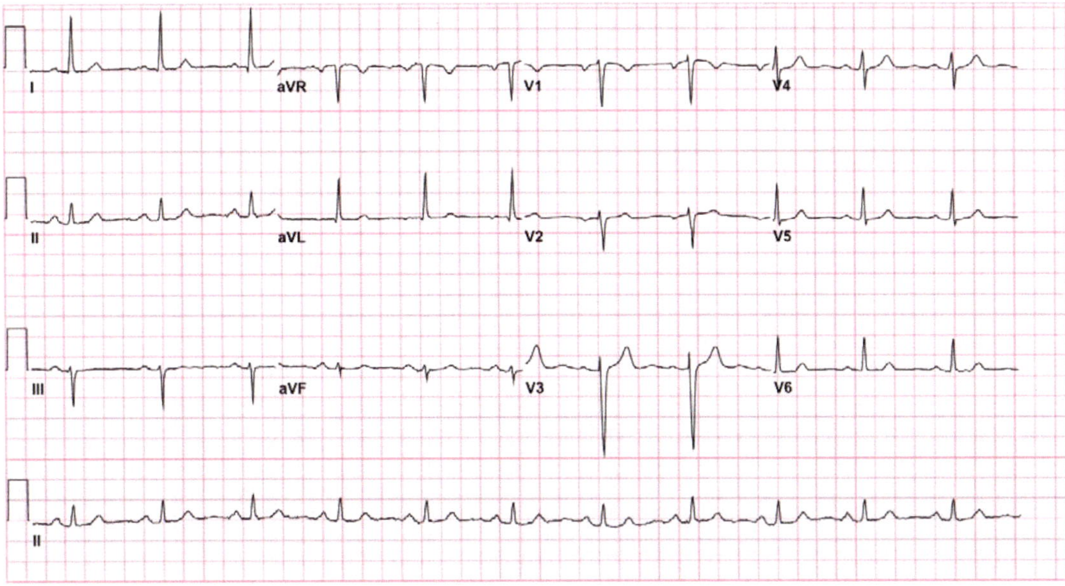

Figure 31.1. Case 1. Resting ECG.

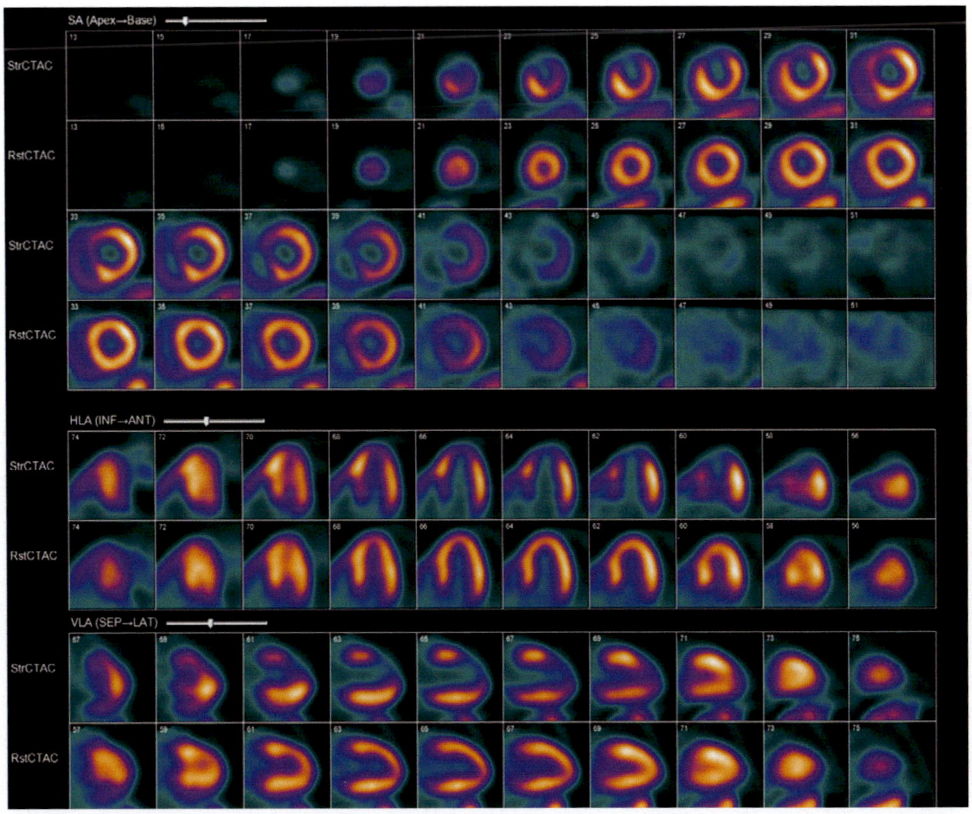

Figure 31.2. Case 1. Stress-rest PET perfusion imaging demonstrating severe reduction of tracer uptake in the mid and apical segments of the anterior wall and apex during stress with improvement at rest, consistent with severe ischemia in the LAD territory.

His BP was 145/89 mmHg and his heart rate was 78 bpm. His chest examination revealed basal crepitation in both lungs. His jugular venous pressure was 3 cm above the sternal angle. He had normal first and second heart sounds with no added sounds or murmurs. The peripheral vascular exam was normal. The initial ECG showed sinus rhythm with ST elevation in the inferior and lateral leads (Figure 31.3). The complete blood count and kidney function were normal. The high-sensitivity cardiac troponin value was 3,898 pg/mL (abnormal >35 pg/mL). The echocardiogram showed normal LV size, systolic function, and wall motion. However, he was noted to have pericardial effusion (▶ Video 31.4).

He was diagnosed with ST-segment-elevation MI. The emergency physician started him on anticoagulation and dual antiplatelet therapy. He underwent an urgent coronary angiogram, which demonstrated nonobstructive disease in the mid LAD (see ▶ Video 31.4). His echocardiogram showed normal LV size, systolic function, and wall motion. However, he was noted to have pericardial effusion (Video 31.5). Subsequently, he underwent CMR, which showed thickening of the pericardium with moderate pericardial effusion (▶ Video 31.6). CMR tissue characterization demonstrated pericardial effusion, edema of the pericardium and nonischemic myocardial injury in the lateral wall of the LV (Figure 31.4).

The patient's diagnosis was changed to acute myopericarditis. He was discharged home on nonsteroidal anti-inflammatory drugs and colchicine.

Acute pericarditis usually mimics ST-elevation MI since the patient presents with acute chest pain and ST elevation on ECG. The diagnosis can be made on an echocardiogram. Pericardial thickening and pericardial effusion suggest the diagnosis of pericarditis. CMR can confirm the diagnosis of acute pericarditis and show myocardial involvement. Pericardial inflammation is confirmed by the presence of pericardial edema and late gadolinium enhancement.

Recently, the entity of myocardial infarction without obstructive coronary artery disease (MINOCA) is increasingly recognized. MINOCA accounts for 5% to 6% of acute MI cases. The findings of ischemic myocardial injury confirm the diagnosis of MINOCA.[5–7]

CASE 3

A 65-year-old man with HIV, diabetes, and hypertension presented to the emergency department complaining of shortness of breath. The shortness of breath started 4 weeks before his presentation and has progressed over time. He now feels short of breath while sitting. He uses three pillows to sleep and wakes up several times at night gasping for air. He did not have chest pain, palpitations, or syncope. His current medications include metformin, lisinopril, and ART.

The clinical examination revealed a BP of 138/70 mmHg. The heart rate was regular at 70 bpm. He had fine crepitations over both lung fields. His jugular venous pressure was 6 cm above the sternal angle. There were normal first and second heart sounds and a third heart

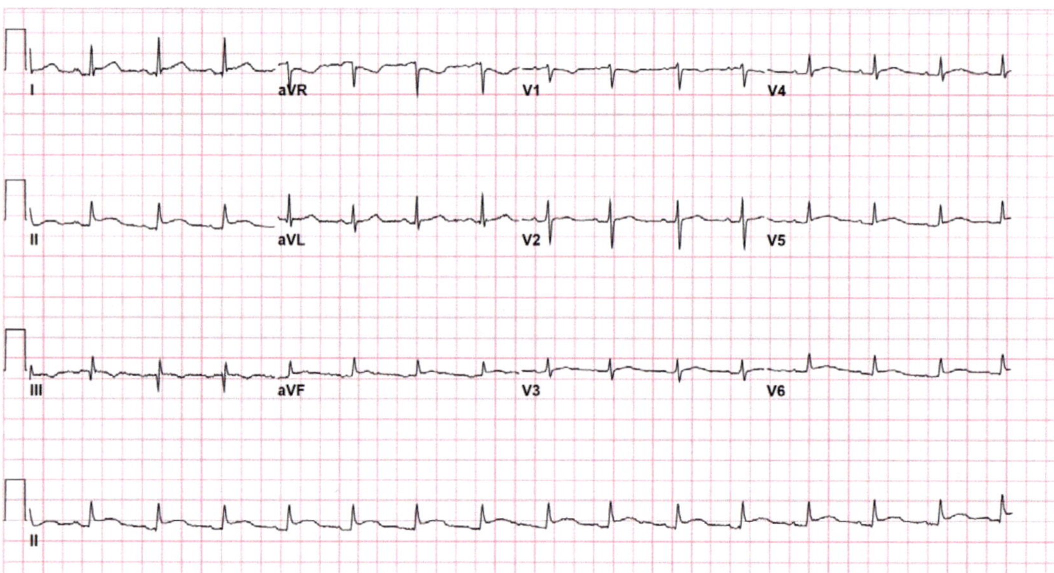

Figure 31.3. Case 2. ECG showing ST elevation in inferior and lateral leads.

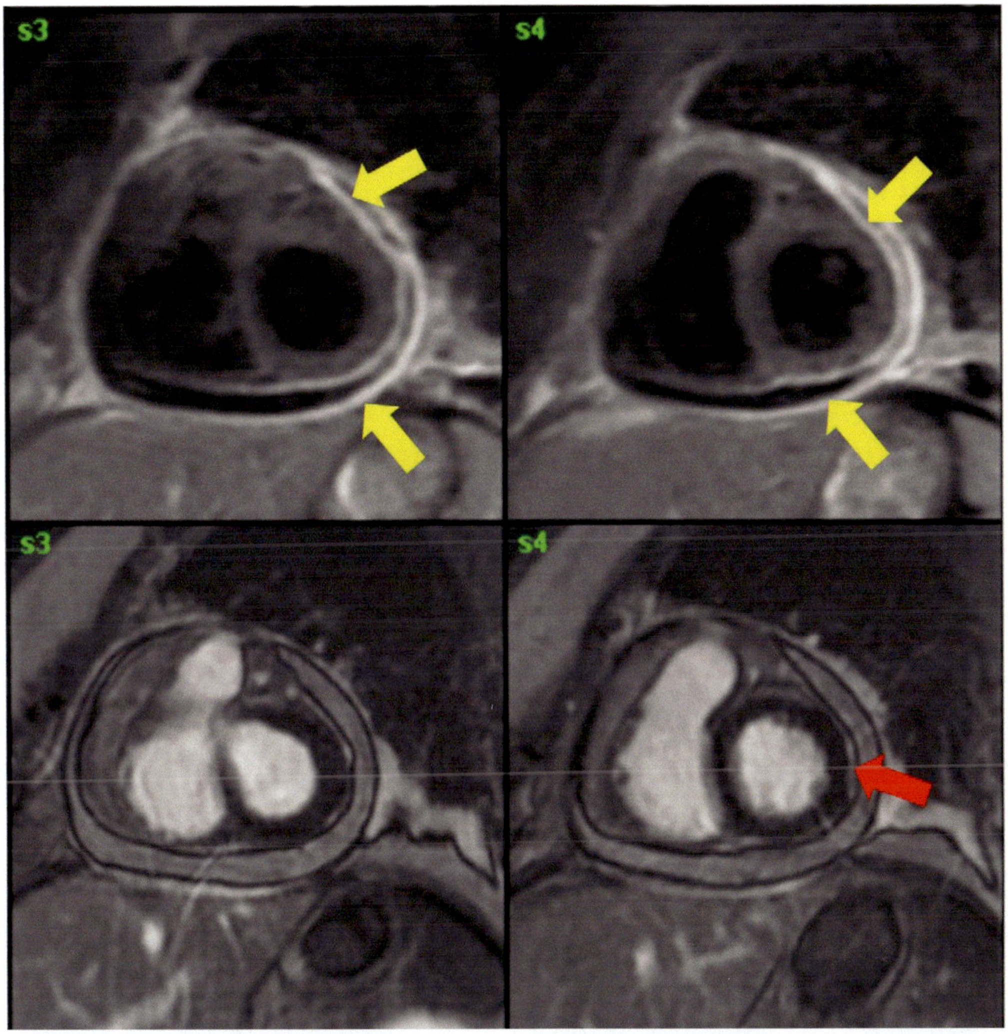

Figure 31.4. Case 2. Edema CMR images (upper panel) showing thickening and edema of the visceral and parietal pericardium (yellow arrows) and delayed myocardial enhancement images showing sub-epicardial delayed enhancement of the lateral wall of the LV.

sound with no murmurs. He has pitting edema up the middle of the legs.

He had normal hemoglobin and renal function. His high-sensitivity troponin value was within the normal limit. B-type natriuretic peptide (BNP) value was 150 pg/mL. The ECG showed normal sinus rhythm with voltage criteria for left ventricular hypertrophy (Figure 31.5). His echocardiogram showed a dilated LV with moderate LV systolic function. The LVEF was estimated to be 35% to 40%. There was global hypokinesia of the left ventricle without significant valvular regurgitation (▶ Video 31.7).

He was diagnosed with heart failure with reduced EF. He was started on intravenous diuresis, an ACE inhibitor, and an aldosterone antagonist. He had an invasive coronary angiography, which showed no epicardial coronary stenoses (▶ Video 31.8). He also underwent CMR, which demonstrated a moderate LV systolic dysfunction with an LVEF of 35% without replacement fibrosis or prior MI (Figure 31.6). The ACE inhibitor was changed to an angiotensin receptor neprilysin inhibitor. The patient was started on beta-blockers when he was euvolemic.

Heart failure is the most common cardiac presentation in HIV. The diagnosis of nonischemic cardiomyopathy is made in cases of heart failure with reduced EF and normal coronary arteries. CMR is increasingly used in the evaluation of patients with heart failure. CMR provides an accurate evaluation of the left and right ventricle EFs. In addition, it provides additional diagnostic and prognostic information. The presence of ischemic myocardial delayed enhancement supports the diagnosis of an ischemic etiology even in the absence of significant CAD. Furthermore, the presence of the delayed enhancement, whether ischemic

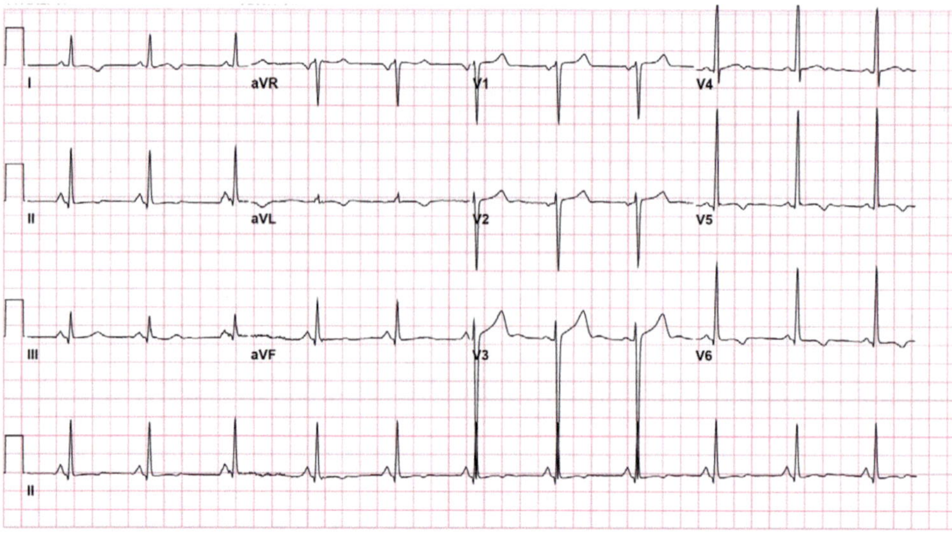

Figure 31.5. Case 3. ECG showing voltage criteria of left ventricular hypertrophy and nonspecific T-wave abnormalities.

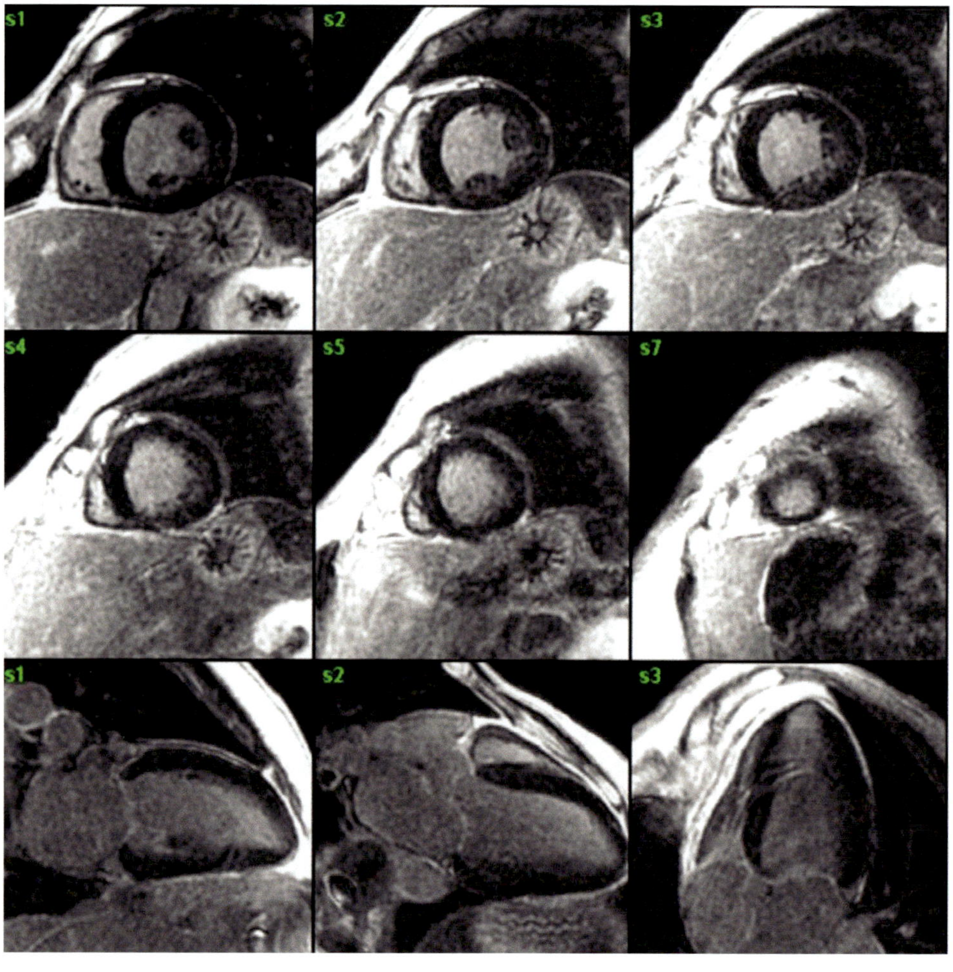

Figure 31.6. Case 3. Delayed myocardial enhancement CMR images showing no replacement fibrosis or prior MI.

or nonischemic, is associated with a higher risk of death, arrhythmia, and hospitalization for heart failure.[8–10]

REFERENCES

1. Hendel RC, Berman DS, Di Carli MF, et al. ACCF/ASNC/ACR/AHA/ASE/SCCT/SCMR/SNM 2009 appropriate use criteria for cardiac radionuclide imaging. *Circulation*. 2009;119:e561–e587.
2. Henzlova MJ, Duvall WL, Einstein AJ, et al. ASNC imaging guidelines for SPECT nuclear cardiology procedures: Stress, protocols, and tracers. *J Nucl Cardiol*. 2016;23:606–639.
3. Aljizeeri A, Ahmed AI, Alfaris MA, et al. Myocardial flow reserve and coronary calcification in prognosis of patients with suspected coronary artery disease. *JACC Cardiovasc Imaging*. 2021;14(12):2443–2452.
4. Bateman TM, Heller GV, Beanlands R, et al. Practical guide for interpreting and reporting cardiac PET measurements of myocardial blood flow. *J Nucl Cardiol*. 2021;28(2):768–787.
5. Antman EM, Anbe DT, Armstrong PW, et al. ACC/AHA guidelines for the management of patients with ST-elevation myocardial infarction—executive summary. *J Am Coll Cardiol*. 2004;44:671–719.
6. Chiabrando JG, Bonaventura A, Vecchie A, et al. Management of acute and recurrent pericarditis: JACC state-of-the-art review. *J Am Coll Cardiol*. 2020;75:76–92.
7. Tamis-Holland JE, Jneid H, Reynolds HR, et al. Contemporary diagnosis and management of patients with myocardial infarction in the absence of obstructive coronary artery disease: A scientific statement from the American Heart Association. *Circulation*. 2019;139:e891–e908.
8. Remick J, Georgiopoulou V, Marti C, et al. Heart failure in patients with human immunodeficiency virus infection: Epidemiology, pathophysiology, treatment, and future research. *Circulation*. 2014;129:1781–1789.
9. 2021 update to the 2017 ACC expert consensus decision pathway for optimization of heart failure treatment. *J Am Coll Cardiol*. 2021;77:772–810.
10. Karamitsos TD, Francis JM, Myerson S, et al. The role of cardiovascular magnetic resonance imaging in heart failure. *J Am Coll Cardiol*. 2009;54:1407–1424.

32.

NUCLEAR IMAGING IN CARDIO-ONCOLOGY

Matthew E. Harinstein and Raymond Russell, III

CASE 1

A 42-year-old woman was referred to the cardio-oncology clinic for the evaluation of a decrease in her LVEF. Six months previously, she was diagnosed with left-sided breast cancer. She is undergoing neoadjuvant therapy with pertuzumab, trastuzumab, and docetaxel. Her echocardiographic LVEF prior to the initiation of therapy was 58%. After 3 months of therapy, her echocardiographic LVEF was 60%. After 6 months of therapy, her echocardiographic LVEF was 50%, although the study was considered suboptimal because of acoustic shadowing caused by a recently placed tissue expander. She underwent gated ERNA. Her calculated LVEF was 49%. The ERNA cine is shown in Figure 32.1 and the LV region of interest (ROI) and background ROI are shown in Figure 32.2.

She reports mild fatigue since starting her neoadjuvant therapy but denies any dyspnea on exertion, paroxysmal nocturnal dyspnea, orthopnea, or peripheral edema. She has no history of heart disease, hypertension, or diabetes. She never smoked. There is no family history of early CAD. Her weight has been stable during her treatment and her body mass index is 24.7 kg/m^2. On physical exam, her blood pressure was 112/76 mmHg and her heart rate was 80 bpm. She had no jugular venous distention. Her lungs were clear to auscultation bilaterally. Cardiac exam revealed a regular rate and rhythm, with a normal S_1 and S_2 and no murmurs, rubs, or gallops. Her abdominal exam was normal. She had no peripheral edema. Her ECG reveals sinus rhythm with normal axis and intervals.

Inspection of the ROIs from the end-diastolic and end-systolic frames of the ERNA (Figure 32.3) reveal that the background (BKG) ROI was placed over a relatively photopenic area. The ROI for the background correction must be carefully chosen to reflect what is considered to be true BKG activity. If it is placed over a photopenic area, such as over a tissue expander, the calculated LVEF will be lower than the true LVEF. In contrast, if the ROI is placed over a "hot spot," such as the spleen, the calculated LVEF will be higher than the true LVEF. The reason for this lies in the calculation of LVEF from ERNA studies. The calculation is LVEF = ((ED counts – BKG counts) – (ES counts – BKG counts))/(ED counts – BKG counts). The numerator can be simplified, resulting in LVEF = (ED counts – ES counts)/(ED counts – BKG counts). Therefore, the BKG counts only affect the denominator and a lower BKG count will result in a larger denominator and subsequently a lower LVEF.

The study was reprocessed with the BKG ROI placed in a more representative area, avoiding both the photopenic region and the spleen. Based on this correction, the calculated LVEF was 54%, indicating the absence of cardiotoxicity. As a result, the patient was able to continue her neoadjuvant therapy with trastuzumab and pertuzumab.

CASE 2

A 52-year-old woman with a history of breast cancer and diffuse large B-cell lymphoma was referred to the cardio-oncology clinic for shortness of breath. Approximately 10 years ago she had been diagnosed with breast cancer, which was estrogen receptor/progesterone receptor (ER/PR) positive, stage I, N1mic M0. She was treated with neoadjuvant chemotherapy with AC (Adriamycin [doxorubicin] and cyclophosphamide) for four cycles. She then underwent 12 cycles of paclitaxel followed by tamoxifen and was on anastrazole, but is no longer taking this drug. Her cumulative anthracycline dose was 240 mg/m^2.

Approximately 5 years later she developed symptoms of unstable angina and was diagnosed with obstructive CAD. Coronary angiography revealed an 80% mid left anterior descending coronary stenosis, for which she had percutaneous coronary intervention with placement of a drug-eluting stent. She completed 12 months of dual antiplatelet therapy and was subsequently treated with aspirin and atorvastatin.

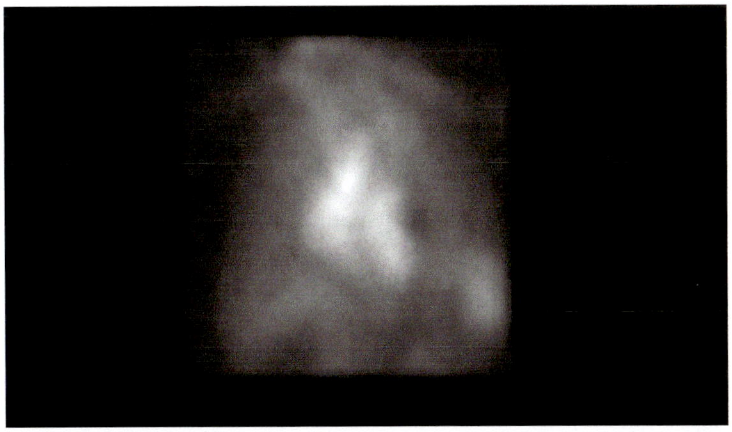

Figure 32.1. Case 1. Equilibrium radionuclide angiocardiogram.

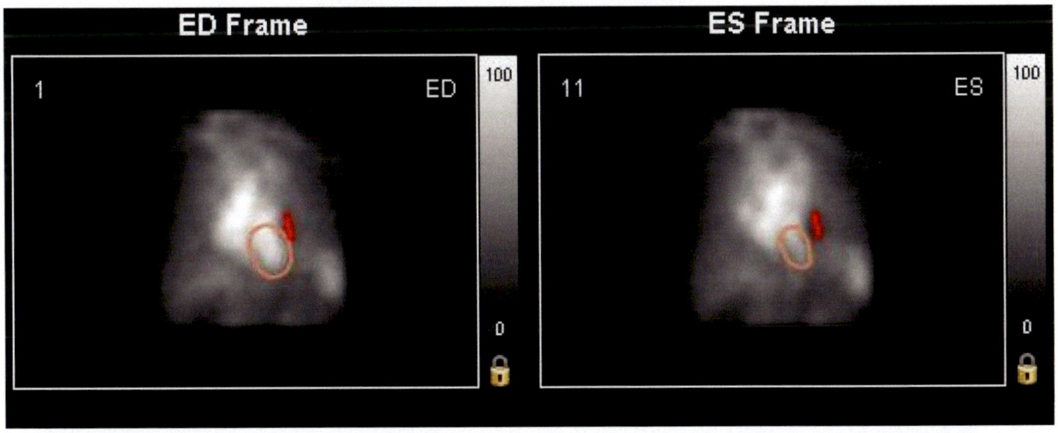

Figure 32.2. Case 1. LV (orange outline) and background (red outline) ROIs for both end-diastolic (ED) and end-systolic (ES) images for the original processing of the patient's ERNA study.

More recently, she was diagnosed with diffuse large B-cell lymphoma. Her treatment plan was R-CHOP (rituximab, cyclophosphamide, doxorubicin, vincristine, and prednisone) therapy for six cycles with four doses of intrathecal chemotherapy. An echocardiogram performed prior to therapy revealed an LVEF of 55–60%. Multigated acquisition scans obtained prior to each dose of R-CHOP revealed a normal LVEF.

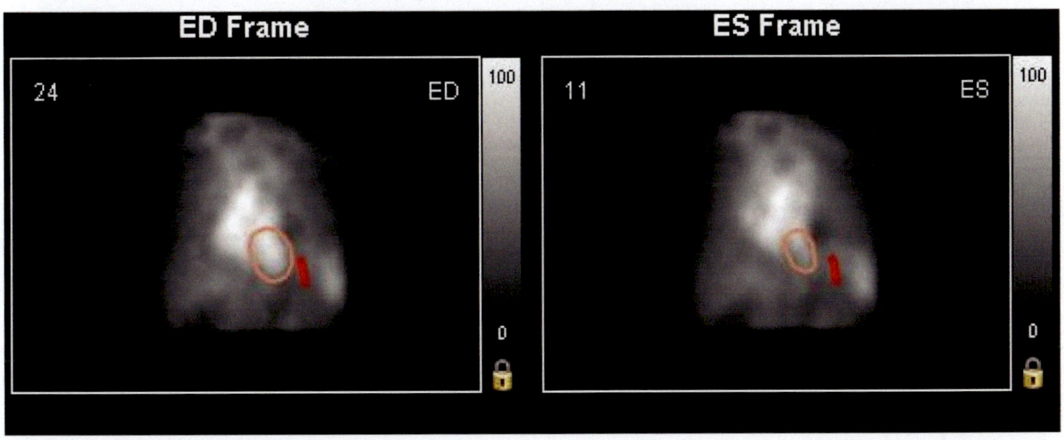

Figure 32.3. Case 1. LV (orange outline) and background (red outline) ROIs for both end-diastolic (ED) and end-systolic (ES) images after moving the BKG ROI to a more representative area.

(A)

(B)

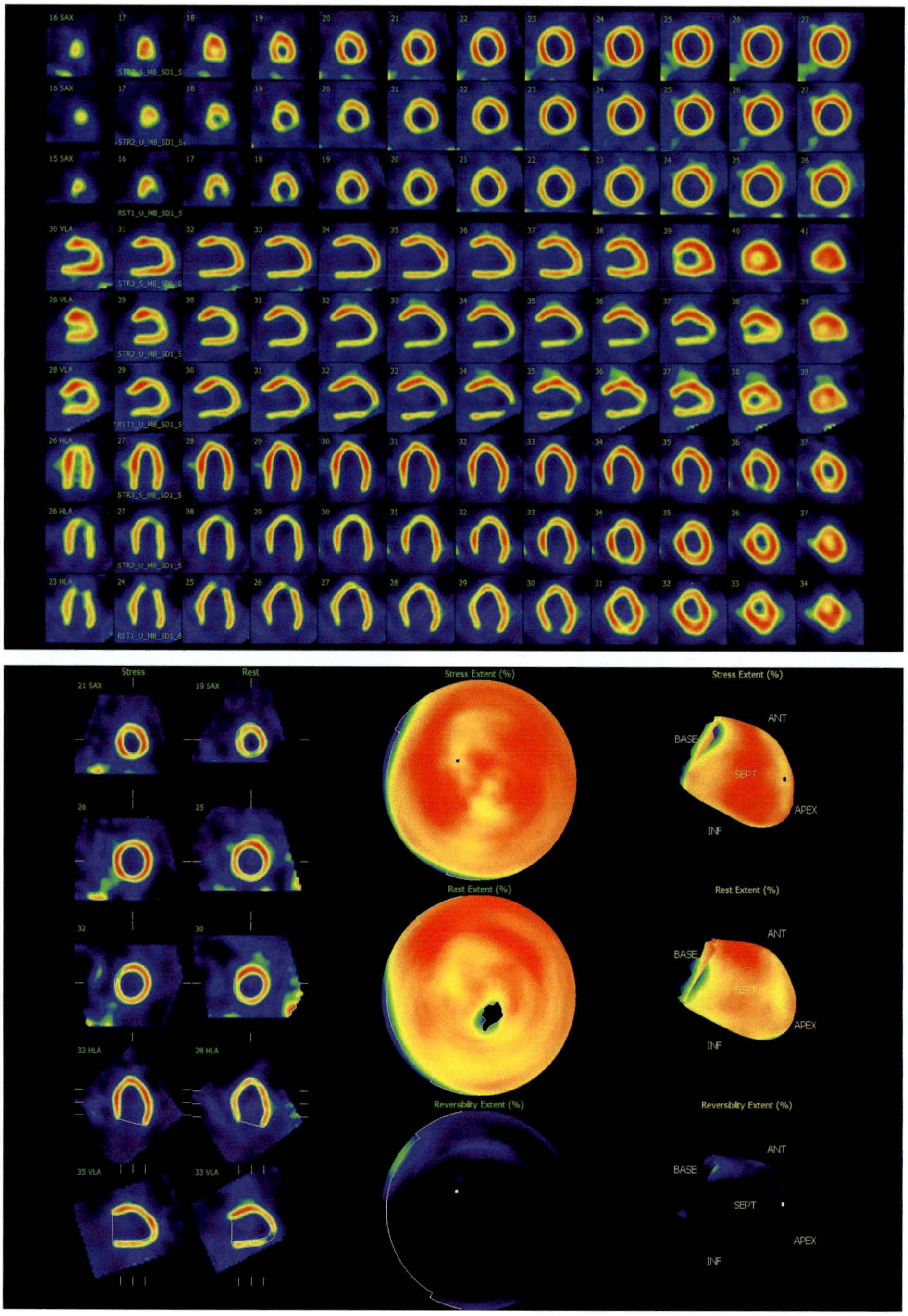

Figure 32.4. Case 2. SPECT perfusion results.

She had completed therapy approximately 8 months prior to presentation and her most recent LVEF, prior to her final dose of chemotherapy, was in the normal range. She reported weakness and fatigue as well as shortness of breath with minimal activity, including walking up a flight of stairs in her home. She also noted lightheadedness and dizziness. Her blood pressure was 104/67 mmHg and heart rate was 56 bpm. Her cardiac exam revealed bradycardia with a regular rhythm, there were basilar crackles in the lung field, and there was no significant lower-extremity edema.

Due to the symptoms and history of CAD, she was referred for a rest–stress pharmacologic SPECT scan. The perfusion images, shown in Figure 32.4, demonstrate no significant ischemia or infarction. The gated results, shown in Figure 32.5, revealed an LVEF of 35%. These findings were more consistent with a nonischemic etiology for her cardiomyopathy.

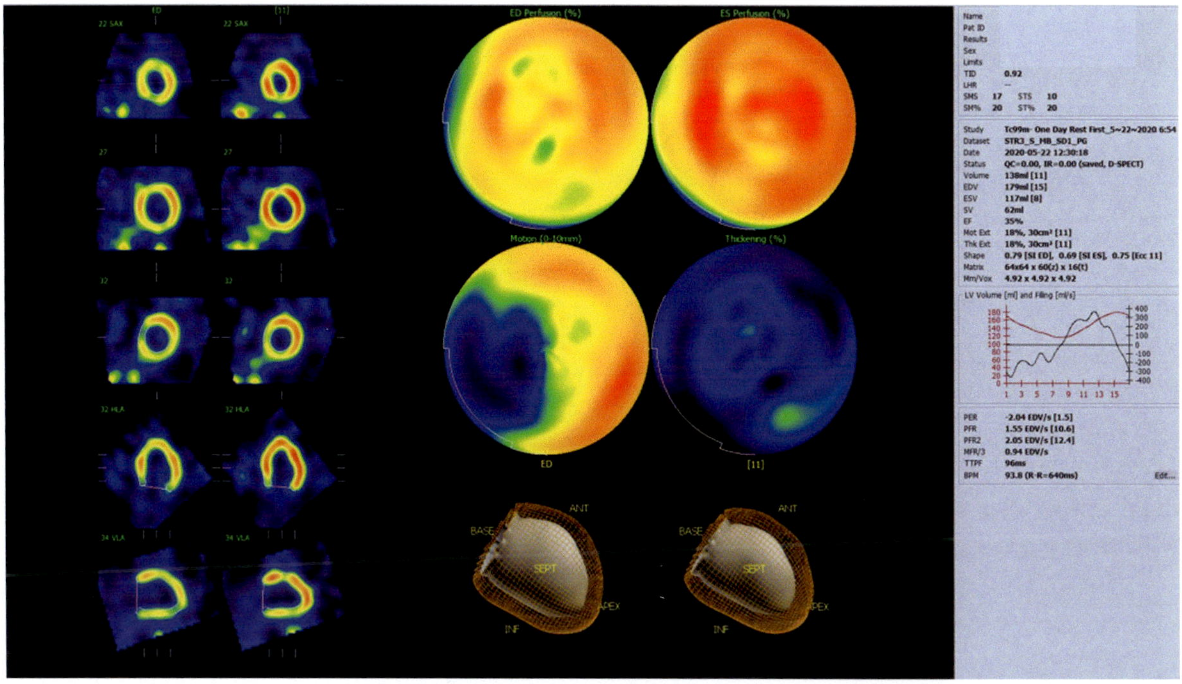

Figure 32.5. Case 2. Gated SPECT results.

This case demonstrates the importance of following recommendations regarding imaging for patients receiving chemotherapy. Patients who receive anthracycline-based regimens should have an LVEF assessment at baseline and prior to each 50-mg/m^2 dose once the total cumulative lifetime dose is greater than 240 mg/m^2 (or equivalent for anthracycline agents other than doxorubicin), as was the case in this patient. Further, assessment of the LVEF should also be performed at the conclusion of therapy and 6 months post-therapy to monitor for the development of cancer therapy–related LV dysfunction. These measures may enable earlier detection of cardiac dysfunction and institution of guideline-directed medical therapy.

CASE 3

A 48-year-old woman was referred for a routine rest SPECT study to evaluate her LVEF while undergoing cancer treatment. She had a history of invasive ductal breast cancer, which was ER/PR positive. The cancer was also HER2/neu positive. She was treated with paclitaxel and trastuzumab weekly for 12 weeks followed by trastuzumab plus tamoxifen with ovarian suppression for 1 year. She had no other significant past medical history and no prior history of cardiovascular disease.

The patient was tolerating her therapy well. At her most recent appointment, she reported no new symptoms and her physical examination revealed no new findings. She had completed her course of paclitaxel and trastuzumab and was now 9 months into her course of trastuzumab, tamoxifen, and ovarian suppression. She had received an assessment of her LVEF every 3 months while on trastuzumab.

Her resting perfusion scan (Figure 32.6) shows no significant perfusion abnormalities. The LVEF, determined by the gated SPECT study, was normal. An anterior still frame of her rotating planar raw cine is shown in Figure 32.7. This image reveals a large photopenic area in the area of the porta hepatis, with displacement of bowel from the mid epigastric region, suggesting the presence of a large mass in the region of the porta hepatis. Further imaging was recommended for correlation.

The patient was subsequently referred for a CT scan of the abdomen and pelvis, which revealed a heterogeneous hypervascular mass in the liver measuring 4.7 cm × 8.3 cm (Figure 32.8). Satellite hypervascular lesions infiltrating surrounding liver tissue were also noted. The pancreas and kidneys were unremarkable.

This case represents the importance of examining all aspects of a SPECT perfusion scan, as extracardiac abnormalities can also be diagnosed. The observation of a potential hepatic mass in the case altered the patient's treatment plan and diagnosed a finding that may have gone otherwise undiagnosed until too late.

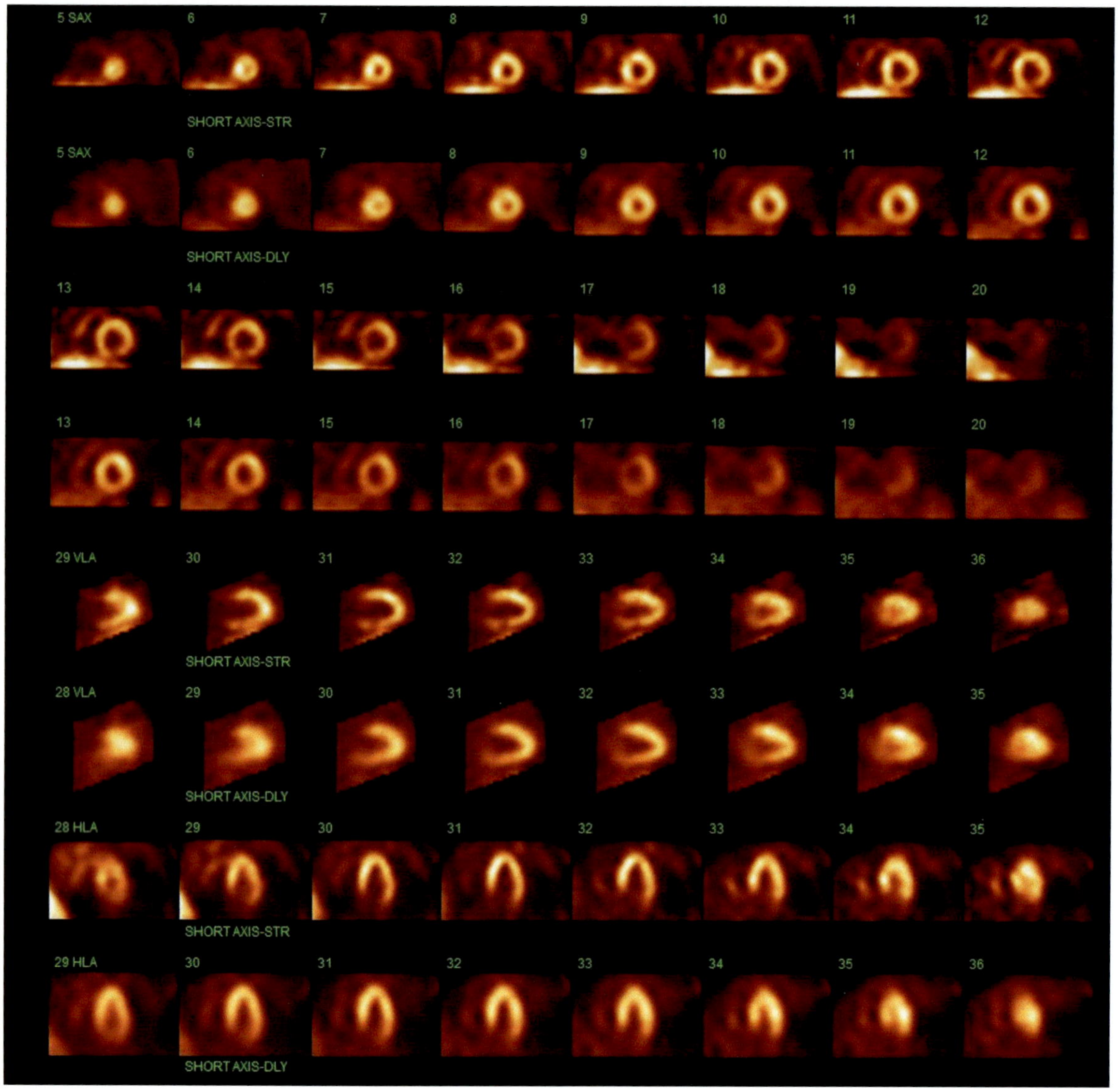

Figure 32.6. Case 3. SPECT perfusion scan demonstrating no significant perfusion abnormalities.

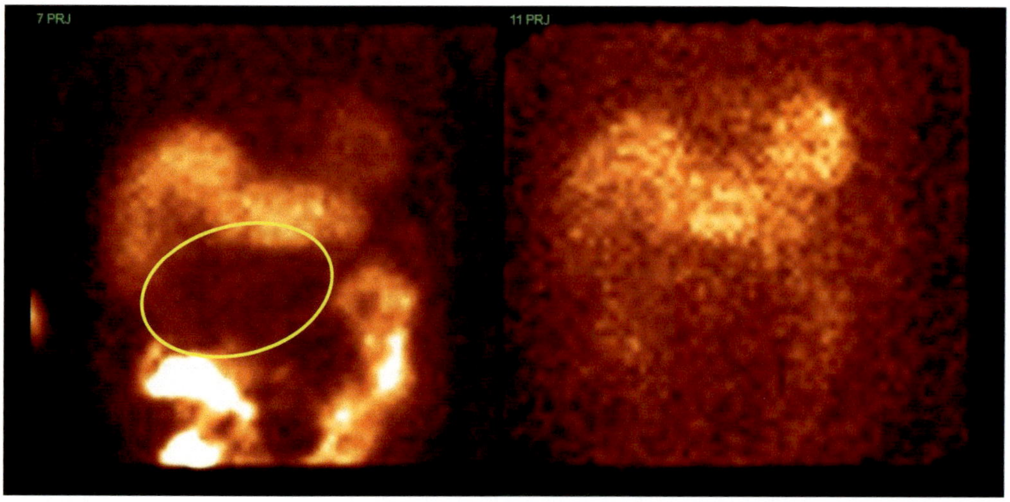

Figure 32.7. Case 3. Rotating planar raw images with photopenic area noting under the liver contour (yellow outline).

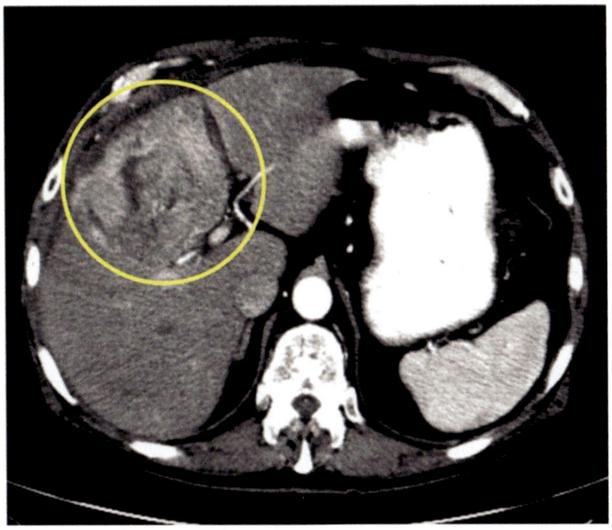

Figure 32.8. Case 3. CT scan demonstrating an intrahepatic mass (outlined in yellow) responsible for the photopenic area on the SPECT scan.

QUESTIONS

1. A 63-year-old woman who was treated for breast cancer with doxorubicin (cumulative dose 240 mg/m^2) is referred to the cardio-oncology clinic for the evaluation of a decrease in her LVEF. Her LVEF prior to the initiation of chemotherapy was 62% by ERNA. Following completion of her chemotherapy, her ERNA-derived LVEF was 47%. She reports dyspnea on exertion but denies chest pain, orthopnea, or paroxysmal nocturnal dyspnea. She has a history of hypertension and diabetes. She underwent a mastectomy and had a tissue expander placed for reconstructive surgery. She does not smoke. She has no family history of early CAD. On physical exam, her blood pressure is 148/92 mmHg and her heart rate is 86 bpm. Her physical exam revealed no murmurs, rubs, or gallops, and her apical pulse was nondisplaced. Her ECG reveals sinus rhythm and a left bundle branch block. In addition to initiation of guideline-directed medical therapy for LV dysfunction, which of the following is the most appropriate next step in her management?
   a. Perform a transthoracic echocardiogram to confirm the decrease in LV function.
   b. Perform a cardiac MR study with gadolinium to evaluate for scarring.
   c. Perform a vasodilator myocardial perfusion SPECT study to evaluate for myocardial ischemia.
   d. Perform an exercise stress echocardiographic study to evaluate for myocardial ischemia.

2. A 45-year-old woman is diagnosed with breast cancer. Her oncologist recommends that she begin a chemotherapy regimen including an anthracycline and trastuzumab. She has a history of hypertension and takes lisinopril. She has no history of CAD or heart failure. At baseline, she can walk 2 miles without symptoms of chest pain or dyspnea. Her ECG revealed normal sinus rhythm with criteria for LV hypertrophy. Prior to the initiation of therapy her LVEF is determined to be 50% by ERNA. She is referred to a cardiologist for assistance in determining the best plan for prevention of cancer therapy–related cardiac dysfunction. Which of the following is the most appropriate preventive recommendation?
   a. Perform ERNA prior to each dose of anthracycline, at the conclusion of therapy, and 6 months after therapy.
   b. Perform ERNA every 3 months.
   c. Continue lisinopril and add metoprolol tartrate.
   d. Perform rest–stress exercise SPECT stress testing prior to initiation of therapy followed by ERNA at the conclusion of therapy and 6 months after therapy.

3. A 65-year-old male is referred to the cardio-oncology clinic for cardiac evaluation. He has a history of diffuse large B-cell lymphoma and is currently receiving treatment with R-CHOP (rituximab, cyclophosphamide, doxorubicin, vincristine, and prednisone). His total lifetime dose of doxorubicin is 250 mg/m^2. He has a history of hypertension and tobacco abuse. During the course of treatment, he was hospitalized once for fluid overload related to heart failure with preserved LVEF. His LVEF by ERNA prior to the initiation of therapy was 60%. His most recent LVEF was 51%. In the office, he reports that he has been having increasing dyspnea on exertion and his chest feels tight when walking up a flight of stairs. On exam, his blood pressure is 146/92 mmHg and pulse 98 bpm. His physical examination is notable for regular rhythm with S_1 and S_2 as well as an S_4. Lung exam reveal basilar crackles bilaterally. There is 1+ bilateral lower-extremity edema. The patient is prescribed furosemide and asked to return in 1 week. Upon return, the edema has improved but the patient notes that the symptoms have not entirely resolved. What is the most appropriate next step in management?
   a. Stop doxorubicin therapy and switch to an alternate regimen.
   b. Continue doxorubicin therapy but administer dexrazoxane prior to treatment.

c. Perform ERNA to assess change in LVEF prior to next dose of doxorubicin.
d. Perform a rest–stress exercise SPECT study.

ANSWERS

1c. The patient had a significant decrease in her LVEF (a decrease of >10% to a value less than the lower limit of normal) in the setting of receiving anthracycline-based chemotherapy. Because she has multiple risk factors for CAD, it is important to exclude ischemia as a potentially reversible cause for her LV dysfunction. A transthoracic echocardiogram is not required as the ERNA has already established a clinically relevant decrease in LVEF. As the physical exam did not reveal any findings to suggest valvular heart disease, a transthoracic echocardiogram is unlikely to provide any information that will change the diagnostic or therapeutic plan. Although a cardiac magnetic resonance study with the administration of contrast may be used to evaluate perfusion and the presence of myocardial scarring, the patient has a tissue expander in place, and it is important to confirm that the injection port on the expander is compatible with magnetic resonance imaging. While a stress echocardiogram would allow for the detection of ischemic heart disease, the presence of a left bundle branch block makes it difficult to identify ischemic dysfunction in the septal segments. Therefore, the most appropriate next step in the evaluation of this patient would be to perform a vasodilator myocardial perfusion SPECT study.

2b. The patient will receive chemotherapy with an anthracycline and trastuzumab. Anthracyclines can cause a type I irreversible cardiomyopathy. The recommended imaging strategy for anthracyclines is to assess the LVEF at baseline and then after a total dose of 240 mg/m^2 of doxorubicin (or equivalent dose of another anthracycline) has been reached, and then when a cumulative dose of 400–450 mg/m^2 is reached, and then prior to each subsequent dose. Additionally, the LVEF should be assessed at the conclusion of therapy and 6 months after completion of therapy. Type II agents, such as trastuzumab, can cause a reversible cardiomyopathy. For trastuzumab, LVEF assessment should take place at baseline, every 3 months during treatment, at the conclusion of therapy, and 6 months after therapy. In this case, the patient had not yet received 240 mg/m^2 of anthracycline; thus, imaging prior to each dose was not necessary. The patient was to receive trastuzumab; thus, she required an ERNA to assess the LVEF every 3 months. The addition of a beta-blocker to ACE inhibitor therapy has not been shown to prevent cancer therapy–related cardiac dysfunction in patients with normal LVEF. This patient has no cardiac symptoms and had good functional capacity, so a stress test is not necessary.

3d. The patient was treated with a chemotherapy regimen that included doxorubicin, which can cause a type I irreversible cardiomyopathy. The patient had a history of HF with preserved LVEF and displayed symptoms consistent with an acute exacerbation. The patient's LVEF had decreased, but the change was not >10% from baseline; thus, discontinuation of doxorubicin on the basis of a change in the LVEF is not necessary. Dexrazoxane is a cardioprotectant drug that chelates iron and is administered prior to each cycle of anthracycline therapy. It may be helpful to limit the chance of cardiomyopathy, but it is not an essential treatment for this patient and is recommended for patients with a total cumulative dose of ≥300 mg/m^2. While the patient should have an assessment of his LVEF prior to his next dose of doxorubicin, he is now exhibiting signs of HF and chest tightness, which did not resolve with treatment for his fluid overload. Thus, given his risk factors, a stress test to rule out myocardial ischemia would be the next best choice in management. Despite the focus on prevention and detection of cardiomyopathy in patients treated with chemotherapy, it is important to recognize that patients may also present with typical causes of cardiac disease, since cancer and heart disease share common risk factors.

33.

RADIONUCLIDE IMAGING IN PATIENTS WITH CONGENITAL HEART DISEASES

Sara L. Partington and Sharmila Dorbala

CASE 1

A 56-year-old man who had tetralogy of Fallot repaired with an RV outflow tract patch and a VSD patch at age 6 presents with dyspnea. He has not had cardiology care since childhood. He has been noticing progressive shortness of breath with exertion over the past few years, but over the last month, he developed retrosternal chest discomfort with exertion that is relieved by rest. On exam, he was mildly hypertensive and euvolemic and had a soft 2/6 systolic ejection murmur and a 2/4 diastolic murmur heard along the left sternal border consistent with pulmonary stenosis and pulmonary regurgitation.

He underwent a ^{13}N-ammonia myocardial perfusion exercise stress test to rule out ischemia as a cause for his chest pain (Figure 33.1A) that demonstrated a fixed perfusion defect in the RV outflow tract, a fixed basal ventricular septal perfusion defect, and large, reversible perfusion defect, consistent with ischemia in the left anterior descending coronary artery territory. He subsequently underwent a CMR that demonstrated severe pulmonary regurgitation, mild pulmonary stenosis, and severe RV dilation, with an RV end-diastolic volume of 208 cc/m^2 (Figure 33.1B) and a moderately decreased RV ejection fraction of 35%. The CMR demonstrated a large region of fibrosis in the RV outflow tract (Figure 33.1C) consistent with a large RV outflow tract patch used to repair his pulmonary stenosis that matched the fixed perfusion defect in the RV outflow flow tract seen on MPI. He underwent an invasive coronary angiogram that confirmed a 90% stenosis of the left anterior descending coronary artery.

Ultimately he underwent a surgical pulmonary valve replacement due to severe pulmonary regurgitation with RV dilation and dysfunction as recommended by ACHD guidelines[1] with a coronary artery bypass graft to the left anterior descending coronary artery.

Tetralogy of Fallot is the most common form of cyanotic heart disease, and long-term survival after surgical repair continues to improve, resulting in many adults with repaired tetralogy of Fallot. The repair for tetralogy of Fallot generally involves relieving RV outflow tract obstruction, often requiring an RV outflow tract patch, and repairing the VSD with a VSD patch. This patch material should be taken into account when interpreting MPI in patients with this congenital heart anatomy.

CASE 2

A 42-year-old male had TGA that was repaired with an atrial switch repair at 6 months of age. The anatomy of TGA is such that the atria and ventricles are in the normal anatomic position, but the aorta originates from the RV and the pulmonary artery from the LV. The atrial switch repair involves creating atrial baffles to direct deoxygenated vena cava blood to the left-sided subpulmonic LV and oxygenated pulmonary venous blood to the right-sided systemic RV. This patient presents with shortness of breath on exertion with some associated chest pain. He is normotensive, there is jugular venous distention, breath sounds are normal with no crackles, and he has 1+ edema to the shins.

He had an echocardiogram demonstrating the pulmonary venous baffle, baffling oxygenated blood to the systemic RV (Figure 33.2A). The systemic RV is severely dilated and dysfunctional (Figure 33.2B). He underwent ^{82}rubidium MPI to evaluate for ischemia as a cause for his chest pain and systemic RV dysfunction (Figure 33.2C). No ischemia was identified.

CASE 3

A 48-year-old woman with pulmonary atresia with an intact ventricular septum and a hypoplastic RV underwent

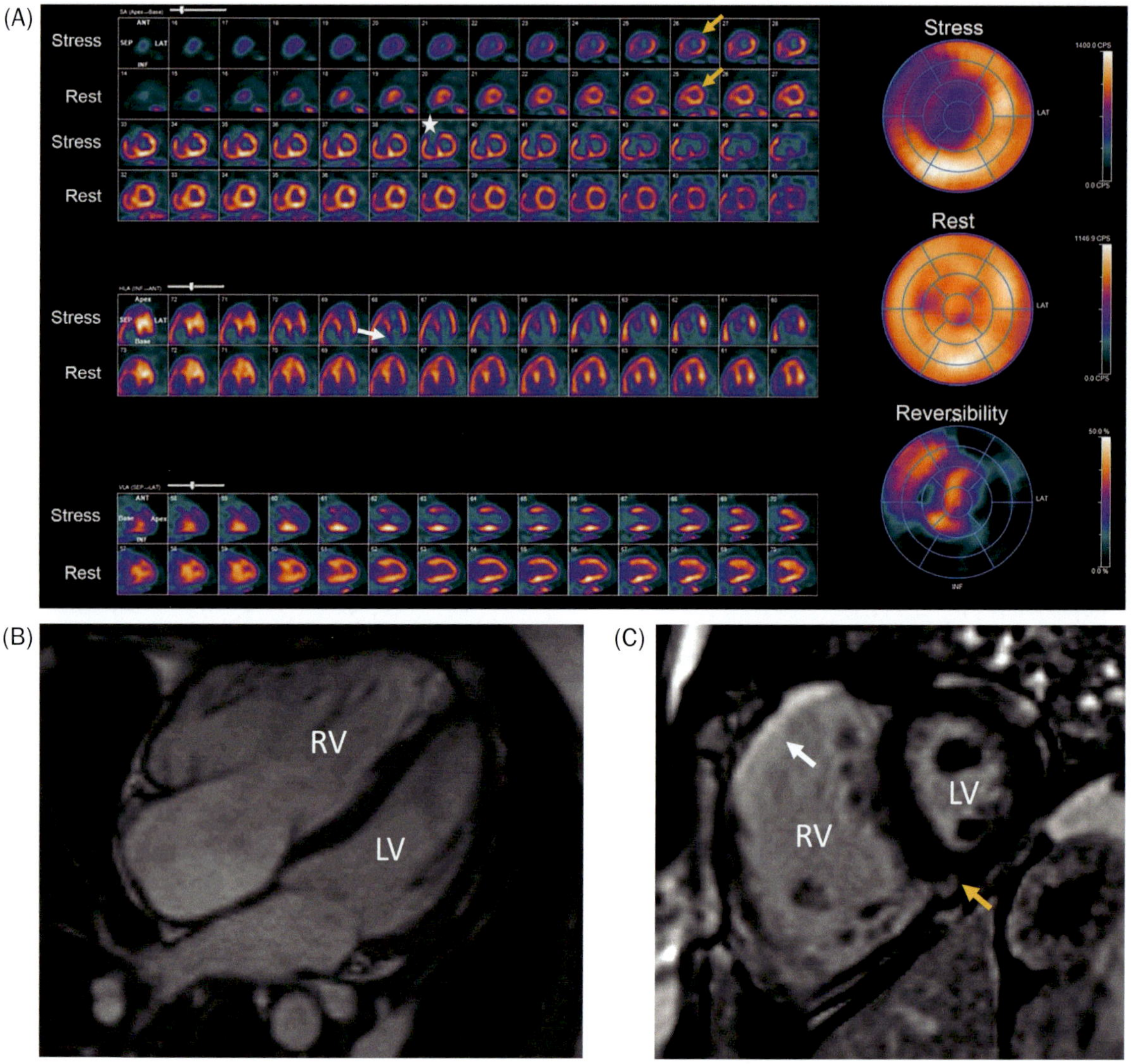

Figure 33.1. Case 1. (A) ^{13}N-ammonia PET/CT study in a patient with repaired tetralogy of Fallot. Stress (top) and rest (bottom) ^{13}N-ammonia myocardial perfusion images in a 56-year-old man who presents with chest pain. There is a fixed defect in the RV outflow tract (star) consistent with an RV outflow tract patch and a fixed defect in the basal ventricular septum (white arrow) consistent with a VSD patch. There is a large and severe perfusion defect in the basal anteroseptal wall, mid anterior wall, mid anteroseptal and infero-septal walls and apex that was reversible (yellow arrow). These findings are consistent with ischemia in the mid left anterior descending coronary artery territory. (B) A steady-state free procession (SSFP) CMR image of a four-chamber view. There is severe RV dilation. (C) Late gadolinium enhancement image in the mid ventricular short-axis position. There is a large region of late gadolinium enhancement representing fibrosis in the RV outflow tract (white arrow) consistent with an RV outflow tract patch. There is also fibrosis at the RV inferior insertion point (yellow arrow), common in tetralogy of Fallot.

a Fontan repair as a child. She presents to the emergency department with palpitations. The Fontan repair ultimately involved connecting her superior and inferior vena cavae to the pulmonary arteries with no subpulmonary ventricle, allowing passive flow to the pulmonary arteries while oxygenated pulmonary venous blood returns to the functionally single ventricle to be pumped to the aorta (see Figure 33.1E in the main textbook). In the emergency department, her palpitations correlate with nonsustained ventricular tachycardia. She is normotensive and euvolemic on exam, with a normal S1 and single S2 with no murmurs.

Her echocardiogram demonstrates a hypoplastic RV and normal LV function with no wall-motion abnormalities (Figure 33.3A). There was concern for myocardial ischemia in the setting of her nonsustained ventricular tachycardia. Patients with pulmonary atresia and intact ventricular septum are at risk for coronary-to-RV fistula that can result in coronary artery obstruction.[2] A nuclear stress test was performed. The patient exercised for 13 minutes on

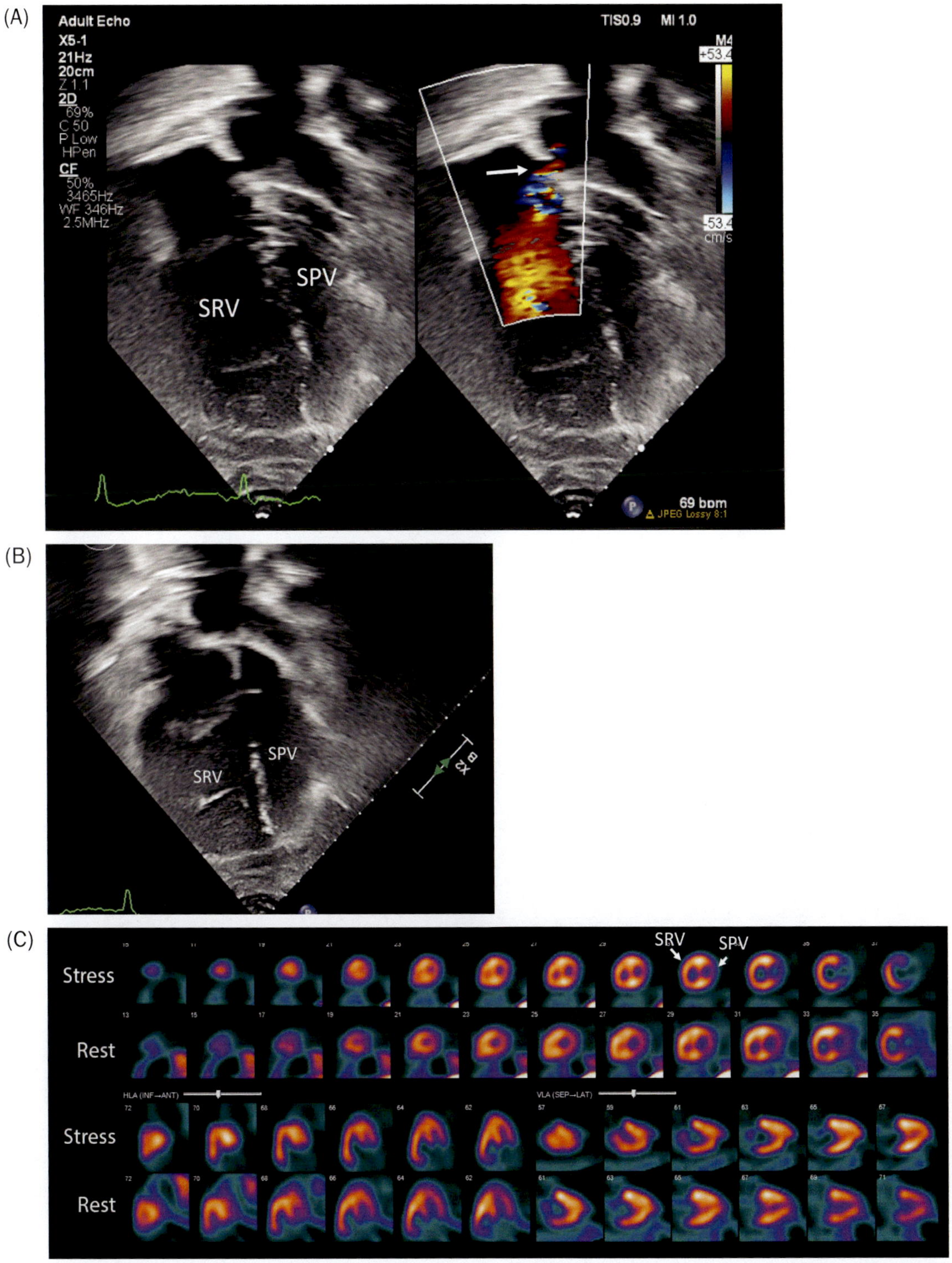

Figure 33.2. Case 2. (A) Echocardiogram four-chamber view in the apex-down format with color Doppler. The images demonstrate a pulmonary venous baffle (arrow) baffling the pulmonary venous blood over the systemic RV. (B) Echocardiogram four-chamber view in the apex-down format. The RV is dilated and appropriately hypertrophied with severe dysfunction. (C) Regadenoson stress (top) and rest (bottom) ^{82}rubidium myocardial perfusion images. The systemic RV is on the right, and it is dilated and appropriately hypertrophied. Myocardial perfusion should be assessed to the right-sided systemic RV. No ischemia is demonstrated. SRV = systemic right ventricle, SPV = subpulmonary ventricle.

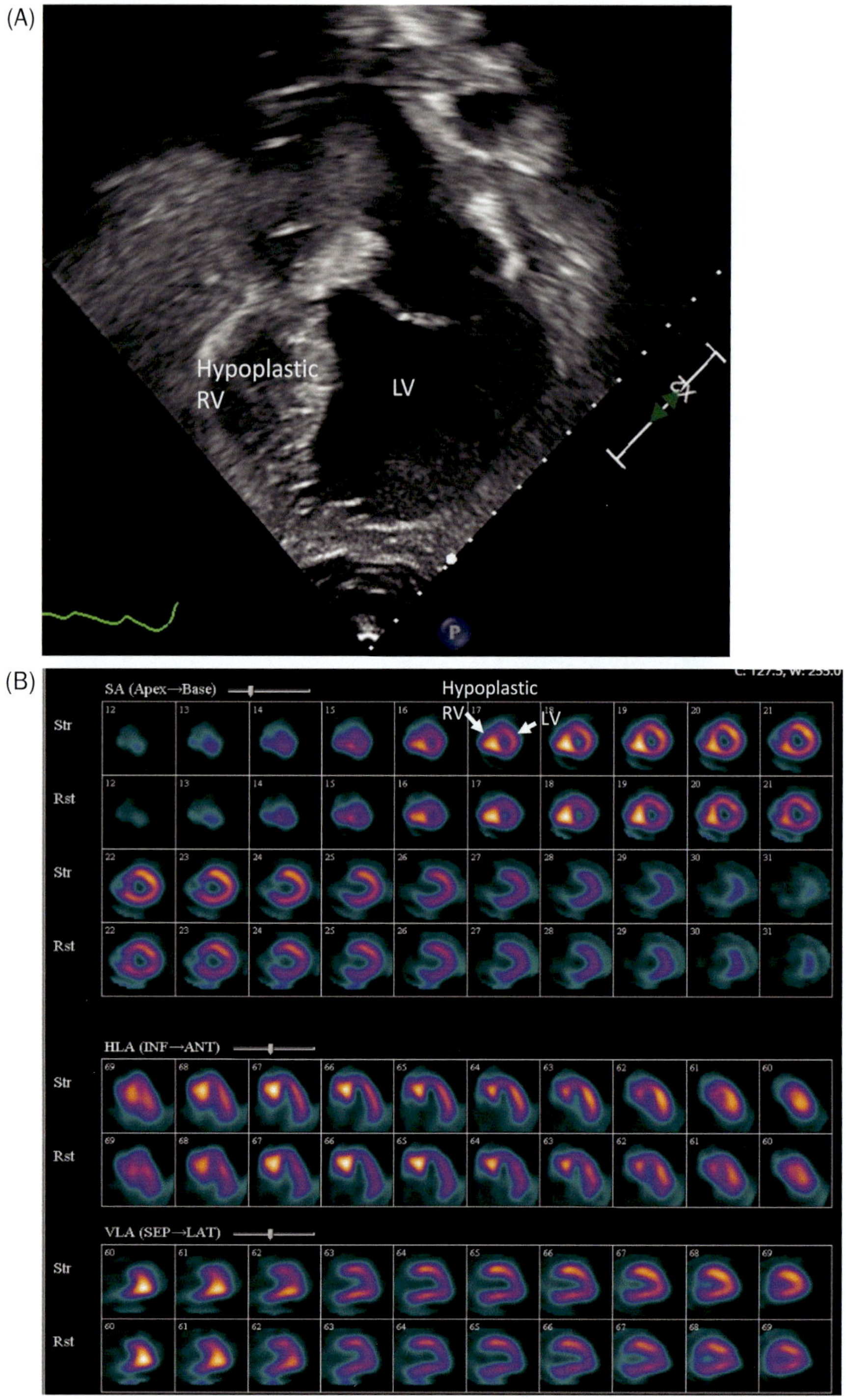

Figure 33.3. Case 3. (A) Echocardiogram four-chamber view in the apex-down format. The images demonstrate a hypoplastic RV and normal LV ejection fraction without any wall-motion abnormalities. (B) Stress and rest ^{99m}technetium images demonstrate a hypoplastic RV with no fixed or reversible perfusion defects.

a modified Bruce protocol and stopped due to dyspnea and had no arrhythmias during exercise but did have some premature ventricular contractions. She reached a peak heart rate of 81% of age-predicted maximum. Stress and rest ^{99m}technetium images were obtained (Figure 33.3B). A hypoplastic RV is seen and no ischemia is identified. She was started on metoprolol for her nonsustained ventricular tachycardia and her palpitations resolved.

REFERENCES

1. Stout KK, Daniels CJ, Aboulhosn JA, et al. 2018 AHA/ACC guideline for the management of adults with congenital heart disease. *J Am Coll Cardiol.* 2019;73:e81–e192.
2. Giglia TM, Mandell VS, Connor AR, et al. Diagnosis and management of right ventricle-dependent coronary circulation in pulmonary atresia with intact ventricular septum. *Circulation.* 1992;86:1516–1528.

34.

PHYSICIAN CERTIFICATION AND LABORATORY ACCREDITATION

Robert C. Hendel, Minnsun K. Park, and Gursukhmandeep S. Sidhu

QUESTIONS

1. Which of the following is true regarding physician certification through CBNC?
   a. Certification is for cardiologists only.
   b. It requires a separate, specialized fellowship.
   c. It requires 4 months of dedicated nuclear cardiology training with 700 hours input.
   d. It can easily be transferred from non-U.S.-based to U.S.-based certification.
2. All of the following are true regarding physician certification except for which answer?
   a. It is a process to achieve professional acknowledgment of dedicated understanding of the field of nuclear cardiology.
   b. The physician certification exam is composed of 160 questions that test competency and knowledge.
   c. It provides for confidence on the part of the patient population by providing quality care for nuclear cardiology practice.
   d. It was established to encourage physicians to maintain prestige and ownership in nuclear cardiology.
3. All of the following are true regarding the accreditation of a nuclear laboratory in the United States except for which answer?
   a. Medicare reimbursement requires a lab to have compliant accreditation.
   b. It provides for quality assurance in reporting and outcome.
   c. It is done every 5 years.
   d. It is an ongoing quality improvement process.

ANSWERS

1c. Cardiology, nuclear medicine, or radiology trainees are all potential candidates for certification under CBNC. Although a separate fellowship in nuclear cardiology may be obtained, it is not a prerequisite for CBNC certification. Part of certification eligibility requirement includes at least 4 months of training as well as a minimum of 700 hours of work experience in nuclear cardiology, including in radiation safety, as well as a minimum of 300 case interpretations under preceptor supervision (per Level II training under COCATS), making c the correct choice. Non-U.S. certification is currently not transferable to a U.S. certificate, and an individual must resubmit the necessary documents and retake the certification examination in order to obtain the U.S. physician certification.

2d. Physician certification is a process by which a physician receives professional recognition for having achieved the necessary knowledge, skills, and experience in a specific field, and one of its purposes is to serve the public by encouraging quality patient care in the practice of nuclear cardiology, making answer choices a and b correct. The initial certification examination contains a total of 160 questions (answer choice c). Answer choice d does not follow any purpose or vision of CBNC and therefore is incorrect.

3c. Accreditation of a nuclear cardiology laboratory is required for CMS reimbursement of nuclear perfusion imaging studies. The IAC process provides a guideline to establish national standards of accreditation in imaging study, reporting, and outcome. The accreditation process is done every 3 years. The procedure is done through independent peer review with a goal of overall quality improvement.

35.

NUCLEAR CARDIOLOGY GUIDELINES AND APPROPRIATE USE CRITERIA

AMERICAN COLLEGE OF CARDIOLOGY, AMERICAN HEART ASSOCIATION, AND EUROPEAN SOCIETY OF CARDIOLOGY

Timothy F. Christian

QUESTIONS

1. A 45-year-old woman with atypical chest pain, mild hypertension, and mild ST-segment abnormalities has a pre-test probability for CAD of 5%. She underwent regadenoson stress testing with rubidium-82 PET perfusion imaging. Assuming that the sensitivity of Rb-82 PET is 90% and the specificity is 80%, what is her approximate post-test probability for having CAD if she has a positive test result (i.e., ischemia in the right coronary artery distribution)?
   a. About 10%
   b. About 20%
   c. About 50%
   d. About 70%
   e. About 90%

2. A 52-year-old female who has hypertension and hyperlipidemia presents to her primary care physician with atypical chest pain, usually non-exertional. Her cardiac exam is normal and there are no carotid bruits present. Her ECG is normal at rest. Heart rate is 72 bpm and blood pressure is 140/90 mmHg. The primary physician orders an exercise ECG. She exercises for 5 minutes on the Bruce protocol, achieving a heart rate of 140 bpm and a blood pressure of 160/90 mmHg. There is a 0.5-mm ST depression at peak exercise and she had no chest pain during exercise. Which one of the following is false?
   a. Her pre-test probability of CAD is 5% to 10%.
   b. The clinical guidelines support ECG stress testing in this case.
   c. The Duke treadmill score is 2.5 (intermediate risk).
   d. Exercise SPECT imaging is not recommended by the guidelines given the absence of chest pain during exercise and <1 mm of ST depression at peak exercise.
   e. The patient has an element of deconditioning.

3. A 42-year-old male is brought to the emergency department with chest pain for 1 week. His risk factors for CAD are confined to a family history, with his father having a myocardial infarction at age 55. He is triaged to immediate computed tomographic angiography, where his calcium score is 660 and there are significant lesions with >75% stenosis in all three coronary territories (Figure 35.1). He is referred to cardiology and undergoes coronary angiography (Figure 35.2). Which one of the following statements is true?
   a. Stress nuclear imaging is inappropriate in this scenario prior to angiography.
   b. Following percutaneous coronary intervention (PCI), the patient should undergo exercise after 6 weeks to detect early restenosis.
   c. Given that the LAD and LCX lesions were successfully stented, delaying intervention on the right coronary artery and obtaining a stress perfusion test is appropriate use.
   d. SPECT MPI will be more accurate than exercise ECG treadmill testing in this population of patients with normal resting ECGs.
   e. The patient should have follow-up exercise perfusion imaging at 1 year following successful coronary artery bypass grafting surgery (CABG).

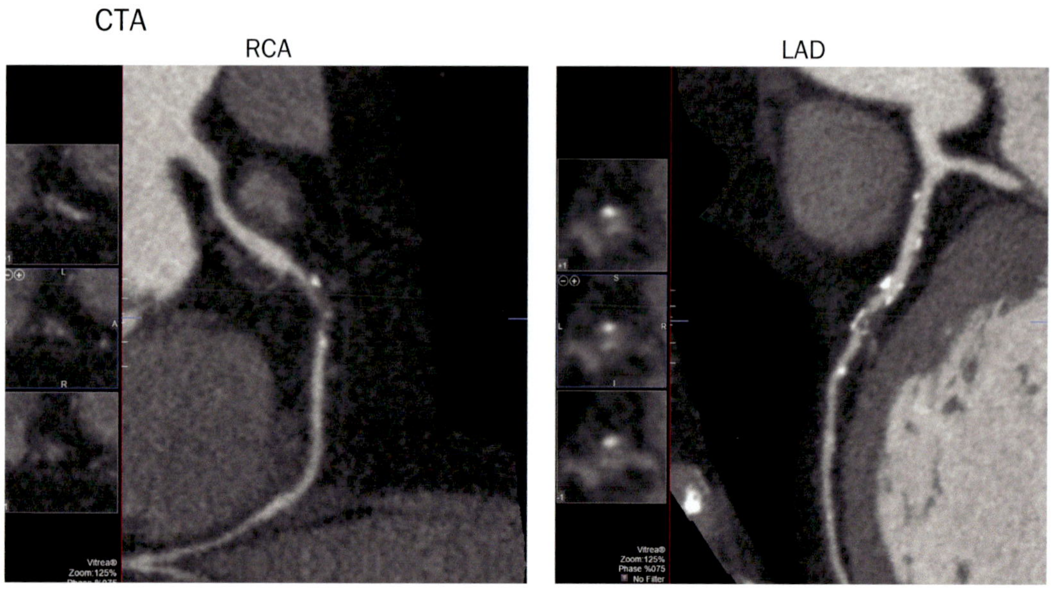

Figure 35.1 Computed tomographic angiography for Question 3.

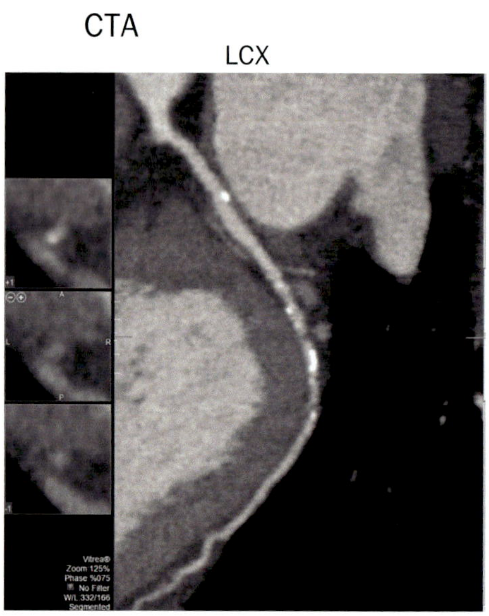

Figure 35.2 Undergoes coronary angiography for Question 3.

ANSWERS

1b. The formula for a positive test using conditional probability involves the sensitivity and specificity of the test and the prevalence of disease in the cohort being tested:

$$(\text{Sensitivity} \times \text{prevalence})/(\text{Sensitivity} \times \text{prevalence}) + [(1 - \text{specificity}) \times (1 - \text{prevalence})]$$

$$0.90 \times 0.05/[(0.90 \times 0.05) + (0.20 \times 0.95)]\text{: or true positives/(true positives + false positives)}$$

$$= 0.19 \text{ or } 19\%$$

2d. Depending on the model used, her pre-test probability for CAD is 5% to 10%, which is intermediate (low risk <5%). Her rest ECG is normal, so the guidelines strongly support ECG exercise stress as first-line diagnostic testing. The Duke score is calculated as duration of exercise in minutes: (5 × ST-depression magnitude) – (4 × chest pain index), which was zero in this case, giving a score of 2.5. The Duke score is trichotomized into low (>5), intermediate (4 to −10) and high (>−11) risk of significant adverse events in the next year. Patients with an intermediate Duke score have a Class 1B indication for stress perfusion imaging. The rapid rise in heart rate is an indication of deconditioning.

3c. The use of stress perfusion imaging in the setting of incomplete revascularization is an "appropriate" use. However, the recommendation is confined to those whose anatomy is favorable to further revascularization. In this specific case, the right coronary artery is a chronic total occlusion and is a difficult revascularization but reasonable to consider if revascularization of the other two arteries has been successful (CABG should have been strongly considered in this case). It is important to note that the appropriate use criteria and guidelines do not address all possible scenarios. The guidelines and criteria do not support routine follow-up testing following percutaneous coronary intervention of <2 years out, nor CABG before 5 years. They do support the use of stress perfusion imaging in patients with a coronary calcium score of >100, particularly with new symptoms.

36.

NUCLEAR CARDIOLOGY REPORT GENERATION

Wael A. AlJaroudi

CASE 1

A 68-year-old Black woman with diabetes, hypertension, obesity, heart failure with preserved LVEF, and controlled asthma presented with shortness of breath and chest discomfort with exertion. The rest ECG was normal. A previous stress MPI test performed 5 years earlier was normal. She exercised for 5 minutes on the treadmill using the Bruce protocol. There were no ischemic changes on the ECG. Her gated SPECT perfusion images are shown (Figure 36.1). The LV end-diastolic volume was 53 mL and EF was 71% with normal wall motion. Rest imaging was not performed.

The report was as follows:

Document type:	Myocardial perfusion stress study
Result date:	-- / -- / ----
Performed by:	--------
Electronically signed by:	------- on -- / -- ---- at --:--

REASON FOR EXAM
Chest discomfort and shortness of breath with exertion, multiple coronary risk factors

RESULTS
Myocardial perfusion imaging:

Ordering provider: -----------------

History: 68-year-old woman with shortness of breath and chest discomfort with exertion. Known to have diabetes mellitus, hypertension, obesity, and heart failure with preserved LVEF.

Location
[site address and contact information]

Measurements:
Height: 62 in,
weight: 198 lbs
Protocol:
Exercise stress test. A standard Bruce protocol was performed with imaging.
ECG at rest: Sinus rhythm. No ST/T-wave changes.

FINDINGS
Test information: The patient's exercise time was 5 minutes, 00 seconds, an estimated workload of 7.1 METs, and the peak heart rate achieved was 89% of her maximal age-predicted.
Measurements: baseline HR, 72 bpm; baseline BP, 137/40 mmHg; peak HR, 136 bpm; peak BP, 142/66 mmHg.
ECG changes: No change from baseline.
Chest pain: No.
Other symptoms: Shortness of breath during exercise.
Blood pressure response: At rest normotensive supine. Stage I systolic hypertension sitting and standing. Appropriate BP increase during effort.
Heart rate response: Normal.
Heart rate recovery: Normal.
Reason for terminating study: Fatigue.

IMPRESSION
Functional capacity: Normal.
ECG interpretation: Negative for ischemia.

IMAGING DATA
Imaging protocol: Stress only.
Acquisition: Gated SPECT.

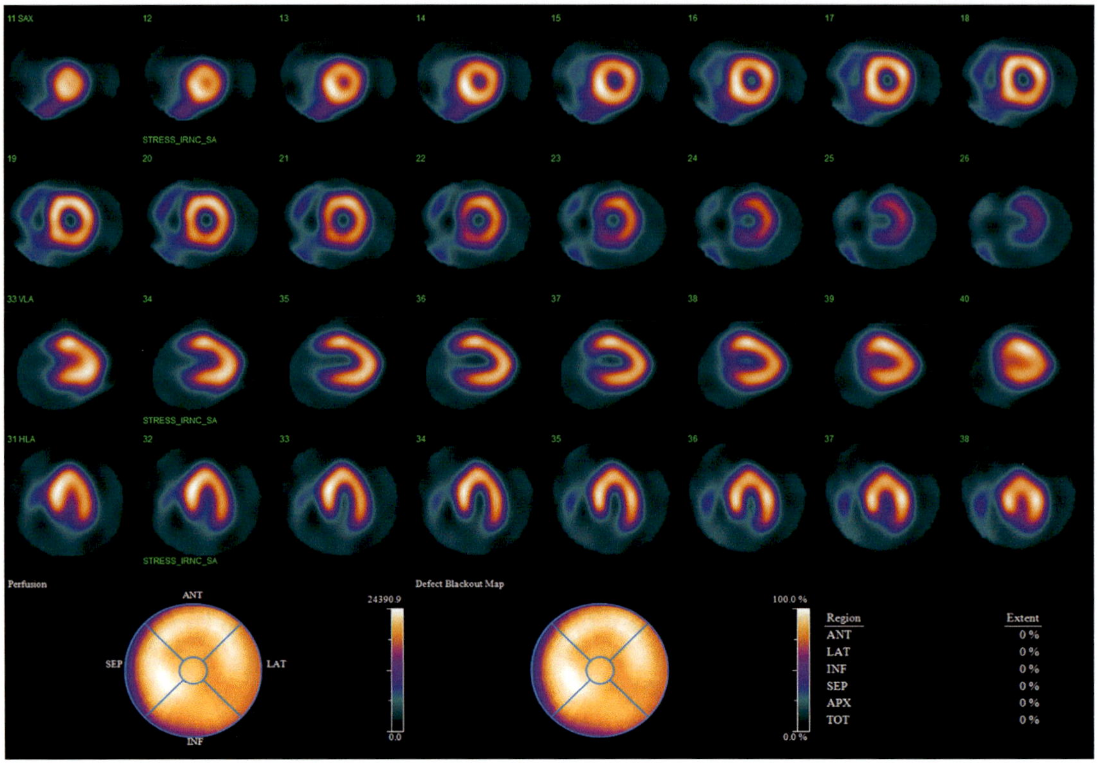

Figure 36.1. Normal stress myocardial perfusion imaging with homogenous tracer uptake.

Radiopharmaceutical: Tc-99m Myoview dose at stress: 10.83 mCi IV.
Attenuation correction: No.
Quality: Adequate.
Artifacts: None.

SPECT images demonstrated uniform tracer distribution throughout the LV myocardium at peak stress.

Wall motion/wall thickening: Normal.
Left ventricular size: Normal.
Left ventricular function: Normal.
Right ventricular size: Normal.
Right ventricular function: Normal.

CONCLUSIONS

1. Normal exercise SPECT myocardial perfusion images.
2. Normal left ventricular systolic function (left ventricular ejection fraction = 71%).
3. Stress ECG response is Negative for ischemia.
4. When compared to the previous study dated -- / -- / ----, there has been no interval change.

CASE 2

A 67-year-old white man with a history of hypertension and hyperlipidemia presented with atypical angina. The physical examination was normal. The rest ECG was normal. He exercised on the treadmill using the Bruce protocol for 7 minutes and 20 seconds and stopped because of shortness of breath. The peak heart rate was 145 bpm, and the peak blood pressure was 180/95 mmHg. The exercise ECG was negative for ischemia. The exercise and rest Tc-99m tetrofosmin gated SPECT images (using same-day exercise/rest protocol) are shown (Figure 36.2). The post-stress LVEF was 70% and the post-rest LVEF was 71%. There were no wall-motion abnormalities.

The structure of the report is similar to that of Case 1. We show pertinent findings that should be included for simplicity:

1. Exercise-rest gated SPECT images reveal a large (40% of LV myocardium using automated 4DM quantitative analysis) and severe perfusion defect in the territory of the left anterior descending artery (involving most of the anterior wall, septum, and apex).

2. The abnormality is mostly reversible, suggesting ischemia.

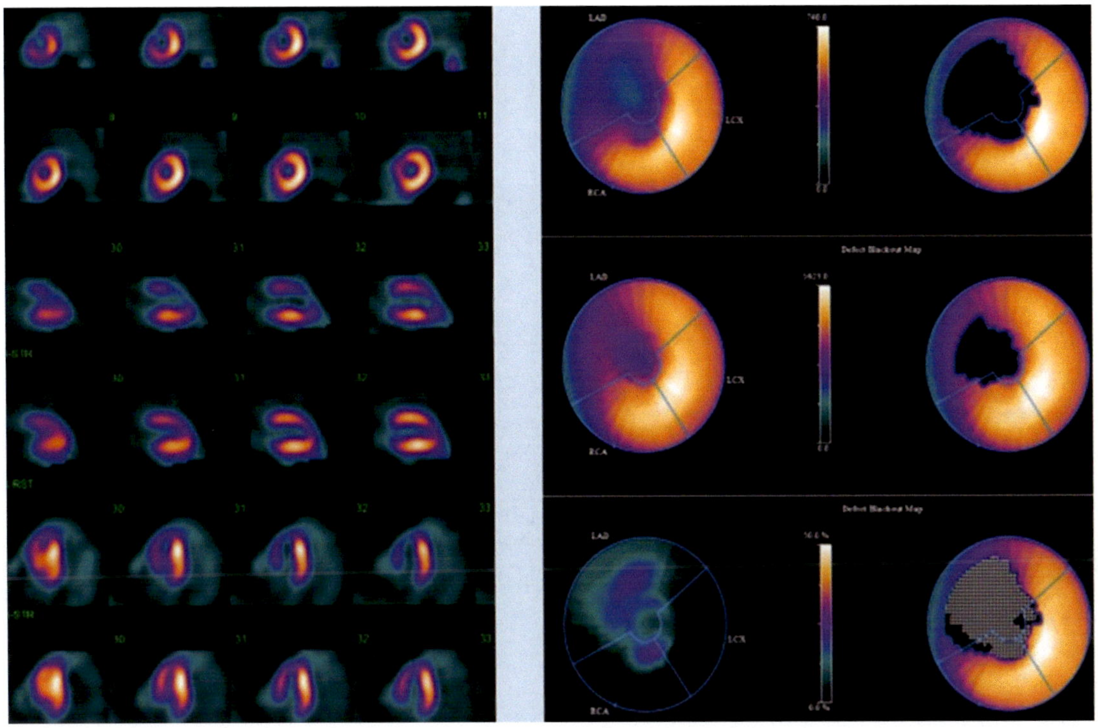

Figure 36.2. Exercise-rest gated SPECT images reveal a large (40% of LV myocardium using automated 4DM quantitative analysis) and severe perfusion defect in the territory of the left anterior descending artery (involving most of the anterior wall, septum, and apex). The abnormality is mostly reversible, suggesting ischemia.

3. The LV function and size are normal.
4. There is no transient ischemic dilation or post-stress stunning.
5. The right ventricular size and function are normal.
6. The rest ECG is normal. There are no ischemic ST shifts during exercise or recovery.
7. There are no prior studies for comparison.
8. Results discussed with Dr. -------- by phone.

CASE 3

A 55-year-old Black woman with a history of heart failure secondary to ischemic cardiomyopathy, uncontrolled diabetes mellitus, hypertension, dyslipidemia, and status post implantable cardiac defibrillator with chest discomfort. She had underwent percutaneous coronary intervention to the LAD 10 years prior followed by stent thrombosis and re-intervention. Her last coronary angiogram from 8 years ago showed patent stent in the LAD and no significant disease in the other vessels. Her LVEF has fluctuated from 20% to 30% over the years. Her ECG at rest was sinus rhythm with left axis deviation, intraventricular conduction delay, with anterolateral and inferior scar. She underwent regadenoson MPI with no significant ECG changes following regadenoson administration (Figure 36.3). The post-stress and post-rest LVEFs were 17%. There were no wall-motion abnormalities. There was diffuse hypokinesis with apical aneurysm. The end-diastolic volume was 322 mL.

The structure of the report is similar to that in Case 1. We show pertinent findings that should be included for simplicity:

1. Abnormal regadenoson SPECT myocardial perfusion images consistent with a large area of scar in the distribution of the left anterior descending and right coronary arteries involving 62% of left ventricular myocardium. There is no transient ischemic dilation or left ventricular stunning.
2. There is a severe perfusion defect of large size in the anterior (mid and distal), inferior (basal, mid and distal), anterior septum (basal, mid and distal), inferior septum (basal and mid) walls and apex of the left ventricle. There is no change in the perfusion defect from stress to rest.

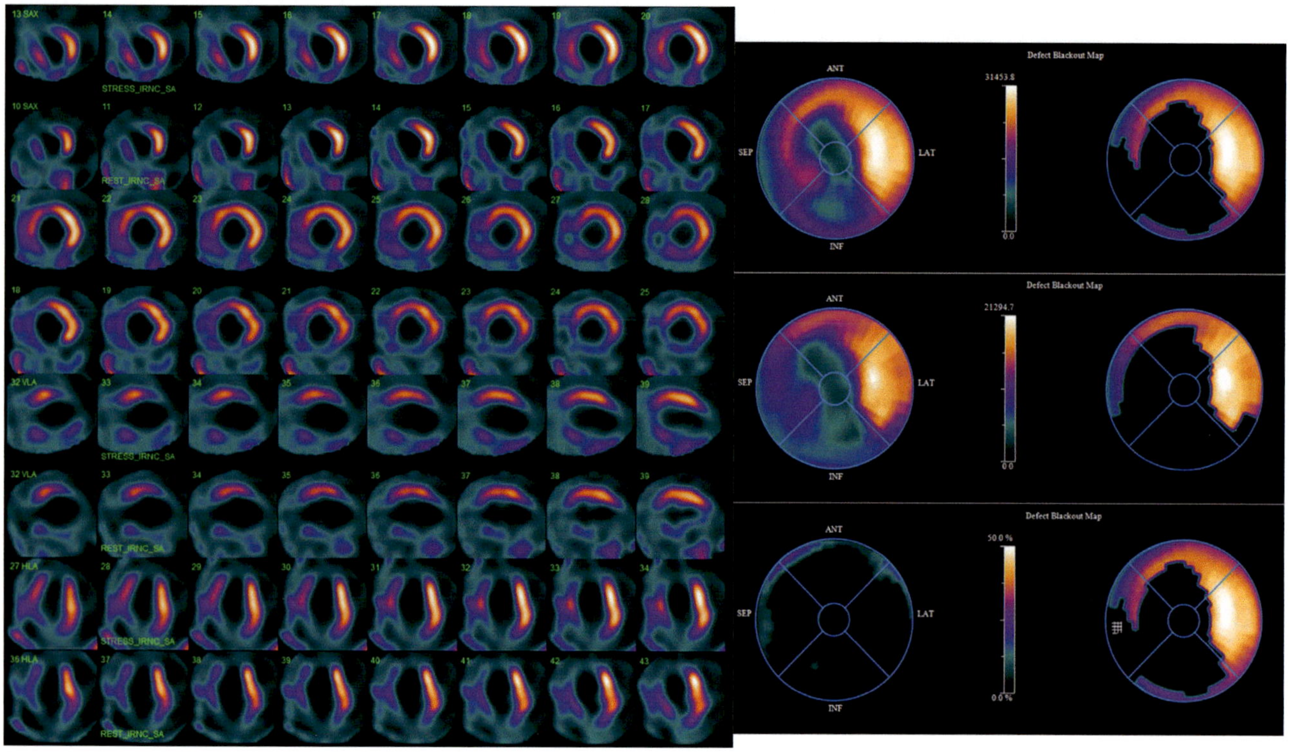

Figure 36.3. Abnormal Regadenoson SPECT myocardial perfusion images consistent with a large area of scar in the distribution of the left anterior descending and right coronary arteries involving 62% of left ventricular myocardium. The left ventricle is dilated. There is no transient ischemic dilation.

3. Severe LV systolic dysfunction (LVEF = 17%). The LV is severely dilated. There is severe and diffuse hypokinesis with apical aneurysm.
4. The right ventricle is of normal size and systolic function.
5. The test is high-risk due to the presence of a large perfusion defect and severely depressed LVEF.
6. There are no prior studies for comparison.
7. Results discussed with Dr. -------- by phone.

QUESTION

1. Which of the following statements in the final impression section of the report is most adequate (four different patients)?
    a. Large fixed perfusion defect involving the basal anterior, mid anterior, distal anterior, mid anteroseptal distal inferoseptal and apex, with partial reversibility
    b. Basal inferior hypoactivity on supine imaging that improves on prone imaging, most likely diaphragmatic attenuation artifact
    c. There is normal myocardial perfusion with a dilated left ventricle with severely reduced global systolic function (EF 28%), and paradoxical septal motion consistent with LBBB.
    d. The prior report indicates the presence of ischemia in the LAD distribution but this is not seen on today's study.

ANSWER

1c. Answer a is incorrect. A better final impression of such a report could read: "Large perfusion defect in the LAD territory (30% of the LV), predominately scar (20% of the LV) with mild ischemia (10% of the LV)." Although naming the segments is good for a database, mentioning the vessel territory is more clinically relevant, particularly in the impression section. Quantification of the perfusion defect size including total, % scar, and ischemia is needed. "Reversible" and "fixed," although technically correct, should be replaced by "ischemia" and "scar," which are more universally understood. Finally, the statement "partial" reversibility is pragmatic as it does not explicitly say what percentage of the defect is ischemic. This is clinically important as it alters the management of the patient.

Answer b is also incorrect. Although such a statement is valid in the main body of the report (findings section), it has minimal value in the final impression and might confuse the referring provider. The final impression needs to be concise and clear: "No evidence of ischemia or scar."

Answer d is also incorrect. Although reporting interval change is crucial, this has to be done using side-by-side comparison of images. A more appropriate impression of this study would state: "There is interval resolution of the ischemia in the LAD territory on side-by-side comparison with the study performed on [date of prior study], likely related to the successful interim revascularization of the corresponding vessel or medical therapy."

Answer c is the most correct. It is important to mention that the perfusion is normal, that the left ventricle is dilated, and that the reduced systolic function is global rather than regional, and to point out the paradoxical septal motion pattern due to LBBB. The patient ended up receiving cardiac resynchronization therapy.

37.

RADIATION CONSIDERATIONS IN IMAGING

Andrew J. Einstein

QUESTIONS

1. Which of the following is correct about stochastic effects of radiation?
   a. They are due to radiation-induced cell death or damage.
   b. They only occur above a threshold dose.
   c. They are also known as tissue reactions.
   d. They do not depend on dose for their severity.
   e. The most common type, cancer, only occurs after a latency period of 10 years.

2. Which of the following principles of radiologic protection applies to patients undergoing nuclear cardiac imaging procedures as well as to staff involved in their care?
   a. Optimization
   b. Dose limitation
   c. Distance
   d. Shielding

3. Use of which of the following studies should be associated with the longest nursing interruption period for a breastfeeding patient?
   a. A MUGA scan performed with 22 mCi of Tc^{99m}-labeled red blood cells in a 38-year-old woman with breast cancer, who is nursing a 4-month-old baby girl
   b. A stress test performed on a CZT camera with 5.1 mCi of Tc^{99m} tetrofosmin at stress and 15.5 mCi of Tc^{99m} tetrofosmin at rest on a 22-year-old woman with familial hypercholesterolemia and chest pain, who is nursing a 17-month-old baby girl
   c. A viability study performed with 2.9 mCi of ^{201}Tl in a 43-year-old woman status post spontaneous coronary artery dissection with myocardial infarction, who is nursing an 11-week-old baby boy
   d. A sarcoidosis PET study performed with 21 mCi of ^{82}Rb and 12 mCi of ^{18}F-FDG in a 19-year-old woman with palpitations and ventricular tachyarrhythmia on a Holter monitor, who is nursing a 7-week-old baby boy.

ANSWERS

1d. Tissue reactions, otherwise known as deterministic effects of radiation, only occur above a threshold dose at which a critical proportion of cells die or are damaged. In contrast, stochastic effects, such as cancer, are caused by mutations and can occur at any dose level; however, the probability of occurring (but not the severity) increases with increased dose. Cancer is indeed the most common type of stochastic effect, but it occurs after a latency period that can be as little as 2 years for hematologic malignancies and 5 years for some solid tumors.

2a. The three fundamental principles of radiologic protection in the international system of radiologic protection are justification, optimization, and dose limitation. Justification and optimization are applicable to both patients and their caregivers. Dose limitation, while essential for health care workers such as nuclear cardiology physicians and technologists, as well as for the general public, is not recommended in the context of patient care, since beyond such a limit patient care could be compromised by disallowing diagnostic testing or treatment involving ionizing radiation. Time, distance, and shielding are practical tenets of radiological protection, not fundamental principles, and maximizing distance for the radiation source and shielding patients from the radiation are not germane to patients who are injected with a radiopharmaceutical.

3c. The International Commission on Radiological Protection recommends that a child should not be breastfed until a radiopharmaceutical is no longer secreted in an amount estimated to give an effective dose of more than 1 mSv to the child, with milk expressed during this interruption period being discarded. For MUGA scans, an interruption period is not essential when red blood cells are labeled in vitro but should be 12 hours with in vivo labeling. In general for most Tc^{99m}-labeled compounds, interruption of breastfeeding is not essential; however, an interruption of 4 hours, during which one meal is discarded, can be advised to be on the safe side. No interruption is recommended for ^{18}F-fluorodeoxyglucose (FDG) or for PET perfusion tracers due to the short half-life. The interruption period does not appreciably depend on the mother's age or baby's age or sex, and administered activity is far less important than the radiopharmaceutical used. Here, the patient receiving ^{201}Tl should have a nursing interruption period of 48 hours, which is longer than that for the other patients.

38.

STATISTICS IN NUCLEAR IMAGING

Charity J. Morgan and Anastasia M. Hartzes

QUESTIONS

1. Researchers have developed a new computer algorithm for automated analysis of MPI and wish to assess the performance of this method for detecting CAD. Three hundred subjects underwent stress MPI and their images were reviewed by both the new algorithm and a board-certified nuclear cardiologist (clinical reference standard). The algorithm returns either a "positive" result (meaning CAD is assumed to be present) or a "negative" result (CAD is assumed to be absent). The results are shown in the table below:

True Disease Status			
Algorithm Result	CAD Present	CAD Absent	
Positive	30	25	55
Negative	6	239	245
Total	36	264	300

   Which of the following is true?
   a. The sensitivity of the algorithm is 82% and its specificity is 88%.
   b. The sensitivity of the algorithm is 55% and its specificity is 98%.
   c. The sensitivity of the algorithm is 17% and its specificity is 10%.
   d. The sensitivity of the algorithm is 83% and its specificity is 91%.

2. ROC curves for two methods (Method A and Method B) of automated analysis of 3D SPECT images are shown in Figure 38.1. According to the AUC, which method performs better?
   a. Method A
   b. Method B
   c. No difference in performance.
   d. Cannot be determined from this figure

3. Refer back to the data from Question 1. Assume that national data suggest that the rate of CAD in the general population is 11.3%. Which of the following is true?
   a. The positive predictive value (PPV) of the algorithm is 12% and its negative predictive value (NPV) is 88%.
   b. The PPV of the algorithm is 54% and its NPV is 98%.
   c. The PPV of the algorithm is 45% and its NPV is 68%.
   d. The PPV of the algorithm is 74% and its NPV is 92%.

4. A study was conducted to assess the prognostic value of the summed stress score (SSS) in cardiac transplant patients. The KM method was used to estimate the survival distributions for time to death. The survival curves are plotted in Figure 38.2. Which of the following is true?
   a. The median survival time for subjects with Low SSS is 5 years and the median survival time for subjects with High SSS is 3 years.

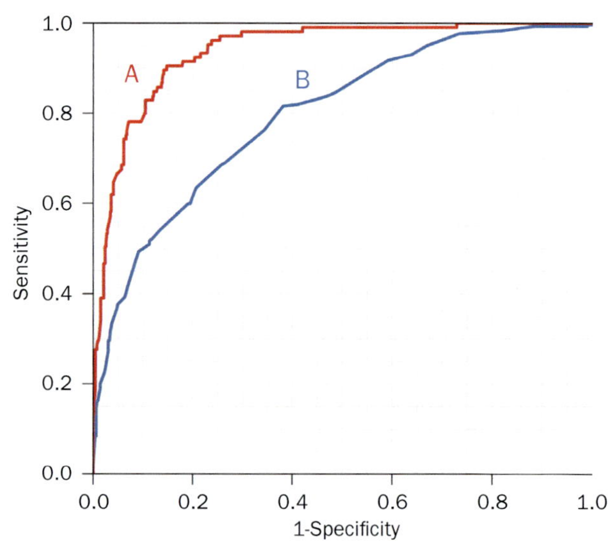

Figure 38.1. ROC curves for two methods of automated analysis of 3D SPECT images.

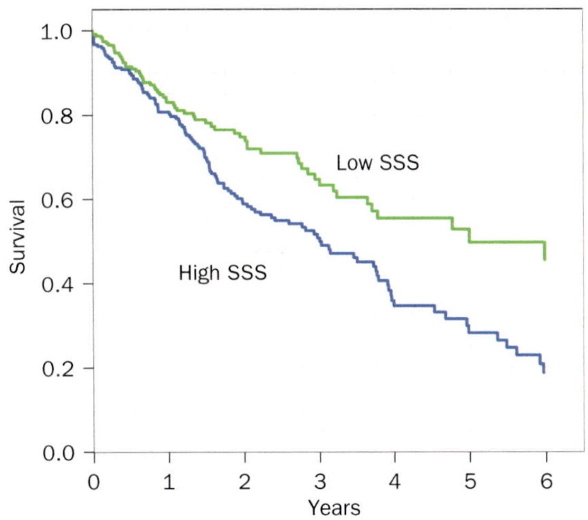

Figure 38.2. Time to death by SSS.

b. The median survival time for subjects with Low SSS is 3 years and the median survival time for subjects with High SSS is 5 years.
c. The median survival time is 3 years for both groups.
d. Median survival times cannot be determined from this figure.

ANSWERS

1d. Recall that sensitivity is the probability that a subject with the disease will test positive and specificity is the probability that a subject without the disease will test negative.

$$\text{Sensitivity} = \frac{TP}{TP + FN} = \frac{30}{30 + 6} = 0.83 \text{ or } 83\%$$

$$\text{Specificity} = \frac{TN}{FP + TN} = \frac{239}{25 + 239} = 0.91 \text{ or } 91\%$$

2a. Recall that ROC curve plots the sensitivity of a diagnostic test against one minus its specificity. Ideally, we would like both sensitivity and specificity to be as close to 100% as possible. The AUC is a measure of the test's performance, with larger areas indicating better performance. The area under the curve for Method A (AUC = 0.94, see shaded area in the Figure 38.3) is greater than that of Method B (AUC = 0.80), so we can conclude that Method A outperforms Method B.

3b. The positive and negative predictive values depend, in part, on the prevalence of the disease. Using the values of sensitivity and specificity calculated in Question 1 and a prevalence of 11.3%, or 0.113, for CAD:

$$\begin{aligned} PPV &= \frac{\text{Sensitivity} \times \text{Prevalence}}{\text{Sensitivity} \times \text{Prevalence} + (1 - \text{Specificity}) \times (1 - \text{Prevalence})} \\ &= \frac{0.83 \times 0.113}{0.83 \times 0.113 + (1 - 0.91) \times (1 - 0.113)} \\ &= 0.54 \text{ or } 54\% \end{aligned}$$

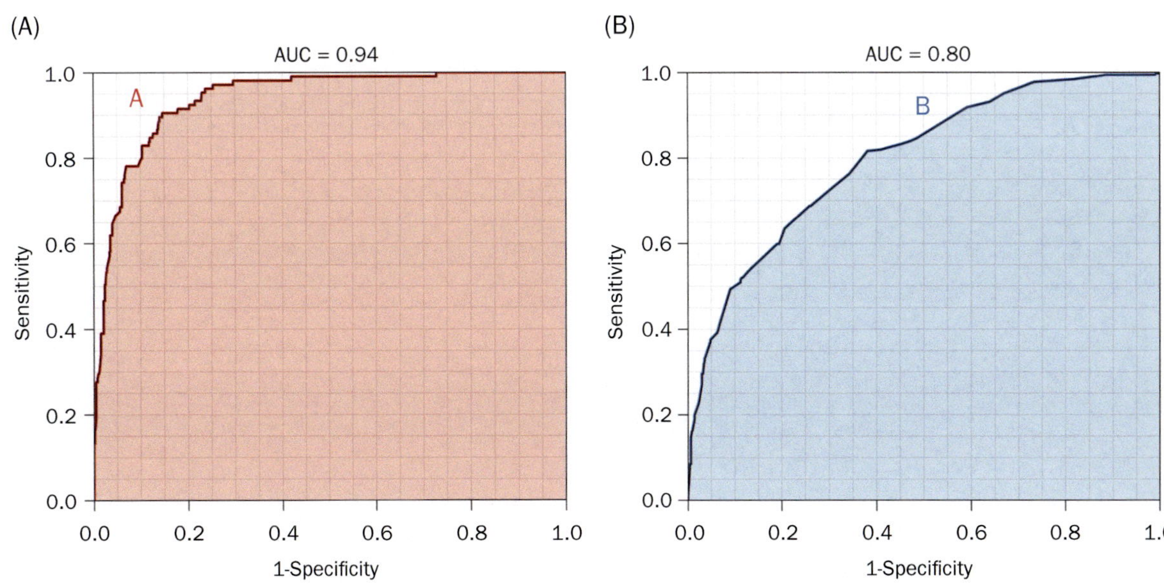

Figure 38.3. AUC for Methods A (red) and B (blue).

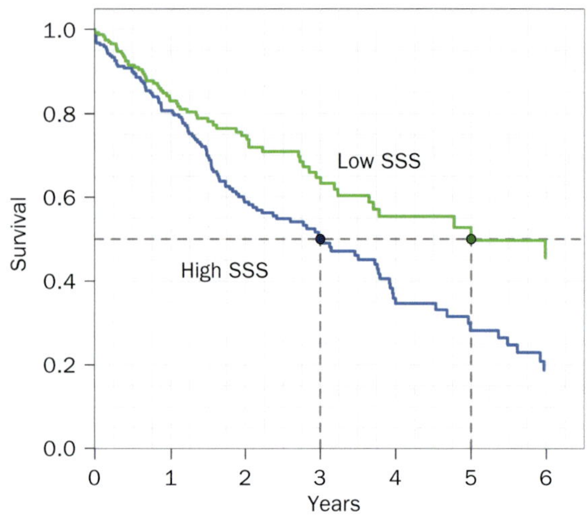

Figure 38.4. Calculating median survival time for Low and High SSS.

$$\text{NPV} = \frac{\text{Specificity} \times (1 - \text{Prevalence})}{(1 - \text{Sensitivity}) \times \text{Prevalence} + \text{Specificity} \times (1 - \text{Prevalence})}$$

$$= \frac{0.91 \times (1 - 0.113)}{(1 - 0.83) \times 0.113 + 0.91 \times (1 - 0.113)}$$

$$= 0.98 \text{ or } 98\%$$

4a. Recall that the median survival time is the time at which we would expect half of the subjects in this population will have had the event being studied. The median survival time can be found by drawing a horizontal line at the survival probability of 50% and determining where that line crosses the survival curve. As can be seen in Figure 38.4, the horizontal line at 50% survival (shown as a gray, dashed line) crosses the survival curve for the Low SSS group at 5 years (indicated with a green circle) and the survival curve for the High SSS group at 3 years (indicated with a blue circle). Therefore, the median survival times for subjects with Low and High SSS are 5 and 3 years, respectively.

39.

NUCLEAR IMAGING IN DEVELOPING COUNTRIES

Amalia Peix, Diana Paez, Joao V. Vitola, Pilar Orellana, and Maurizio Dondi

These three cases are typical of patients from emerging economies—particularly Case 1, a patient whose only risk factor is a family history of premature coronary artery disease (CAD), not rare in certain ethnicities, and Case 3, a patient with heart failure due to delayed assessment of his CAD.

CASE 1

A 32-year-old man has atypical chest pain but a positive family history for CAD (his mother had a myocardial infarction at age 55 years). He denies other risk factors, such as hypertension, diabetes, smoking, and hyperlipidemia. He achieved 14 METs on the Bruce protocol and denied chest pain but had a 2-mm horizontal ST depression in the recovery period in the lateral leads. His Duke score was +4 (intermediate risk).

QUESTION

1. Which of the following is most appropriate?
   a. The pain is not angina. Reassurance is appropriate.
   b. SPECT imaging is recommended.
   c. Coronary angiography is recommended.
   d. Repeat testing with pharmacologic stress is recommended.

ANSWER

1b. SPECT MPI (Figures 39.1A,B) showed severe reversible perfusion defect involving the entire anteroseptal region and apex; this is consistent with disease in the left anterior descending artery (LAD). There is transient ischemic dilatation. There is mild hypokinesia in the anteroseptal region and apex post exercise (myocardial stunning). There is a drop in the left ventricular ejection fraction (LVEF) from 57% post-rest to 51% post-exercise. A subsequent invasive coronary angiography, after MPI results, showed an occluded LAD proximally with collateral filling from the right coronary artery (Figure 39.1C, arrow). Patients with a family history of premature CAD are at high risk. Stress SPECT MPI adds prognostic and diagnostic value to treadmill testing in these patients. Though unusual, large ischemia could be observed in patients who achieve high METs during exercise. The presence of transient ischemic dilatation, transient wall-motion abnormality, and a drop in post--exercise EF are indicative of large ischemia, as demonstrated by MPI.

CASE 2

A 57-year-old man with diabetes, hypertension, and dyslipidemia is scheduled for vascular surgery. He also has degenerative disease in both knees that limits his physical activity. He underwent computed tomographic coronary angiography (CTA), which demonstrated mild-moderate atherosclerosis in all three coronary arteries (Figure 39.2A). His coronary artery calcium score was 180, which is 85% compared to patients of same age, gender, and race.

QUESTION

2. Which of the following statements is most appropriate?
   a. Most CTAs show severe CAD in patients with peripheral vascular disease.
   b. Patients with abnormal CTA findings should be referred routinely to invasive coronary angiography.

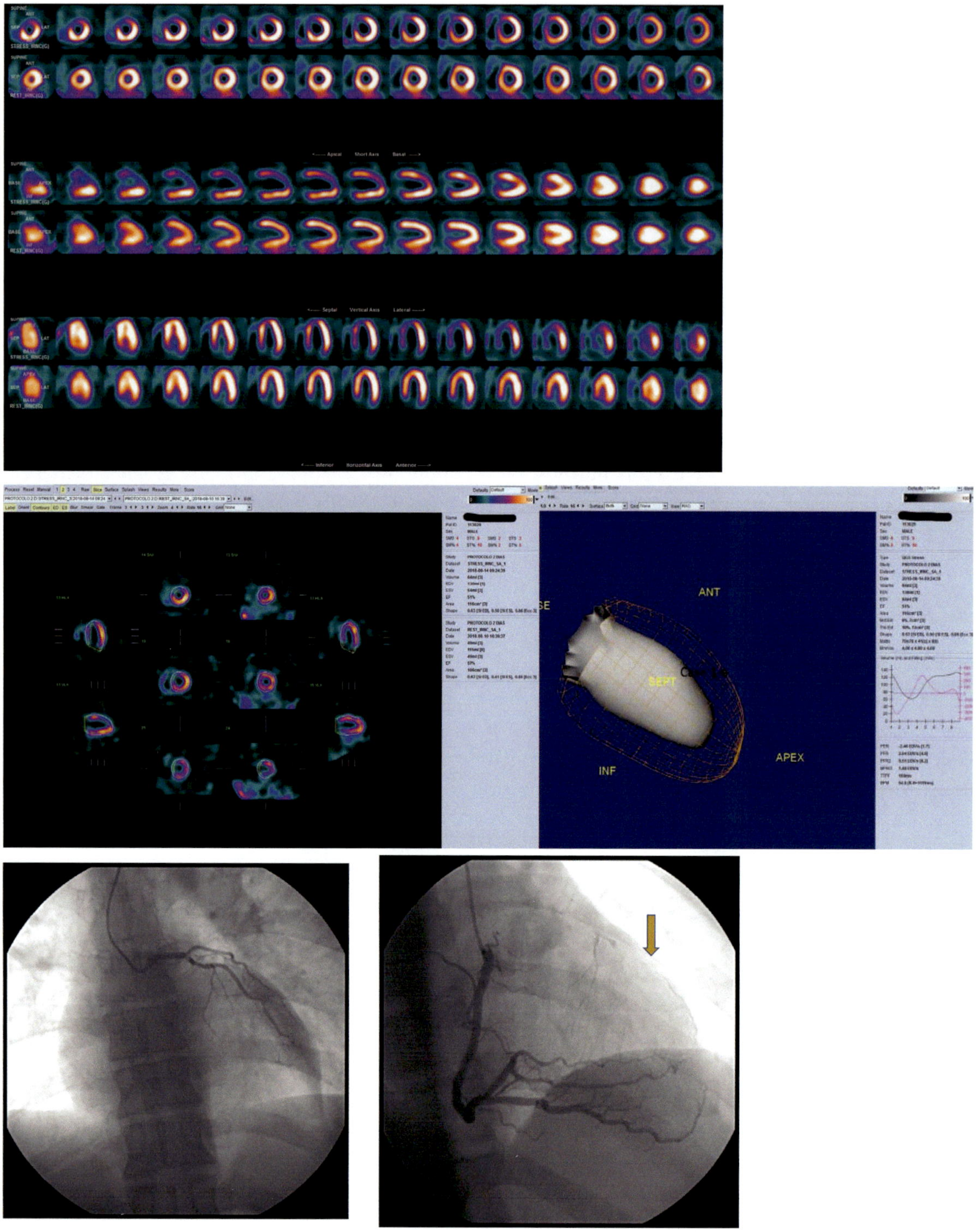

Figure 39.1. Case 1. (A, B) SPECT MPI showed severe reversible perfusion defect involving the entire anteroseptal region and apex; this is consistent with disease in the left anterior descending artery (LAD). There is transient ischemic dilatation. There is mild hypokinesia in the anteroseptal region and apex post exercise (myocardial stunning). There is a drop in the left ventricular ejection fraction (LVEF) from 57% post-rest to 51% post-exercise. (C) A subsequent invasive coronary angiography, after MPI results, showed an occluded LAD proximally with collateral filling from the right coronary artery (arrow).

(A)

(B)

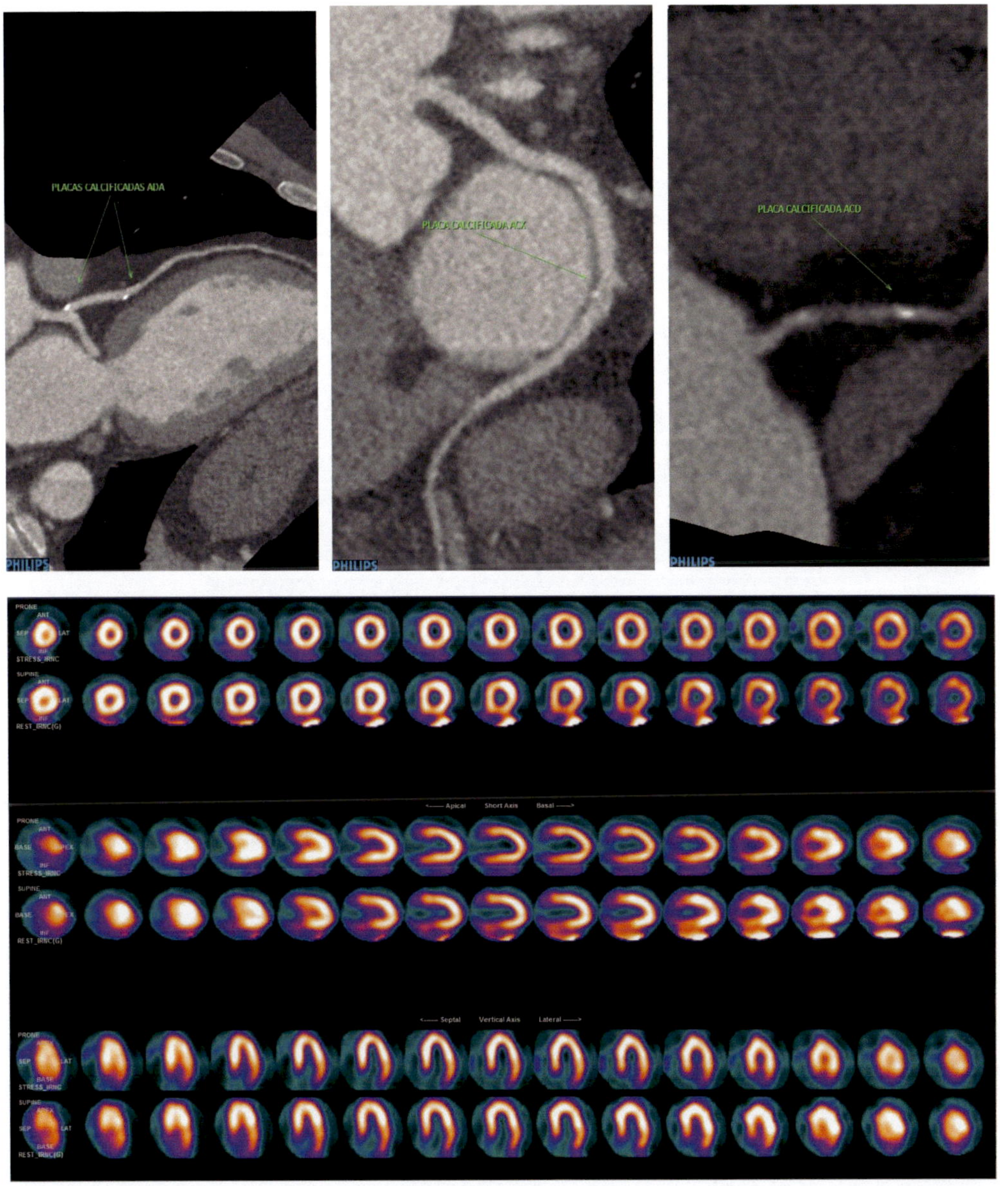

Figure 39.2. Case 2. (A) CTA demonstrated mild-moderate atherosclerosis in all three coronary arteries. (B) SPECT MPI showed a normal perfusion pattern and left ventricular systolic function with an EF > 70%.

c. Pharmacologic stress SPECT MPI might be helpful in patients with indeterminate CTA findings.
d. CTA should never be used for preoperative risk assessment.

ANSWER

2c. He subsequently underwent adenosine SPECT MPI, which showed a normal perfusion pattern and left ventricular systolic function with an EF > 70% (Figure 39.2B). Vascular surgery was performed without adverse events. When CTA is used as a first-line test, it is often helpful to exclude CAD since its negative predictive value is very high. CTA may also identify patients with CAD who may or may not have myocardial ischemia. The coronary artery calcium score is a useful screening tool but needs to be examined in relation to a population of similar age, gender, and race. Intermediate scores are not very reassuring.

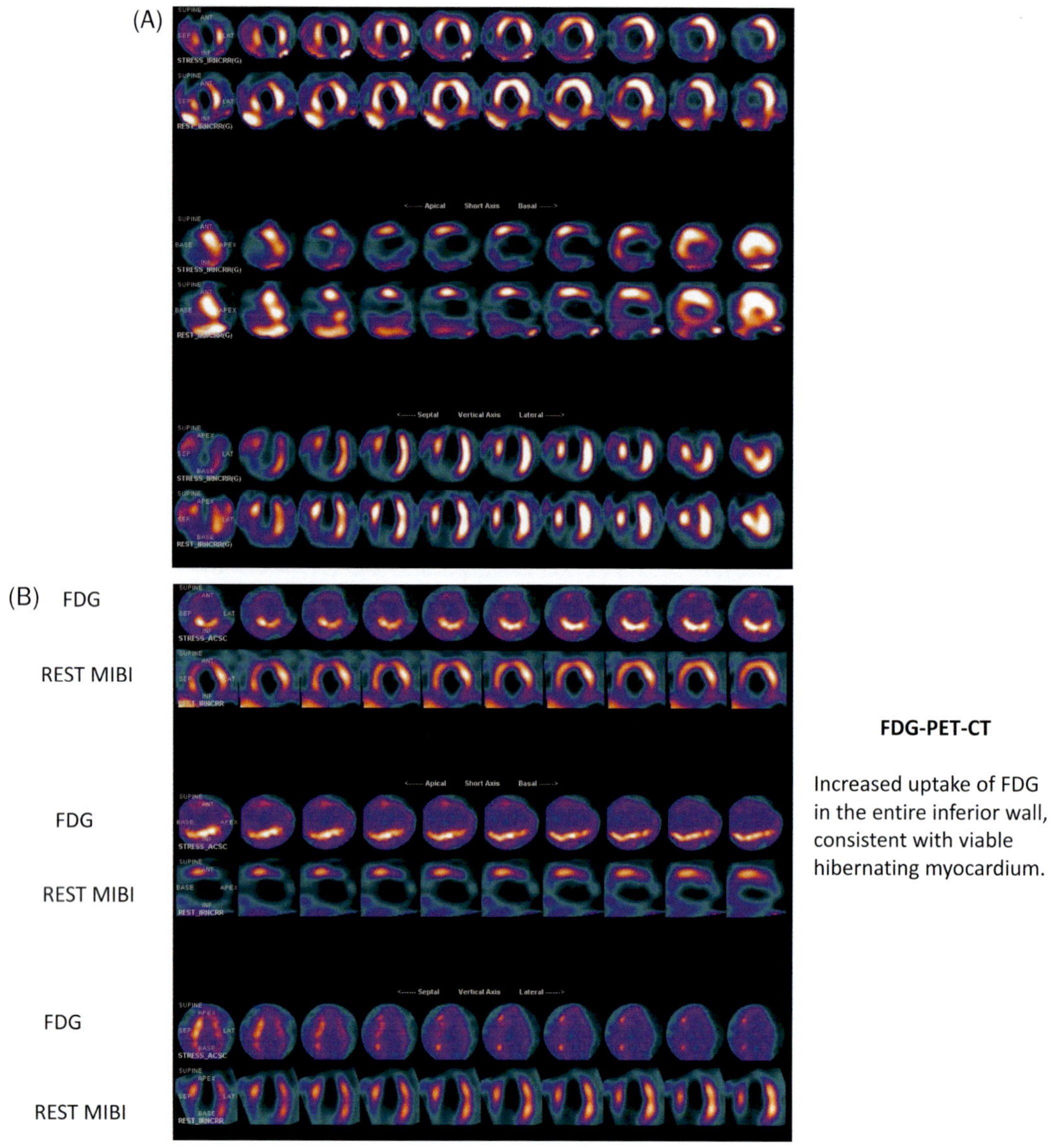

Figure 39.3. Case 3. (A) Stress and rest SPECT MPI findings. The left ventricle is dilated. There is moderate to severe anterior, septal, and inferior abnormality with some reversibility. The gated images demonstrated a severely dilated left ventricle and diffuse hypokinesis with an EF of 28% post-stress and 26% post-rest. (B) FDG PET accompanied by rest SPECT perfusion study (FDG PET, top panels; perfusion SPECT, bottom panels). There is increased uptake of FDG in the entire inferior wall, consistent with viable hibernating myocardium in that wall (mismatch pattern).

CASE 3

A 60-year-old man presented with heart failure symptoms but no angina. He has had hypertension, diabetes, and prior myocardial infarction and is active smoker. He underwent stress/rest SPECT MPI for assessment of myocardial viability. He then had an F-18 FDG PET study. Coronary angiography revealed severe (90% diameter stenoses) of all three vessels with reasonable runoff. The left ventricular systolic function was depressed on transthoracic echocardiography, with an ejection fraction of 25%. Stress and rest SPECT MPI findings are shown in Figure 39.3A, and the FDG PET accompanied by rest SPECT perfusion study is shown in Figure 39.3B (FDG PET top panels and perfusion SPECT bottom panels).

QUESTION

3. Which of the following statements is most appropriate?
   a. The images are consistent with primary dilated cardiomyopathy.
   b. The perfusion defects are in one vascular territory.

c. The left ventricular dilation is out of proportion to the degree of perfusion defects.
d. The FDG uptake was most helpful in the inferior wall, where a clear evidence of mismatch (decreased perfusion but preserved metabolism) is noted.

ANSWER

3d. The stress/rest SPECT MPI (see Figure 39.3A) shows a dilated left ventricle. There is moderate to severe anterior, septal, and inferior abnormality with some reversibility. The gated images demonstrated a severely dilated left ventricle and diffuse hypokinesis with an EF of 28% post-stress and 26% post-rest. The FDG PET (see Figure 39.3B) showed increased uptake of FDG in the entire inferior wall, consistent with viable hibernating myocardium in that wall (mismatch pattern). This case illustrated the role of nuclear imaging in the assessment of heart failure patients. Often the clinician is interested in knowing whether the patient has dilated or ischemic cardiomyopathy and whether coronary revascularization is beneficial. Evidence of hibernation on imaging (mismatch pattern) is very useful to determine whether the myocardium is likely to recover with coronary revascularization.

40.

ESSENTIALS OF NUCLEAR CARDIAC IMAGING

ASK THE EXPERTS

Ami E. Iskandrian, Fadi G. Hage, Pradeep Bhambhvani, and Ernest V. Garcia

QUESTIONS

1. The impact of noninvasive imaging on outcomes was first rigorously defined by:
   a. Echocardiography
   b. Computed tomography
   c. Nuclear cardiology
   d. Magnetic resonance imaging

2. If the exposure rate for a point source of activity is 32 R/h at 1 meter, what is the exposure rate at 4 meters?
   a. 32 R/h
   b. 8 R/h
   c. 3.6 R/h
   d. 2 R/h

3. How will increasing the axial field-of-view (along the table) of a 3D PET system impact MPI?
   a. Sensitivity will be increased in the area of the heart.
   b. Time-of-flight information will be lost.
   c. Resolution will be improved.
   d. There will be no difference if the axial field of view is extended beyond the heart.

4. To quantify glucose utilization with FDG with a one-tissue compartment, imaging duration should be restricted:
   a. To shorten the end-time so that phosphorylation in negligible.
   b. To delay the start-time until after phosphorylation is complete.
   c. To delay the end-time to include phosphorylation.
   d. To shorten the end-time to include dephosphorylation.

5. An 80-year-old asymptomatic patient with known CAD is referred for SPECT MPI for assessment of prognosis and management. He has a history of an inferior NSTEMI that was treated medically at an outside institution. He is on aspirin and a beta blocker. The patient underwent a resting MPI followed by treadmill exercise FPRNA and SPECT MPI. The following results were obtained: On the rest MPI, a small inferior perfusion abnormality with summed rest score 4; on the exercise MPI, peri-infarct ischemia inferiorly with summed stress score 9 and summed difference score 5; peak exercise LVEF, 54%. How would you assess the patient's risk of death and nonfatal MI?
   a. Low risk of death and nonfatal MI
   b. Low risk of death but intermediate risk of nonfatal MI
   c. Increased risk of death and nonfatal MI
   d. Increased risk of death and intermediate risk of nonfatal MI

6. The average Tc-99m SPECT MPI study is a:
   a. Low-dose procedure (≤3 mSv)
   b. Moderate-dose procedure (3–20 mSv)
   c. High-dose procedure (20–50 mSv)
   d. Very-high-dose procedure (>50 mSv)

7. A 65-year-old woman with a past history of hypertension, type 2 diabetes, and high cholesterol and a family history of CAD presents for stress testing prior to knee replacement surgery. She has not been very active in the past 6 months due to knee pain and denies any exertional chest pain or shortness of breath. Her resting ECG has normal sinus rhythm with a normal axis and intervals with nonspecific ST and T-wave changes. Her resting BP was 145/75 mmHg and a HR of 72 bpm. She undergoes regadenoson stress with a peak effect BP of 130/70 mmHg and HR of 92 bpm. ECG demonstrates 0.5 to 1 mm of ST depression in leads II, III, and aVF. SPECT imaging finds a medium-sized,

mild-to-moderate-intensity perfusion defect in the inferior wall from apex to base. Rest images show improvement in this defect. Gated images find normal LV function at rest and stress. Which of the following is the highest-risk finding in this SPECT study?
   a. Increased LV volume with stress compared to rest
   b. A summed difference score of 4
   c. Stress LVEF 54% and rest LVEF 55%
   d. ST depression with vasodilator stress

8. The regulated variable for matching myocardial oxygen supply with demand is:
   a. Coronary venous oxygen saturation
   b. Coronary venous adenosine concentration
   c. Coronary venous AMP concentration
   d. Coronary venous potassium concentration

9. Measurements of myocardial blood flow can readily be combined with standard PET MPI. Which of the following statements is *false*?
   a. Does not entail an increase in radiation burden to the patient
   b. Requires start of the image acquisition immediately prior to the radiotracer injection
   c. Precludes the assessment of regional LV function
   d. Allows conversion of regional myocardial radiotracer concentrations into quantitative regional myocardial blood flows

10. How does CZT SPECT imaging for MBF differ from conventional SPECT MPI?
   a. Larger doses of SPECT radiotracers are required for better count density and improved time–activity curves.
   b. CT attenuation correction is necessary for better image resolution.
   c. Dynamic SPECT imaging is required during the radiotracer injection at rest and during stress, in addition to the usual delayed static imaging.
   d. 201Tl is the preferred radiotracer due to its better uptake/flow kinetics compared to ^{99m}Tc tetrofosmin and ^{99m}Tc sestamibi.

11. The reason that ST depression in the inferior leads is less reliable in predicting ischemia during exercise testing is:
   a. Right coronary artery ischemia is difficult to determine with exercise testing.
   b. The Ta wave of atrial repolarization can lower the ST segment, resulting in ST depression that is not secondary to ischemia.
   c. Inferior ST depression is rarely observed with exercise testing.
   d. The statement is incorrect: ST depression in the inferior leads reliably predicts ischemia.

12. Which of the following statements is correct for vasodilator gated SPECT MPI?
   a. The increase in myocardial blood flow is dependent on the increase in double product (HR and BP).
   b. The presence of a reversible perfusion defect indicates myocardial ischemia.
   c. The sensitivity of the test is higher in patients with three-vessel disease than one-vessel disease.
   d. The HR response is coupled to the degree of drop in BP.

13. AV block from adenosine infusion administered for MPI:
   a. Is usually due to right coronary artery ischemia.
   b. Occurs before coronary vasodilatation.
   c. Is a marker of sick sinus syndrome.
   d. Occurs after coronary vasodilatation.
   e. Both a and b

14. The combination of exercise with adenosine during stress MPI is used to:
   a. Increase myocardial blood flow.
   b. Decrease target-to-background activity.
   c. Decrease side effects.
   d. Increase liver activity.

15. Which of these perfusion defects may be due to LBBB during exercise MPI?
   a. Antero-septal scar
   b. Infero-lateral ischemia
   c. Antero-septal ischemia
   d. Multivessel ischemia

16. A 55-year-old man with atypical angina is referred for an exercise stress SPECT MPI. He has a past medical history of hypertension treated with lisinopril 10 mg daily. He does not have any family history of CAD. His physical exam is unremarkable, and a baseline ECG is within normal limits. During the procedure, he achieves a maximal workload of 12 METS, develops an upsloping ST-segment depression of 0.5 mm in inferior leads at peak stress, and has no anginal symptoms. Based on this information, how likely is this patient to have ischemia affecting >10% of the myocardium on MPI?
   a. 0–2%
   b. 5–7%
   c. 10–12%
   d. 15–17%

17. Which of the following statements is most appropriate in patients with type 2 diabetes mellitus?
    a. MPI using Tc-99m radionuclides is not useful in patients with diabetes since it is always abnormal due to microvascular disease.
    b. MPI with N-13 ammonia during upright exercise is the most common imaging modality in these patients.
    c. Gated SPECT MPI using Tc-99m radionuclides provides useful information for patient management.
    d. The HR response during vasodilator stress testing is often supernormal due to sympathetic overactivity.

18. When assessing a patient preoperatively, which one of the following is true?
    a. All patients planning to undergo moderate- or high-risk surgery should undergo cardiac stress testing.
    b. Guidelines provide clear mandates for the management of all patients.
    c. Tools such as the Revised Cardiac Risk Index (RCRI) have proven helpful in guiding decision-making.
    d. The presence of one or more risk factors using commonly used risk calculators should lead to stress testing.

19. In addition to multivessel obstructive coronary disease, which of the following conditions can be associated with impaired global MFR?
    a. Severe LV dysfunction
    b. Renal failure
    c. Incomplete response to dipyridamole
    d. All of the above

20. Which of the following noninvasive tools can be used to diagnose coronary microvascular dysfunction?
    a. Exercise ECG
    b. Non-contrast CT
    c. PET
    d. Coronary CT angiography

21. What is the minimum FDG uptake (%) in a hypoperfused region that may result in a significant recovery in systolic function and improved clinical outcome after revascularization?
    a. 20%
    b. 90%
    c. 50%
    d. 70%

22. A 67-year-old woman with heart failure and severe LV systolic dysfunction (EF 30%) has a history of CAD on a recent coronary angiogram showing the presence of two-vessel disease (occlusion of the RCA and 70% stenosis of LCx). Her ECG showed a left bundle branch block with a QRS duration of 140 msec. Accordingly, a stress/rest ^{99m}Tc-tetrofosmin SPECT scan was performed for functional evaluation. Phase analysis was also performed on rest gated images, and the phase standard deviation (SD) and histogram bandwidth (HB) were computed. Which of the following findings would support cardiac resynchronization therapy as a valuable therapeutic option to improve cardiac function?
    a. Large inferior and infero-lateral myocardial scar with no inducible ischemia. On phase analysis, SD 55 degrees and HB 165 degrees, with the region of latest myocardial activation located at the level of the inferior wall.
    b. Large area of inducible ischemia involving the inferior and lateral walls. On phase analysis, SD 55 degrees and HB 165 degrees, with the region of latest myocardial activation located at the level of the lateral wall.
    c. No inducible ischemia with a small inferior scar. On phase analysis, SD 55 degrees and HB 165 degrees, with the regional of latest myocardial activation on the lateral wall.
    d. Large lateral inducible ischemia with a small inferior scar. On phase analysis, SD 35 degrees and HB 70 degrees.
    e. No evidence of inducible ischemia or scar. On phase analysis, SD 35 degrees and HB 70 degrees.

23. Global myocardial uptake of ^{123}I-*m*IBG is customarily assessed by measuring which of the following?
    a. Decrease in tracer counts per pixel between early and delayed images
    b. Intensity of tracer uptake on tomographic images
    c. Ratio of counts per pixel in the heart to counts per pixel in the mediastinum
    d. Tracer uptake in the lung

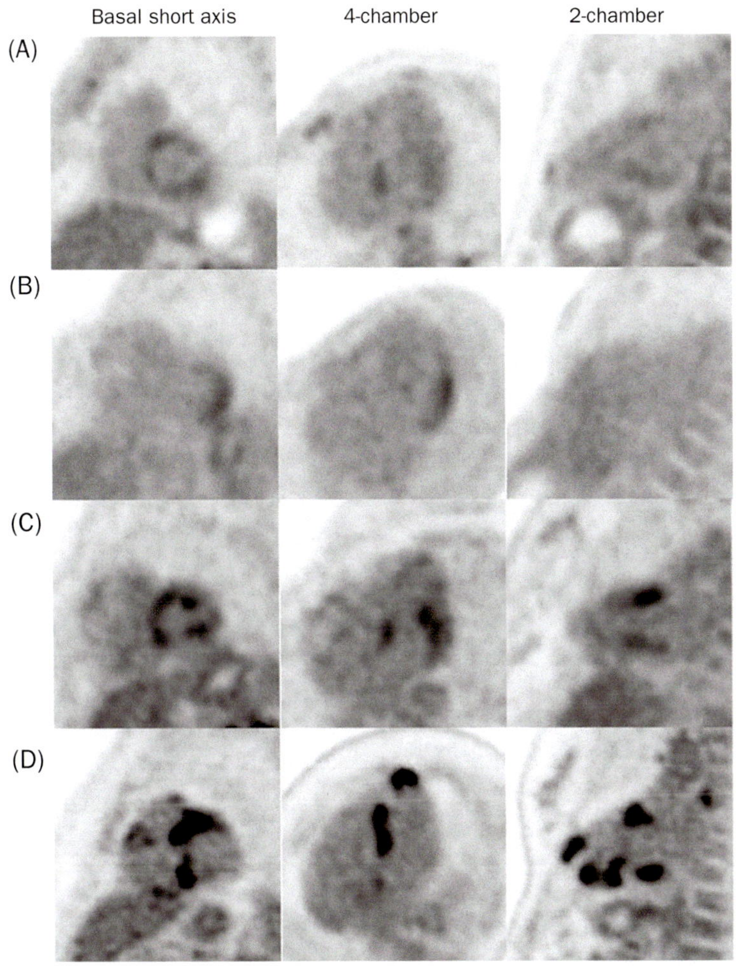

Figure 40.1. Image for Question 24.

24. Which one of the following cardiac patterns of FDG uptake (Figure 40.1) is most likely to represent cardiac sarcoidosis?

25. What is the gold standard for the diagnosis of cardiac amyloidosis and its subtypes? Choose the best answer.
    a. Cardiac MRI
    b. Echocardiogram
    c. ECG
    d. Endomyocardial biopsy
    e. Tc99m pyrophosphate

26. Radiolabeled-leukocyte scintigraphic SPECT imaging affords a high specificity for the diagnosis of prosthetic valve endocarditis, and it may be added in which of the following situations?
    a. ^{18}F-FDG PET/CT findings definite for prosthetic valve endocarditis
    b. 18F-FDG PET/CT with normal findings to rule out prosthetic valve endocarditis
    c. ^{18}F-FDG PET/CT with equivocal findings for the diagnosis of prosthetic valve endocarditis
    d. 18F-FDG PET/CT with apparent FDG uptake around the prosthetic valve but not observed on non–attenuation-corrected PET images

27. Which one of the following statements is accurate regarding atherosclerotic plaque imaging?
    a. Given the role of inflammation in plaque rupture, imaging molecular markers of inflammation may allow the identification of high-risk carotid plaques.
    b. Identification of individual vulnerable plaques offers a low positive predictive value for acute coronary syndrome.
    c. The small size of the plaques, vicinity to blood pool, cardiac motion, and partial volume effect are barriers to accurate noninvasive molecular imaging of coronary plaques.
    d. All of the above

28. A 72-year-old woman presents with exertional chest pain. Her BMI is 32. She is in persistent atrial fibrillation with HR 96, and had a pacemaker implanted 10 years ago for intermittent symptomatic bradycardia. She has hypertension and chronic kidney disease with a glomerular filtration rate of 25 mL/min. What is the best approach to determining the etiology of chest pain?
    a. Vasodilator PET
    b. Vasodilator stress CMR
    c. CT coronary angiography
    d. Dobutamine stress echocardiography

29. A 60-year-old male with a history of hypertension and type 2 diabetes requiring insulin presented with acute chest pain and dyspnea for the last 2 hours that started while gardening. On examination, his HR was 85 bpm regular, and BP was 80/55 mmHg. He had one episode of nonsustained conscious VT on telemetry while in the emergency department. Figure 40.2 shows his ECG. A bedside echocardiogram showed an akinetic mid to apical septal, mid to apical anterior, basal to mid anteroseptal, and apical inferior wall (Movie B). The most likely lesion on invasive angiogram is:
    a. Occluded proximal LAD
    b. Occluded LCx
    c. 70% lesion in RCA
    d. 70% lesion in proximal LAD, 50% lesion in circumflex, 50% lesion right coronary

30. The first-line modality to exclude suspected CAD in a 55-year-old female patient with atypical angina is which of the following?
    a. Invasive coronary angiography because of the high pretest probability for CAD
    b. CCTA if the patient is suitable and adequate local expertise is available
    c. Cardiac magnetic resonance imaging (cMRI) in any case
    d. SPECT MPI because it yields the highest negative predictive value
    e. PET MPI because it offers the highest negative predictive value

31. AI techniques that use predefined features but no other specific rules to make decisions or predictions are referred to as which of the following?
    a. Machine learning
    b. Convolutional autoencoder
    c. Convolutional neural networks
    d. Expert systems

32. Which of the following statements is most appropriate among patients with cardiomyopathy and low LVEF?
    a. LV volumes are not predictive of fatal arrhythmias.
    b. Effective biventricular pacing does not reduce arrhythmic risk.
    c. The burden of sympathetic denervation predicts the risk of sudden cardiac death.
    d. Dyssynchronous myocardial contraction is not present in patients who receive ICD therapy.

33. A 55-year-old male with diabetes and hypertension was recently diagnosed with HIV and started on antiretroviral therapy. He presented to his family physician complaining of occasional shortness of breath on minimal exertion without chest pain or palpitations. Clinical examination was normal apart from morbid obesity (BMI = 45). The resting ECG showed voltage criteria for LV hypertrophy with

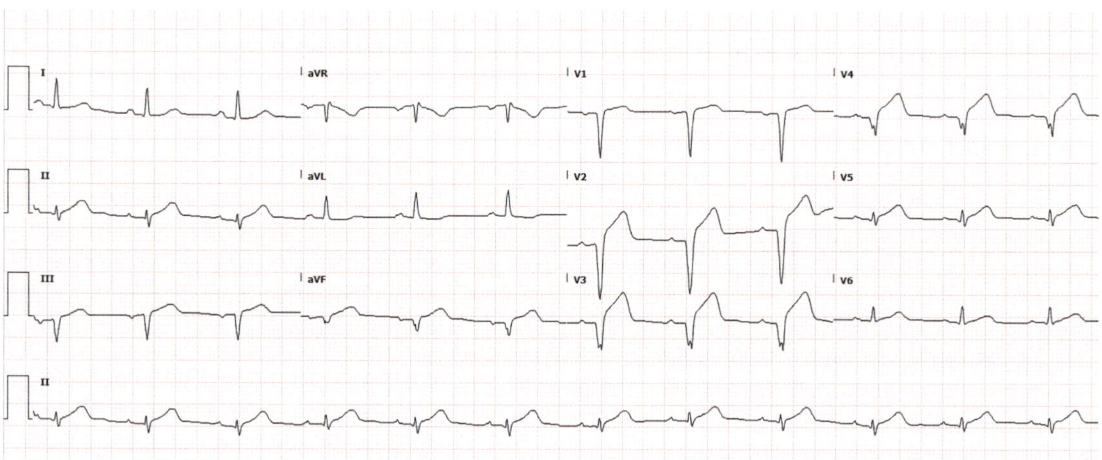

Figure 40.2. Question 29. ECG showing sinus rhythm with anterior Q waves in leads V1 to V4 with associated ST-segment elevation, and inferior Q waves in leads III and aVF.

strain pattern. An echocardiogram showed normal LV systolic function without significant valvular pathology. What is the best modality to rule out CAD in the patient?
  a. SPECT MPI with exercise
  b. SPECT MPI with vasodilator
  c. PET MPI with vasodilator
  d. Invasive coronary angiography

34. A 48-year-old patient presents to the outpatient primary clinic for routine follow-up. He has a history of hypertension and acute myeloid leukemia at age 12. His cancer was treated with a chemotherapy regimen of asparaginase, cytarabine, doxorubicin, etoposide, and mitoxantrone in addition to radiotherapy. The cumulative anthracycline dose was 350 mg/m^2. His LVEF was within the normal range at the initiation and conclusion of treatment. The patient takes enalapril for blood pressure, but no other medications. He exercises 5 days per week by walking on the treadmill. He denies chest pain, shortness of breath, or palpitations. On physical examination his BP is 148/90 mmHg and HR is 68 bpm. The cardiac examination reveals a regular rhythm with a normal S1 and S2. His lungs are clear, his abdomen is soft and nontender, and his legs reveal no edema. An ECG revealed normal sinus rhythm with criteria for LV hypertrophy and normal voltage. In addition to increasing the enalapril to optimize BP control, what is the next best step in his management?
  a. Obtain a gated blood pool SPECT study using a solid-state camera.
  b. Continue current management and follow up in 1 year.
  c. Add aspirin and statin therapy given the patient's history of receiving radiotherapy.
  d. Obtain a technetium pyrophosphate scan.

35. What is the preferred modality of stress testing in an adult with complex congenital heart disease?
  a. Exercise stress test
  b. Vasodilator stress test
  c. Dobutamine stress test
  d. Pacing stress test

36. The rest ECG and SPECT perfusion images obtained at rest, exercise, and adenosine (on different days) shown in Figure 40.3 most likely represent which of the following?
  a. Severe stenosis of the left main coronary artery
  b. Breast attenuation artifact
  c. Prior myocardial infarction
  d. Normal pattern due to left bundle branch block

37. Quality assurance and improvement programs strive for all of the following *except*:
  a. Appropriate patient selection
  b. Imaging testing protocols and procedures
  c. Imaging quality and reporting
  d. Comparison with other nuclear laboratories

38. Which scenario will generate the *least* incremental value following a stress perfusion SPECT study?
  a. A 45-year-old woman with two risk factors for CAD and atypical chest pain
  b. A 60-year-old male with hypertension and noncardiac chest pain
  c. A 65-year-old male smoker with typical chest pain walking up hill, relieved by rest
  d. A 40-year-old male with hyperlipidemia and a history of syncope
  e. A 55-year-old woman with type 2 diabetes and no symptoms

39. Which of the following is a recommended dose-optimization strategy for nuclear cardiology?
  a. Use of PET rather than SPECT for all patients undergoing MPI
  b. Routine performance of stress-only imaging
  c. Use of a high-efficiency camera with reduced administered activity
  d. Use of filtered backprojection

40. Which of the following statements is most appropriate for patients with cardiac amyloidosis?
  a. The ECG almost always shows LV hypertrophy.
  b. Most patients are young since the disease is congenital.
  c. Most patients present with heart failure and low LVEF.
  d. 99mTc-PYP is helpful to identify cardiac amyloidosis and guide management.
  e. All the answers above are correct.

ANSWERS

1c.

2d. Radioactive exposure decreases at $1/r^2$, where r is the distance to the point source. If the exposure is 1 R/hr at 1 meter it will be 1/(2*2) at 2 meters, and so forth. Thus:

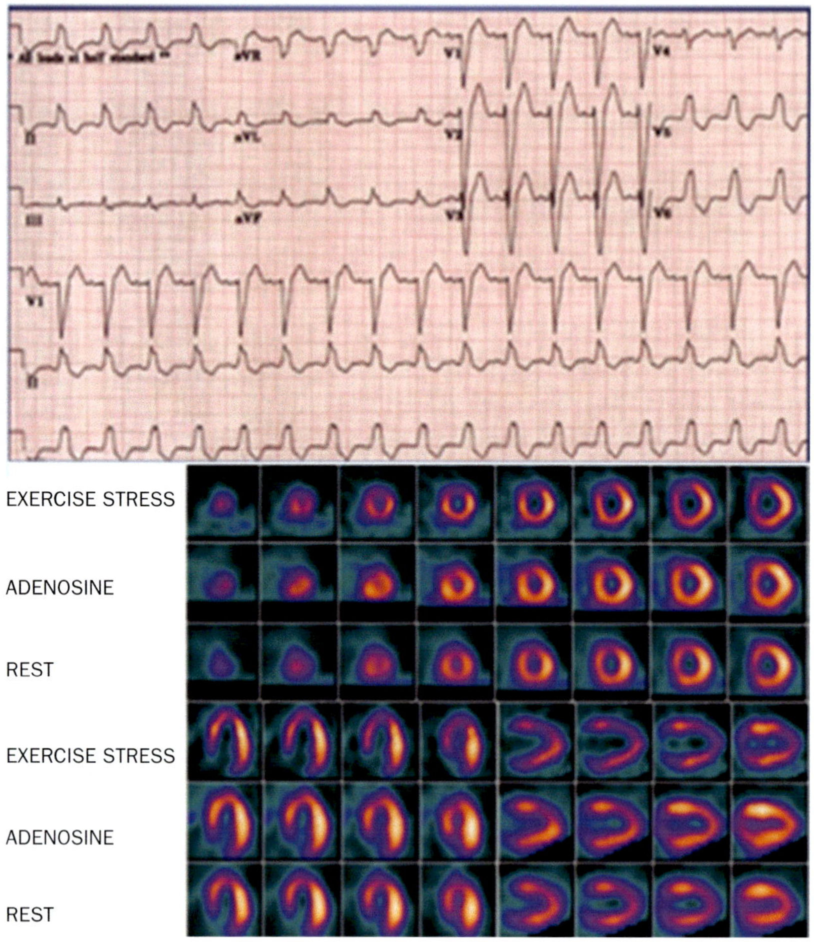

Figure 40.3. Image for Question 36. Top figure is 12-lead ECG. Bottom figure is SPECT MPI using Tc-99m at peak exercise, during adenosine infusion, and at rest.

- 32 R/h at 1 meter
- 32/(2*2) = 8 at 2 meters
- 32/(3*3) = 3.6 at 3 meters
- 32/(4*4) = 2 at 4 meters

3a. Increasing the axial field of view increases the sensitivity of a 3D PET system in the center of the field of view. If the patient is properly positioned with the heart in the middle of the field of view, this will increase the sensitivity over the heart. There will be no impact on the use of time of flight and little impact on resolution.

4a. Complete FDG kinetics are modeled using a two-tissue compartment model in which the second compartment models the phosphorylated form. Since a one-compartment model cannot represent phosphorylation and dephosphorylation, dynamic imaging times should be truncated to when these processes are negligible.

5a. Peak exercise LVEF is the strongest radionuclide predictor of subsequent mortality and, while also predictive of nonfatal MI, SPECT MPI is a more powerful predictor of nonfatal MI. An SDS of 5 gives him a <1% risk of MI at 1 year, so this patient is at low risk of death with a peak exercise LVEF >50% and low 1-year risk of nonfatal MI.

6b. The average Tc-99m SPECT MPI study performed on a conventional SPECT camera using guideline-directed doses for a 1-day low-dose rest (8–12 mCi) and high-dose (24–36 mCi) stress protocol results in an effective dose of 8.4–12.6 mSv. Some Tl-201 protocols such as a stress or rest (2.5–3.5 mCi) with reinjection (1–2 mCi) protocol or a dual-isotope Tl-201 rest (2.5–3.5 mCi) and Tc-99m stress (8–30 mCi) protocol can result in an effective dose of over 20 mSv if the higher dose range is used. The use of high-efficiency solid-state cameras and stress-only protocols can also potentially result in effective doses of less than 3 mSv.

7a. TID in the setting of ischemia is a high-risk finding. A summed difference score (SDS) of 4 translates to 6% ischemia, which would not fall into the high-risk category. With LVEF assessed with SPECT imaging, the stress LVEF is 45 minutes post-stress and is imaged at rest. Because of the timing, LVEF is not expected to increase as with PET

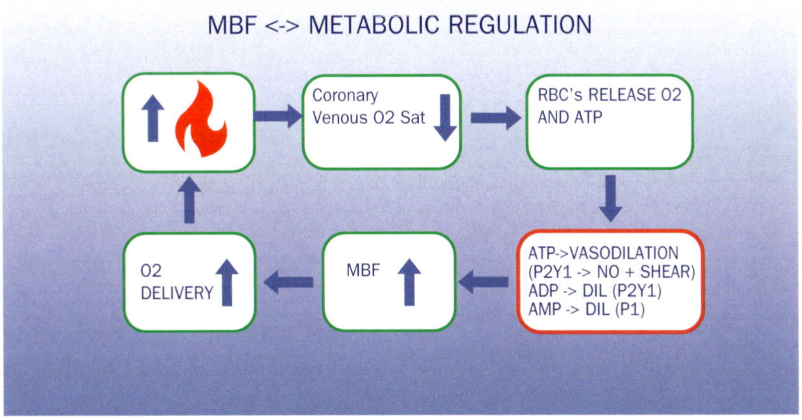

Figure 40.4. Mechanisms involved in the augmentation of MBF in response to an increase in myocardial oxygen demand (flame). Coronary venous oxygen saturation declines and RBCs release both ATP and oxygen. ATP in turn initiates an ascending vasodilation via endothelial P2Y1 receptor agonism and subsequent nitric oxide release with relaxation of arteriolar pre-capillary smooth muscle and thus an increase in MBF. ATP also is metabolized to ADP and AMP, both of which participate in vascular relaxation. In addition, ADP stimulates RBC receptors, which inhibit further ATP release once MBF has increased sufficiently to meet myocardial oxygen demand and a new steady state has been attained.

imaging, and only a substantial decrease in LVEF is prognostically significant. The prognostic implications of ST-segment changes vary depending on the presence or absence of perfusion defects.

8a. The current consensus opinion based on an abundance of experimental evidence is coronary venous oxygen saturation, which is taken as the best integrated measure of myocardial metabolic activity and hence in the normal coronary circulation is the signal for changes in myocardial blood flow (Figure 40.4). The other metabolites all have been investigated in detail and at present have not been shown to play a determining role. Red blood cell release of both ATP and oxygen, in particular ATP, stimulates an ascending vasodilation, which, in coordination with its breakdown products ADP and AMP and endothelial nitric oxide, increases myocardial blood flow in response to a decline in coronary venous oxygen saturation.

9c.

10c. Dynamic MPI of the radiotracer injection is required for generation of the blood (arterial input) and tissue time–activity curves for kinetic modeling to calculate MBF. Incorrect answers:

a. MBF imaging is performed with usual doses of SPECT radiotracers and can be done with reduced low doses.[1,2]
b. Reasonably accurate SPECT MBF measurement is possible without CT attenuation correction, and most CZT camera systems are not equipped with CT.
d. Although ^{201}Tl has better uptake/flow kinetics than ^{99m}Tc tetrofosmin and ^{99m}Tc sestamibi, MBF measurement results are similar with all three radio tracers due to the greater noise in the ^{201}Tl images related to the lower injected radiotracer dose.

11b. Just as depolarization and repolarization of the ventricle are represented on the ECG by the QRS and T wave, respectively, atrial depolarization is reflected in the P wave and atrial repolarization in the "Ta wave." The Ta wave is usually directed in the opposite direction than and lasts longer than the P wave. With exercise, the P and Ta waves increase in size and duration, allowing the Ta wave to extend into the ST segment. As P-wave amplitude is greatest in the inferior leads, Ta waves are more likely to extend into and lower the ST segment in the inferior leads. When ST depression occurs in the inferior leads, the negative deflection of the Ta wave is the more likely cause than myocardial ischemia.

12c. Answer a is incorrect as the increase in myocardial blood flow is dependent on the degree of vasodilation of small vessels due to direct effect of adenosine and is unrelated to double product. This is a major difference when compared to exercise. Answer b is incorrect as in most patients the perfusion defect is due to a difference in peak hyperemic areas (less in the territory of the diseased coronary artery than in normal or less severely diseased coronary arteries) without accompanying myocardial ischemia. In the minority of patients, myocardial ischemia is present with vasodilator stress due to coronary steal. Answer c is correct, but that does not mean that all three diseased coronary arteries will always have perfusion defects. On average, one-third of

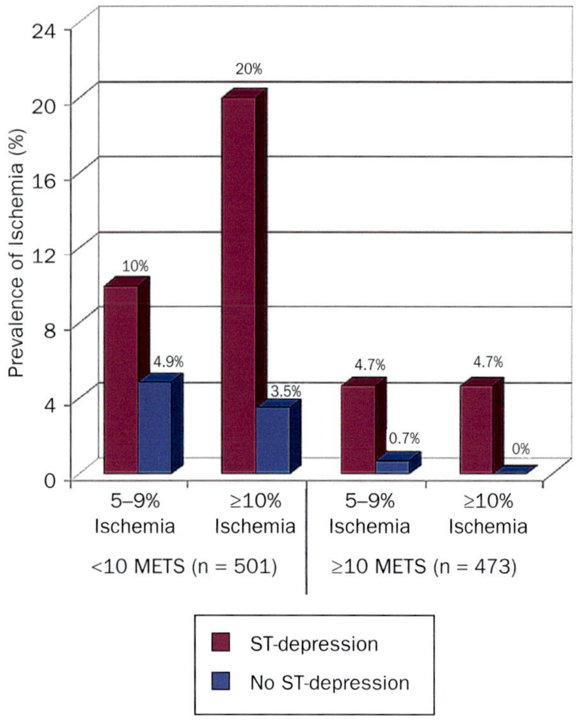

Figure 40.5. Answer 16. Prevalence of ischemia on myocardial perfusion imaging based on functional capacity and ECG changes. METS, metabolic equivalents. Reproduced with permission from Bourque et al. *Journal of the American College of Cardiology* 2009;54:538-45.

patients will have a one-vessel disease pattern, one-third will have a two-vessel disease pattern, and the remaining third will have a three-vessel disease pattern. Only <10% will have no perfusion defects. In reality, measuring coronary hemodynamics also shows that not all three diseased coronary arteries are physiologically important—the well-known saga of differences between anatomy and physiology! Answer d is incorrect. The HR response is due to direct sympathetic stimulation and is not a reciprocal response to a decrease in BP. That is why the HR response has important prognostic relevance, because it tests the integrity of the autonomic system.

13d. This has relevance as the radiotracer could be injected rather than canceling the test.

14c. Myocardial blood flow is maximal with the vasodilator adenosine and does not increase further with exercise; the target-to-background ratio increases rather than decreases due to a decrease in liver activity.

15c. Perfusion defects due to left bundle branch block are reversible (ischemia) and in the territory of the left anterior descending artery.

16a. The predictive value of high exercise capacity (defined as ≥10 METs) for detection of myocardial ischemia was evaluated in a cohort of 1,056 patients. Four hundred seventy-three patients achieved a high workload, and among those with no ischemic ST changes, the prevalence of ischemia affecting >10% of the myocardium was 0% (Figure 40.5). Upsloping ST elevation of 0.5 mm does not meet criteria for ischemia. Therefore, this patient's likelihood of having significant ischemia on MPI is very low.

17c. Not all diabetic patients have microvascular disease, and even in the presence of microvascular disease MPI may be normal. On the other hand, perfusion defects on MPI could also be an expression of epicardial disease. Gated SPECT MPI provides useful information about perfusion, viability, and LV geometry and function, taking a central role in risk assessment of patients with diabetes. In many subjects with diabetes exercise capacity is impaired, and pharmacologic stress may be the only option for testing. The HR response to adenosine and regadenoson in diabetic patients is often blunted due to autonomic neuropathy.

18c. When evaluating patients prior to planned surgery, risk stratification tools and risk calculators, such as the RCRI, should be used to help determine which patients should be considered for stress testing. Such tools incorporate factors such as surgical risk; known CAD or current ischemic chest pain; past or present heart failure; a history of prior stroke or transient ischemic attack; and diabetes. Each is given 1 point and the score is totaled. Those with a total RCRI score of 0 or 1 are at low risk for major adverse cardiovascular events and can usually proceed without further cardiac testing.

19d. Globally reduced MFR is often attributable to multivessel coronary disease, caused by a reduced capacity to increase blood flow during stress in all three coronary territories. Alternatively, conditions associated with microvascular dysfunction, such as severe LV dysfunction and renal failure, should also be considered as potential explanations for a reduced global MFR. Inadequate response to dipyridamole could also result in a lack of flow increase at stress, resulting in globally reduced flow reserve, and needs to be verified; this should be a consideration particularly when the change between rest and stress MBF is zero or minimal (i.e., MFR is ~1.0 and homogeneous throughout all coronary territories), with no other indications of ischemia or high-risk findings. A full hemodynamic response to dipyridamole is often associated with an HR increase of at least 10 bpm and a decrease in systolic BP of at least 10 mmHg. The absence of any hemodynamic changes or symptoms typically attributable to the side effects of dipyridamole may further support the possibility of an incomplete dipyridamole response in this specific setting. Additionally, quantitative calculation of a "splenic response ratio," measuring the relative reduction in radiotracer activity concentration in the spleen at stress compared to rest (using the liver as a reference), is another described means of assessing the adequacy of dipyridamole response and may provide additional prognostic information*. If an incomplete response to dipyridamole is suspected despite a caffeine-free period of at least 24 hours prior to the test, consideration can be given to a repeat study with an alternative stress agent such as dobutamine.

20c. The coronary microcirculation is too small to be directly imaged in vivo and must be evaluated indirectly by perturbing function. PET with blood flow quantification represents the gold standard for noninvasive diagnosis of coronary microvascular dysfunction.

21c. Answer c is correct, as a maintained FDG uptake in a hypoperfused region of at least 50% is necessary for a potential recovery in systolic function and improved clinical outcome after coronary revascularization. An FDG uptake of <50% is commonly considered as nonviable; thus, answer a is incorrect. Answers b and d are not correct, as 90% and 70% FDG uptake reflects predominantly viable myocardium but not the "minimum" of ≥50% FDG uptake needed for potential functional recovery and improved clinical outcome after restoration of coronary flow.

22c. It is well established that in patients with severe LV systolic dysfunction (EF < 35%), cardiac resynchronization therapy (CRT) is clinically effective when the pacing lead is positioned on the latest-contracting viable myocardial region. In these patients, the evaluation of regional myocardial viability is of great value since the presence of extensive myocardial scar is associated with far less benefit from CRT. When mechanical dyssynchrony is revealed by phase analysis, cutoff values of 45 degrees for SD and 135 degrees for HB have been shown to predict the response to CRT. Answer a is incorrect because the region of latest mechanical activation is located on a scar. As for answer b, given the presence of significant inducible ischemia, coronary revascularization should be attempted before assessing the need for CRT. Answers d and e are incorrect because no dyssynchony was revealed.

23c. Global myocardial uptake of ^{123}I-*m*IBG is the ratio of count per pixel in the heart to the counts per pixel in a region of interest (a 7 × 7 pixel box has been recommended) in the upper mediastinum, and is known as the heart-to-mediastinum ratio. The decrease in counts between early and delayed images, known as the washout, likely reflects a combination of neuronal integrity and systemic and local adrenergic tone. For tomographic images, regional defects are assessed. Tracer uptake in the lungs can reduce image quality and make ^{123}I-*m*IBG studies difficult to interpret.

24d. This is a classic example of multifocal FDG uptake involving most of the interventricular septum from base to apex, as well as the right ventricular free wall. You can also appreciate focal uptake posterior to the heart in the two-chamber view, most likely representing a mediastinal FDG-avid node. This patient was diagnosed with biopsy-proven sarcoidosis. Subjects A, B, and C actually correspond to healthy volunteers who failed to make the metabolic switch despite their following the ketogenic diet for at least 24 hours, reinforced with prolonged fasting. Pattern A corresponds to FDG uptake limited to the base of the LV, often referred to as the "basal ring" sign; pattern B is limited to the lateral wall; and pattern C is trickier, as it represents heterogeneous uptake along the LV, including the papillary muscle. However, please notice the difference in appearance with respect to patient D, which is more lobulated and has clear-cut segmental areas of complete suppression of normal myocardium between segments exhibiting intense FDG uptake. Cardiac MRI and/or MPI if available can be very helpful to spatially co-localize imaging findings.

25d. Endomyocardial biopsy remains the gold standard for the diagnosis of cardiac amyloidosis. In the presence of an abnormal free light chain assay or a monoclonal protein, histologic confirmation of the amyloid type is required, regardless of the grade of myocardial uptake of the bone tracer. The presence of amyloid in non-cardiac sites such as the abdominal fat pad, bone marrow, and so forth, along with typical cardiac MRI or echocardiographic findings. may be sufficient to diagnose cardiac amyloidosis. However, given the range of sensitivities, a negative fat pad biopsy is insufficient to exclude the diagnosis. Cardiac MRI or echocardiography alone cannot make the diagnosis of cardiac amyloidosis. In the right clinical setting, and without an abnormal free light chain assay or a monoclonal protein, Tc99m pyrophosphate scintigraphy has high diagnostic accuracy for TTR cardiac amyloidosis. However, as already mentioned, if abnormal free light chain assay or a monoclonal protein is present, then Tc99m pyrophosphate scintigraphy cannot distinguish between TTR and AL cardiac amyloidosis.

26c. ^{18}F-FDG PET/CT has a high sensitivity for the detection of prosthetic valve endocarditis but a relatively low specificity. This is contrasted with the relatively low sensitivity but high specificity of radiolabeled-leukocyte scintigraphic SPECT imaging for the diagnosis of prosthetic valve endocarditis. Thus, if ^{18}F-FDG PET/CT demonstrates equivocal findings for prosthetic valve endocarditis, then adding radiolabeled-leukocyte scintigraphic SPECT is of further help for a more definite diagnosis or to rule out prosthetic valve endocarditis. Answers a and b are incorrect, as radiolabeled-leukocyte scintigraphic SPECT does not add further information when ^{18}F-FDG PET/CT is definite in its interpretation. Answer d is incorrect, as apparent FDG uptake around the prosthetic valve that is no longer present on non-attenuation-corrected PET images is seen as artifactual on the PET/CT. This is because the FDG signal in the proximity of high-density regions such as a metal device or prosthetic valve may be erroneously elevated owing to an attenuation over-correction based on the CT captured metal density.

27d. Nearly three-quarters of acute coronary syndromes are caused by plaque rupture. A thin fibrous cap, extensive inflammation, a large necrotic core, and a paucity of vascular smooth muscle cells are among the structural and biologic features of vulnerable plaques prone to rupture. Accordingly, imaging plaque inflammation may provide valuable information regarding the propensity for rupture. However, the plaque phenotype is a dynamic process, and the majority of vulnerable plaques never rupture, or their ruptures remain asymptomatic. Therefore, the detection of individual vulnerable plaques by molecular imaging has an inherently low positive predictive value for acute coronary syndrome. This issue may be addressed by focusing on plaque vulnerability (for instance, as a global score in the entire heart) rather than imaging individual plaques. However, in the case of carotid plaques, the presence of high-risk features may help risk stratify the lesions and possibly predict cerebrovascular accidents. The small size of the plaques relative to the spatial resolution of nuclear imaging techniques (~4–6 mm for PET, ~8–10 mm for SPECT), vicinity to blood pool, cardiac motion, and partial volume effect, as well as uptake by cardiomyocytes (in the case of ^{18}F-FDG), are major barriers to accurate imaging of coronary plaques.

28a. This vignette exemplifies an important clinical advantage of stress testing with SPECT or PET imaging, which is the wide applicability of radionuclide imaging irrespective of body habitus, cardiac rhythm, renal function, the presence of implanted cardiac devices, or allergy to iodinated contrast. These clinical conditions are often present in the stress testing population and preclude the use of other stress imaging modalities. This clinical effectiveness is an important attribute of radionuclide imaging. In this patient, the ability to quantify myocardial blood flow with vasodilator PET offers the added advantages of ensuring that the patient has responded to the coronary vasodilator, excluding balanced myocardial ischemia due to multivessel diseases and offering powerful prognostic information.

29a. The ECG changes with the regional LV wall-motion changes on echocardiogram are highly suggestive of a ST-elevation myocardial infarction secondary to an occluded proximal LAD. The inferior Q waves are due to a large LAD (type III or IV) that supplies the apical inferior wall.

30b. In this middle-aged female patient with atypical chest pain, the pre-test probability is very low. A test with a high negative predictive value such as CCTA is the best choice in this setting. Therefore, the other answers are incorrect.

31a. Machine learning techniques use predefined features but no other specific rules. The other answers are incorrect:

Answer b: Convolutional autoencoders are algorithms that reproduce the input layer into the output layer, with inner hidden layers with reduced dimensions. This leads to selection of only the most critical information to separate out signal from noise.

Answer c: Convolutional neural networks (a subtype of deep learning) make predictions directly from imaging data, without being programmed to detect specific features.

Answer d: Expert systems algorithms generate predictions using a combination of observed data and heuristic rules obtained from human experts.

32c. Prospective studies have shown that LV end-diastolic volume (PAREPET) and burden of sympathetic innervation (ADMIRE-HF) are independent predictors of fatal arrhythmias. LV dyssynchrony is prevalent among patients with heart failure and reduced EF, and observational data suggest ventricular tachyarrhythmia occurs with a significantly higher frequency among those with dyssynchrony. Effective resynchronization therapy with biventricular packing reduces (even ameliorates) dyssynchrony and confers protection against arrhythmic events.

33c. The patient has an intermediate likelihood of CAD and therefore needs further risk stratification. This obese patient with symptoms on minimal exertion is unlikely to exercise long enough for a diagnostic test. Vasodilator MPI is recommended in patients who cannot exercise adequately. PET MPI has been shown to be superior to SPECT in obese patients. In addition, ASNC and SNMMI guidelines recommend the use of PET if vasodilator MPI is planned. Invasive coronary angiography is reserved for patients with a high likelihood of CAD and those with a high likelihood of requiring intervention. Therefore, vasodilator PET MPI is the best option for evaluating CAD in this patient.

34a. The patient has a history of childhood cancer and received treatment with an anthracycline-based regimen. Because the total dose of anthracycline received was greater than 240 mg/m^2, the patient should have biyearly assessment of LVEF to monitor for later-stage development of cancer therapy–related cardiac dysfunction. Since the patient has not had an assessment of the LVEF since completion of therapy, it should be assessed at this time. Imaging with a solid-state camera will reduce the radiation exposure to the patient, which is particularly important given the frequent testing the patient will require over the course of his lifetime. Continuing current management only is not correct because the patient needs to have an assessment of his LVEF; if findings are abnormal, the medical regimen will need to be altered. At this stage, there is no indication for aspirin and statin therapy. The patient has not presented with other signs of amyloidosis and the ECG revealed normal voltage, so there are no specific signs to suggest that a technetium pyrophosphate scan should be obtained at this stage.

35a. A symptom-limited exercise stress test is the preferred test for evaluation of ischemia in patients with complex congenital heart disease. Many of these patients have dynamic obstruction, and vasodilator stress may not elicit ischemia if there is a compressive mechanism to the ischemia. Exercise stress also provides usual physiologic information, including HR, BP, oxygen saturation, ECG changes, and arrhythmia in response to exercise. A pharmacologic stress test is an alternative when fixed obstruction or atherosclerosis is the suspected mechanism of ischemia.

36d. The reversible antero-septal abnormality is seen with exercise due to high HR but not during adenosine, where the maximum HR is lower.

37d. Quality improvement processes provide for improvement in all aspects of nuclear cardiology, from the use of appropriate use criteria to patient selection, test selection, performance, interpretation, and reporting. The goal is to achieve an acceptable national standard of care. The process is blinded through rigorous peer review; the information is confidential and is not shared with other nuclear laboratories.

38c. Incremental value = post-test probability minus pre-test probability. This relationship is a curve where the maximal incremental information is at a pre-test probability of 50% (a flip of a coin). The closer the pre-test probability gets to either extreme (0 or 100%), the less either a positive or negative result changes the probability of disease. Scenarios a, b, d, and e are all intermediate-risk patients where stress imaging is indicated. Scenario c is a patient with a very high probability of disease. Neither a positive nor a negative stress perfusion result will change that, and this patient is best referred directly to angiography.

39c. Use of PET is an outstanding dose-reduction approach; however, current PET protocols do not routinely enable exercise stress testing, which provides important diagnostic and prognostic information, so there remains a role for SPECT MPI in many patients. Stress-only imaging is typically only applicable for patients with normal perfusion, function, and so forth on stress-first imaging. Use of high-efficiency cameras, incorporating cadmium-zinc-telluride or cesium-iodide detectors, together with reduction of administered activity, is a recommended dose-optimization strategy. Image reconstruction methods using iterative reconstruction, typically with the ordered subsets expectation maximization algorithm, are preferred to filtered backprojection and can enable reduction in administered activity.

40d. A variety of ^{99m}Tc-labeled diphosphonate and PYP (bone-avid) compounds can be used to diagnose ATTR cardiac amyloidosis with high sensitivity and specificity. The explanation for this differential uptake in ATTR versus AL cardiac amyloidosis is unknown, but it has been suggested that the preferential uptake by ATTR may be a result of higher calcium content. The management is different according to the subtype. Thus, answer d is correct. A thick LVe and diastolic dysfunction on echocardiography raises the possibility of cardiac amyloidosis. However, despite the thick LV on echocardiography, patients with amyloidosis may not show classic hypertrophy findings on ECG such as tall "r" waves on V5 and V6. In fact, often the ECG shows low (or normal) voltage (thus, answer a is incorrect). There are three main subtypes of amyloidosis: light chain amyloidosis (AL), caused by a plasma cell dyscrasia; senile systemic amyloidosis (wtATTR); and hereditary (familial) amyloidosis (mATTR). In cardiac amyloidosis most patients are elderly at disease onset, around the sixth decade of life (thus, answer b is incorrect). Cardiac amyloidosis frequently present with congestive heart failure and preserved EF. Angina also occurs due to intramyocardial vessel infiltration (thus, answer c is incorrect).

REFERENCES

1. Acampa W, Assante R, Mannarino T, et al. Low-dose dynamic myocardial perfusion imaging by CZT-SPECT in the identification of

obstructive coronary artery disease. *Eur J Nucl Med Mol Imaging*. 2020;47(7):1705–1712.

2. Pang Z, Wang J, Li S, et al. Diagnostic analysis of new quantitative parameters of low-dose dynamic myocardial perfusion imaging with CZT SPECT in the detection of suspected or known coronary artery disease. *Int J Cardiovasc Imaging*. 2021;37(1):367–378.

BIBLIOGRAPHY

Bami K, Tewari S, Guirguis F, et al. Prognostic utility of splenic response ratio in dipyridamole PET myocardial perfusion imaging. *J Nucl Cardiol*. 2019 Dec;26(6):1888–1897. doi:10.1007/s12350-018-1269-9

Bourque JM, Holland BH, Watson DD, Beller GA. Achieving an exercise workload of ≥10 metabolic equivalents predicts a very low risk of inducible ischemia: Does myocardial perfusion imaging have a role? *J Am Coll Cardiol*. 2009;54:538–545.

Harnett DT, Hazra S, Maze R, et al. Clinical performance of Rb-82 myocardial perfusion PET and Tc-99m-based SPECT in patients with extreme obesity. *J Nucl Cardiol*. 2019;26:275–283.

Hendel RC, Berman DS, Di Carli MF, et al. ACCF/ASNC/ACR/AHA/ASE/SCCT/SCMR/SNM 2009 appropriate use criteria for cardiac radionuclide imaging. *Circulation*. 2009;119:e561–e587.

Jacobson AF, Lombard J, Banerjee G, Camici PG. ^{123}I-mIBG scintigraphy to predict risk for adverse cardiac outcomes in heart failure patients: Design of two prospective multicenter international trials. *J Nucl Cardiol*. 2009;16:113–121.

Lee KL, Pryor DB, Pieper KS, et al. Prognostic value of radionuclide angiography in medically treated patients with coronary artery disease: A comparison with clinical and catheterization variables. *Circulation*. 1990;82:1705–1717.

Sharir T, Germano G, Kang X, et al. Prediction of myocardial infarction versus cardiac death by gated myocardial perfusion SPECT: Risk stratification by the amount of stress-induced ischemia and the post-stress ejection fraction. *J Nucl Med*. 2001; 42:831–837.

Slomka PJ, Miller RJH, Isgum I, Dey D. Application and translation of artificial intelligence to cardiovascular imaging in nuclear medicine and noncontrast CT. *Semin Nucl Med*. 2020;50:357–366.

Taqueti VR, Dorbala S, Wolinsky D, et al. Myocardial perfusion imaging in women for the evaluation of stable ischemic heart disease: State-of-the-evidence and clinical recommendations. *J Nucl Cardiol*. 2017;24:1402–1426.

INDEX*

For the benefit of digital users, indexed terms that span two pages (e.g., 52–53) may, on occasion, appear on only one of those pages

Tables, figures, and boxes are indicated by *t*, *f*, and *b* following the page number

* Index entries from the sixth edition of Nuclear Cardiac Imaging : Principles and Applications

Q

R

S

T